I0115072

WEIGHT
SUCCESS
FOREVER

The 4 Steps to Creating It

John D. Correll

Fulfillment Press
U.S.A.

Weight Success Forever: The 4 Steps to Creating It

Fulfillment Press | U.S.A.

Copyright © 2021 by John Correll • All rights reserved. No part of this book may be digitally stored or retrieved, or be reproduced, distributed, or transmitted, in any form or by any means, without expressed written permission from the author. The only exception is reviewers may quote short excerpts in a review.

Printed in United States of America
ISBN: 978-1-938001-82-6 (for paperback) ~ 978-1-938001-83-3 (for hardcover)
Amazon URL: amazon.com/dp/1938001834

Version: TXT 2021-06 (12) | COV 2021-06 (3)
Cover, infographics, text creation, formatting, editing and proof reading by John Correll
Photo on back cover by Bill Bacheler

Fulfillment Press specializes in the creation and publication of educational media for career and life fulfillment. The name Fulfillment Press is a publishing imprint and registered DBA, or assumed name, of Correll Consulting, LLC. The name Weight Success Method™ is a trademarked name used by Correll Consulting, LLC to denote the weight management method described in this book. World Weight Success Empowerment Series™ is also a trademarked name and is used by Correll Consulting, LLC to denote a book/E-book series.

John Correll enjoys walking, biking, sight-seeing with his grandson, creating photographs, book publishing, and reading American history and positive psychology. More on him can be found at: correllconcepts.com/correll_bio.htm
(Note: This is not the same John Correll who creates the excellent kids' books.)

Dedicated to the Readers of this book. ~ May you live out your life in your desired weight range and strive to become the finest person you're capable of being and help others to do the same … and derive peace, joy, and fulfillment as a result.

Special thanks to my wife and life partner Janet for triggering my initial search for the cause of why a few people are succeeding at creating healthy-weight living while most are not.

Disclaimer: Before beginning any diet or weight management program, or making a major change to a present dietary program, a licensed physician should be consulted. If any information in this book should contradict or conflict with any prescription or advice of your physician or chosen dietary program, we recommend you ignore and do not apply whatever that conflicting information contained in this book might be. This book is not a dietary guide. It does not recommend a particular dietary program. It aims at a general audience. The Weight Success Method and other methods, suggestions, and statements contained in this book derive from the author's personal experiences, perspectives, and conclusions. They do not derive from scientific testing; therefore, it should not be assumed that these methods, suggestions, and statements will work for every person and in every situation. The author and publisher shall have neither liability nor responsibility to any person or entity with respect to any loss or damage caused, or alleged to have been caused, directly or indirectly, by the information contained in this book.

For additional resources and books by John Correll, go to: correllconcepts.com

Consulting Service – If your company or organization would like a keynote speaker or would like assistance in implementing the principles of the Weight Success Method in a customized program for clients or staff, go to: correllconcepts.com/consulting.pdf

---

NOTE: If, in addition to this printed book you'd also like to have a free digital version on your computer, tablet, and/or smartphone, go to **http://correllconcepts.com/wsf.pdf** and download a free PDF version for your personal use.

In essence, the surest way to create Weight Success Forever is this.

> **1** – Read Chapter **1** of this book.
> **2** – Do the ten STARTUP Actions.
> **3** – Start the five DAILY Actions.
> **4** – Keep doing <u>all five</u> Daily Actions <u>every</u> day ... forever.*

* Typically takes less than 8 minutes of dedicated time per day.

If you're one who desires to succeed at putting your life on the track of lifelong healthy-weight living, and do it more easily and enjoyably than you've likely ever thought possible, this *Weight Success Forever* book is for **YOU.**

This book presents numerous new concepts. Some of these concepts are central to succeeding at healthy-weight living. These key concepts are restated throughout the book. This restatement is **INTENTIONAL.**

Table of Contents

SUCCESS is:

The act of creating a desired life-enhancing situation <u>and</u> deriving benefits, enjoyment, and fulfillment from it.

WEIGHT SUCCESS is:

Living most or all of one's days in one's desired healthy-weight range <u>and</u> deriving benefits, enjoyment, and fulfillment from it. To succeed at creating Weight Success forever you must apply a Weight Success METHODOLOGY.

A WEIGHT SUCCESS METHODOLOGY is:

an action plan that consists of specific actions that, when performed by you, cause a maximal number of success drivers to be included in your weight success pursuit, which in turn results in easiest possible creation of lifelong Weight Success.

The WEIGHT SUCCESS METHOD presented in this book is the most effective Weight Success Methodology we know.

CHAPTER 1: Weight Success Method (5 Parts)

The Weight Success Method and how to do it, presented in five parts (A–E).

THIS CHAPTER 1 contains five parts, which are labeled as this:

This Chapter 1 contains about everything you need for creating lifelong weight success. But if a situation should arise in which you have a question that needs answering or a problem that needs resolving, look to Chapters 2–27 (p. 42–168). They are the *Backup Resource* chapters.

Almost no one enjoys being overweight, but most of us are; almost all of us would like to live non-overweight, but most of us don't achieve it. This is the head-scratcher of the 21st century.

WEIGHT SUCCESS
—— is the GOAL ——

WEIGHT SUCCESS METHOD™
—— is the MEANS ——

Goal+Means+Action=WEIGHT SUCCESS™

WEIGHT SUCCESS = Living most or all of one's days in one's desired healthy-weight range AND deriving benefits, enjoyment, and fulfillment from it.

Part 1-A: How the Method Came About and Why It Works

A FIRST STEP to succeeding at weight control and healthy-weight living is to know the main ways people live their life as pertains to weight management. In modern society most persons live out their life in one of these — or a variation of one of these — *six weight journey scenarios*. Which one will you live?

Scenario 1: Luck-out — The person effortlessly spends their entire life living at their healthy weight. Their metabolism and rate of calorie consumption are perfectly matched for life. It's a *rare* lucky coincidence.

Scenario 2: Oblivious — At some point the person begins gaining weight. This weight gain is slow but unceasing. It's so slow the person seldom notices the change from month to month. So they never apply a serious preventive measure ... which results in slow, unceasing weight gain for life.

Scenario 3: Fail and Quit — At some point the person begins gaining weight. Eventually they decide to "do something about it." This leads them to pursue "weight control." It takes the form of either (a) an exercise program or (b) a dieting program. Sooner or later, the program "fails" them or they tire of it, so they quit it. They never seriously try again ... which results in weight gain for life.

Scenario 4: Yo-yo — At some point the person begins gaining weight. So they go on a diet. This results in them losing weight. After achieving their weight loss goal they celebrate and go back to "normal living." But the lost weight returns. Still, they're persistent. So, again they go on a diet — and again they lose weight and again it returns. They repeat this process multiple times in their life. We call it yo-yo dieting or yo-yo life.

Scenario 5: Weight Success Action — At some point the person begins gaining weight. They decide to do something about it. So they undertake an exercise program. And, for a while it "works," or at least "helps out." But eventually they realize that the only lasting solution is to manage their eating. So they enact a diet and take their weight down to their healthy weight. Then they make one of the

most impacting decisions of their life. They decide that living the rest of their life at their healthy weight is a *mandatory* feature of their life.

This decision causes them to pursue weight control in a different way than most do. Intentionally or non-intentionally, knowingly or not, they begin doing weight success actions every day. And, because they're doing this *they create healthy-weight living for most or all of the rest of the days of their life.*

> **TWO KEY DEFINITIONS:** (1) A *success action* is an action that contributes to creating a certain desired life-enhancing situation. ~ (2) A *weight success action* is an action that contributes to creating weight success, or contributes to living the rest of one's life in one's desired healthy-weight range and deriving benefits, enjoyment, and fulfillment from it. (Keep this definition in mind.)

Scenario 6: Anorexia — At some point the person begins gaining weight. One day they look in a mirror and what they think they see horrifies them, even if they're only slightly overweight. They decide they must lose weight so they won't "be fat." So they reduce food intake and lose weight. But every time they look in a mirror they see only a "fat person," even when they're no longer overweight. So they keep eating less and losing more weight, until they die! What causes this? Astounding as it is, their mindset — or beliefs and views — is what causes them to perform the actions that result in the tragic outcome of scenario 6! In short, it's because of this dynamic:

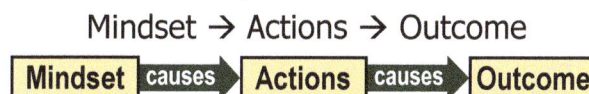

Mindset → Actions → Outcome

Mindset [causes] → Actions [causes] → Outcome

Now here's the key point. *Mindset* is also what causes people to perform the actions that result in scenarios 2, 3, and 4 ... and *mindset* is also what causes them to perform the actions that result in scenario **5.** Please keep this in mind.

How This Book and the Weight Success Method Came About

It happened like this.

It was summer of '79. For several years I had been grappling with weight gain. My two chief weapons were "one-week diets" and "watching what I ate." Both were annoying — neither effective. Then I decided that exercise might be my salvation. So in July 1979 at age 35 I took up bicycling. I figured it would enable me to eat as much as I wanted without gaining weight. And, for many years it did, *as long as* I was logging over a hundred biking miles a week at vigorous speed.

But then, around 2000 something happened. I was 56 years old, and the happy scenario of eating as much as I liked and burning up these calories with vigorous cycling was no longer working. Two things caused this situation. First, at age 56 I had less muscle mass than at age 35, which resulted in burning fewer calories during biking. Second, I was biking fewer miles and at a slower speed at 56 than at 35, which further resulted in burning fewer calories.

So in 2000 I discovered, to my horror, that I was now gaining weight in spite of bicycling. I was back into the same bad situation I was in in 1979. I was gaining weight and had no easy antidote for it. It was a bummer. But it triggered one of the most gratifying discoveries of my life: the discovery of a method for maintaining my weight exactly where I want it to be *without* pain, hassle, and yo-yo dieting ... and, if necessary, without exercise.

I initially dubbed it "Weight Freedom Method" and later called it "Healthy-weight Method." Finally I adopted the name *Weight Success Method.* And how has this method worked out? Fantastically well! By applying the Method *since 2007* I've been maintaining my weight in my healthy-weight range for nearly every day since. And, most importantly, it has happened easily and enjoyably — and has also brought personal epiphanies and fulfillment.

> **Note:** If you'd like to know exactly *why* the Method is enjoyable, go to Ch. **17** at page 103.

Now, I know some people think the reason I'm living in my healthy-weight range is my body automatically maintains itself at that weight. But that's incorrect. I'm just like everyone else. My body doesn't perform such an incredible feat. I know for a fact it will readily gain at least a pound a week if I let it. For this to happen all I need do is eat just a little more food, or a few more calories per day. If I did that, my body would gain at least a pound a week and in 30 months weigh over 300 pounds.

In short, the Weight Success Method works, and because it does I wrote this book. And, how long has it been working? The note below hung on my bulletin board for the entire year of 2019. It indicates **12** years of living in my healthy-weight range.

Which means, each New Year's Eve I update the note with a new note that displays the next higher number. Believe me, it's a *great* way to kick off each year. I see the note *every* day of the year. I get a good feeling from it every day. Now here's the final point: *If I can do it, you can do it.* There's nothing special about me. I'm convinced what's working for me will work for you, too.

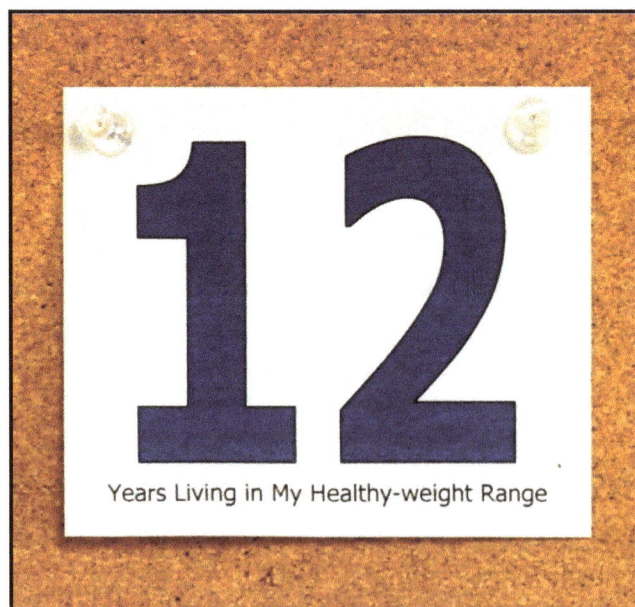

Years Living in My Healthy-weight Range

Who Can Benefit from the Method

You can benefit from the Weight Success Method presented in this book in any of four ways. First, if you've lost weight and are now at your desired weight and want to *easily stay* that way, apply the Weight Success Method and you'll make the weight loss stick for life.

Second, if you're presently in the process of losing weight and you want to do it more *easily* and *enjoyably,* do the Method in combination with the dietary program you're now pursuing and losing weight will become easier and more enjoyable.

Third, if you've never been overweight and you want to ensure you easily stay *non*-overweight the rest of your life, start doing the Method and you'll easily prevent yourself from ever becoming overweight and, thereby, live in your healthy-weight range the rest of your life.

Fourth, if you're overweight and you want to (a) reduce your weight to your desired healthy-weight range and then (b) live in your healthy-weight range the rest of your life, do the Method and it'll happen — and most likely it'll happen more easily and enjoyably than you ever imagined.

The Salient Distinguishing Factor

In the world of dieting and weight control this book stands apart from others. It's because of a certain key distinguishing factor. What most distinguishes this book from all others is:

This book pursues weight control — a.k.a. healthy-weight living — with a
Success Methodology

We define *success methodology* as: an action plan that pertains to a certain type of pursuit and consists of specific actions that, when performed by a person, cause a maximal number of success drivers to be included in that pursuit, thereby resulting in easiest possible creation of the desired situation or outcome associated with the pursuit.

This book presents a success methodology for creating *weight success.* Or, expressed in detail, it presents a success methodology for living most or all of the rest of your days in your desired healthy-weight range while also deriving benefits, enjoyment, and fulfillment from it. This methodology is what distinguishes this publication from all others.

As previously stated, the name of the success methodology is *Weight Success Method.*

Some people might refer to this book as a "diet book." But that would be an inaccurate description. It's not a diet book; it's a Weight Success Empowerment Book. Meaning, it's a book that empowers people to succeed at achieving weight success by giving them an effective methodology that, when applied, results in the inclusion of *success drivers* into their weight success pursuit — which, in turn, results in them succeeding at living most or all of the rest of their days in their desired healthy-weight range <u>and</u> deriving benefits, enjoyment, and fulfillment from it.

Success Drivers

So, what is a success driver? We define a *success driver* as: a condition or activity that, when present, increases the likelihood of a person succeeding at a certain pursuit — or, more specifically, increases the likelihood of a person performing actions that foster creation of a certain desired situation or outcome associated with the pursuit.

So, when success drivers are present, success at a pursuit usually happens — and often happens more easily and enjoyably than what one expects. Conversely, when success drivers are absent, success usually doesn't happen or if it does happen it involves inordinate time and effort. So ...

Success Drivers ➔ Success at a Pursuit
<u>No</u> Success Drivers ➔ <u>No</u> Success

Which means, by installing and maintaining success drivers in a significant personal life-enhancing pursuit we make each day be a Success Day — that is, a day that contributes to creating a certain desired outcome associated with that pursuit. This is the *essential dynamic* by which success is achieved in every significant personal endeavor or pursuit — including the pursuit of lifelong healthy-weight living. In infographic form the dynamic looks like this (next page).

A certain significant life-enhancing pursuit

+ plus

Success drivers included in the pursuit

↓ results in

Making each day be a **Success Day** — that is, a day that contributes to creating the desired outcome associated with that pursuit

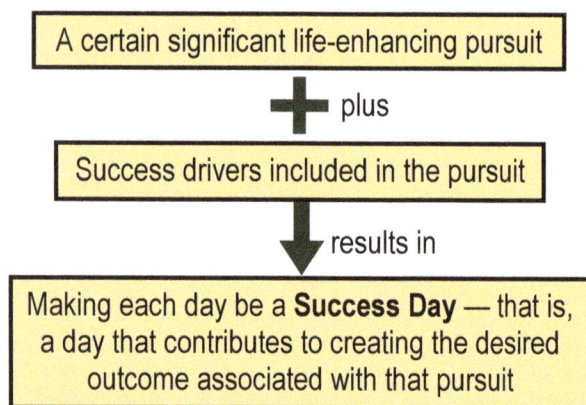

There are 19 main success drivers in the pursuit of weight success. They're the drivers I regard as being most effective for creating success in almost any significant personal pursuit, including the pursuit of weight control and healthy-weight living. The more drivers that are included, the more easily one achieves the desired outcome or goal. Here are those 19 main success drivers.

1 – Achievement goal
2 – Failure cause awareness
3 – Goal-achieving mindset
4 – Enjoyment of process
5 – Motivating reason
6 – Mandate decision
7 – Feedback system
8 – Reminder system
9 – Goal-achieving knowledge
10 – Essential Success Actions
11 – Desire
12 – Focus
13 – Self-communication
14 – Progress tracking and response
15 – Self-reinforcement
16 – Setback surmounting
17 – Persistence
18 – Goal-achieving relationships
19 – Whole-mind involvement

> **Note:** For a full description of these success drivers, go to Ch. **19** at page 117.

Now, this long list might look daunting. But don't be put off by its length or seeming complexity. Installing and maintaining these success drivers in your weight success journey is *easy* to do if you take the right approach. This right approach is the success methodology we call *Weight Success Method.* Doing the ten Startup Actions (p. **14**) of

the Method helps install Success Drivers #1–9 into your weight success pursuit. Doing the five Daily Actions (p. **22**) helps install and maintain Success Drivers #10–19 into your weight success pursuit.

To sum up, by doing the Weight Success Method you will automatically include most or all of the 19 success drivers into your weight success journey, which will result in you succeeding at more easily creating lifelong weight success. In infographic form it looks like this.

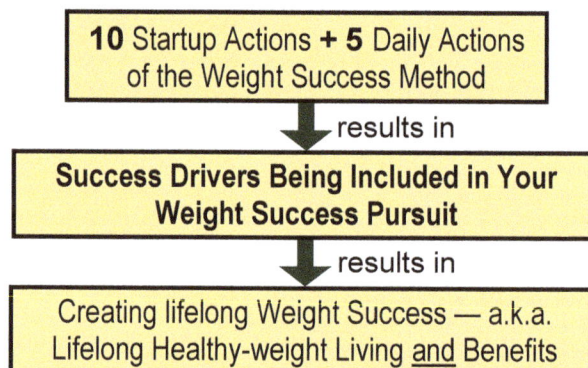

10 Startup Actions **+ 5** Daily Actions of the Weight Success Method

↓ results in

Success Drivers Being Included in Your Weight Success Pursuit

↓ results in

Creating lifelong Weight Success — a.k.a. Lifelong Healthy-weight Living <u>and</u> Benefits

So, when pursuing weight <u>reduction</u> do the Weight Success Method. This causes success drivers to be included in your weight *reduction* pursuit. After achieving your desired weight and going into weight <u>maintenance</u>, continue doing the Weight Success Method. This causes success drivers to be included in your weight *maintenance* pursuit.

> For additional introductory info on the Weight Success Method and what makes it unique and powerful, go to Ch. **2** at page 43.

The Secret Discovered

Research tells us that about **90** percent of the times when people lose weight they eventually gain it back. Numerous sources substantiate this number. Here, for example, is one such source:

https://healthblog.uofmhealth.org/health-management/weighing-facts-tough-truth-about-weight-loss

So, for every 100 persons who have lost weight and succeeded at achieving a certain desired weight, at least 90 of them have *failed* at maintaining that desired weight. This is a sad situation, indeed. It's a situation that forces a seminal question: WHY is it that, as of year 2020, at least 90 percent of the people who set out to achieve lifelong weight control eventually fail at it, and only ten percent succeed at it?

For several decades now researchers have been seeking to uncover the factors that have been causing this situation. For easy reference I call these factors **_fat-promoting factors._** They are factors that promote overeating and/or weight gain, or that make it easier for a person to overeat and/or gain weight. These researchers have been looking everywhere and have come up with an amazing compilation of fat-promoting factors.

Several years ago I decided to make myself knowledgeable of these sinister forces. So in December 2015 I conducted some Internet research. I compiled a list of the factors that weight scientists and researchers have "discovered" are a "cause" of overeating and/or weight gain. Here it is.

As of December 2015, here's what researchers have identified as a "cause" of overeating and fat gain: genes, hormones, heredity, body chemistry, brain function, gender, age, menopause, lifestyle, too slow rate of metabolism, expanded appetite or food cravings, decreased smoking, anxiety, stress, depression, lack of sleep, lack of fiber, lack of fatty acids, eating at the wrong time, skipping breakfast, eating foods in the wrong sequence, eating too fast, eating foods derived from grains, eating foods containing "hidden carbs," low-fat foods, salt, sugar, artificial sweeteners, potato chips, food advertising, fast-food restaurants, availability of packaged foods made with too much sugar, artificial additives in food, low cost of food due to agricultural innovation, taste buds insensitivity, too little exercise, working night shifts, unhealthy friends and family, glamorization of overweight- ness, criticism of overweightness, hearing people talk about body weight, thinking you're overweight, too many plus-sized models, yo-yo dieting, age and weight of your mother when you were born, level of carbon monoxide in the atmosphere, indoor temperature too high, lack of air conditioning during hot months, living near a noisy highway or railway or airline flight path, doing repeated decision-making at work, certain environmental factors that promote eating, endocrine disrupting chemicals such as bisphenol A and phthalates, certain environmental chemicals such as flame retardants, types of bacteria in your intestine, increasing abundance of food in modern society, certain viruses such as adenoviruses, and certain drugs such as medications that treat depression, heartburn, diabetes, inflammation, allergies, hypo- thyroidism, hypertension, contraception, and men- tal illness. Yes, every one has been cited as a factor causing overeating or overweightness.

And, amazingly, the list keeps growing! As previously stated, the above array of fat-promoting factors is current as of _December 2015._ It's much larger as of the date you're reading this, because since 2015 the obsessive quest to "discover" new scapegoat fat-promoting factors has been surging onward.

Not surprisingly, this "science of fat-promoting factors" is super-seductive. When I first encoun- tered it it seemed like some of these factors pertained to me. It seemed like they might be the cause of my overeating and weight gain. Finally, I realized that this "discovering fat-promoting factors craze" is creating one of the craziest, most harmful national delusions in history. It's the _"I can't control my weight"_ delusion. This is a _very_ dangerous thing. It's dangerous because it leads to the copout conclusion "There's no point in me even trying."

So, don't be sucked into the growing fat- promoting factors movement. Don't let the media hype that publicizes it make you believe you don't control your destiny when it comes to healthy- weight living. Because, you _do_ control it.

Sure, some of these fat-promoting factors might promote overeating and make it easier to gain weight. But not a one _causes_ a person to overeat or be overweight. Overeating and over- weightness are caused by one thing only: overper- formance of a certain 3-action process, the process of opening our mouth, inserting food into our mouth, and swallowing the food — a process that happens to be _totally controllable_ by each of us. Our failure to recognize and act on this truth is a main factor preventing our succeeding at creating healthy-weight living.

So, we now return to our starting question: Why is it, as of 2020, that 90 percent of the people who set out to achieve lifelong weight control eventually fail at it, and only ten percent succeed at it?

After much thought I finally realized what's happening. It has little or nothing to do with fat-promoting factors. Rather, the ten percent who are succeeding at lifelong weight control are pursuing weight control in a *different way* than the ninety percent who are failing at it. Specifically, those who are <u>succeeding</u> at weight control *are doing weight success actions every day.* Those who are <u>failing</u> at weight control are <u>not</u> doing weight success actions every day <u>or</u> are not doing enough weight success actions every day.

So, what exactly is a weight success action? Any action that contributes to creating weight success we call a *weight success action.* And, *weight success* is: Living most or all of one's days in one's desired healthy-weight range <u>and</u> deriving benefits, enjoyment, and fulfillment from it.

One of the purposes of this book is to set forth a host of potent weight success actions, which we'll be doing in upcoming sections of this book. But at this point you might like some specifics. So here are some specific actions that are weight success actions: the ten Startup Actions (p. 14) of the Weight Success Method, the five Daily Actions (p. 22) of the Method, the actions described in the Weight Success Benefits Directive (p. 32), and any of the actions prescribed in Chapters 2–27.

Now, distilled to simplest form, here's the key to succeeding at creating lifelong weight success. I've dubbed it Weight Success Secret, for short.

> **The Weight Success Secret is:**
> To succeed at lifelong healthy-weight living,
> *do <u>Weight Success Actions</u> every day.*

By doing Weight Success Actions every day you create Weight Success Days — that is, days that contribute to creating weight success. So, how does one create Weight Success Actions? *Enact a success methodology that, when performed each day, installs success drivers into your daily weight success pursuit.*

Interestingly, this dynamic — the process of daily enacting a success methodology that installs success drivers into a particular pursuit — is the basic dynamic by which success is achieved in virtually every type of significant human endeavor. (Note: This dynamic can happen knowingly <u>or</u> non-knowingly, deliberately <u>or</u> by accident.) Pertaining to the pursuit of weight success, it's my opinion that the most effective success methodology is the Weight Success Method.

The Weight Success Method comprises two parts: (1) ten STARTUP actions and (2) five DAILY actions. You do the ten startup actions at the beginning of your weight success journey. Then, after that, you do the five daily actions each day for the rest of your life. No, it's not time-consuming. Doing all five actions typically takes *less than* eight minutes of dedicated time per day.

Note: If you'd like more introductory info on the Weight Success Method, go to Ch. **2** at page 43.

Most people think the first step to healthy-weight living is to change the way one eats. Actually, the first step is to change the way one THINKS — or how one conceives of one's <u>self</u>, of one's <u>mind</u>, of one's <u>life</u>, and of
how healthy-weight living works. (This book explains.)

Part 1-B: Summation of the Method in One Page

HERE'S THE essence of the Weight Success Method.

Weight Success Actions are It!

An action that contributes to you creating weight success we call a *Weight Success Action.* To create lifelong weight success, do Weight Success Actions *every day.* This is the secret to lifelong healthy-weight living. To accomplish it, do these actions — which are the key <u>Weight Success Actions</u>.

FIRST, do these ten *Startup Actions.*

1. Realize that the *real cause* of overweightness is the act of consuming more calories than what your body is metabolizing (p. 14).

2. Identify your desired healthy-weight *range* (p. 14).

3. Identify your desired weight success *benefits* (p. 15).

4. Make weight success a *mandatory* feature of your life (p. 15).

5. Hold the desire and belief that weight success *will* happen and happen *easily* (p. 15).

6. Make your *top* eating priority to be healthy-weight calorie consumption (p. 17).

7. Adopt a bona fide dietary program that fits *you* (p. 19).

8. Set up a *fail-proof* reminder mechanism (p. 20).

9. Obtain a *good* scale (p. 20).

10. Commit to doing *Weight Success Actions* <u>every</u> day (p. 20).

SECOND, after doing the ten Startup Actions, do these five *Daily Actions* each day (which typically takes <u>less than</u> **8** minutes of dedicated time per day).

1. Correctly weigh yourself each day (p. 22).

2A. Each time your daily weight reading is a <u>desired</u> reading, praise yourself (p. 23),
    - OR -

2B. Whenever your daily weight reading is an <u>undesired</u> reading, enact immediate corrective action (p. 26).

3. Each day, direct your mind — including subconscious mind — to act on your eating directions, and also visualize one of your weight success benefits (p. 28).

4. Each day, say your Healthy-weight Goal at least 25 times (p. 34).

5. Each time you eat, apply guided eating (p. 35).

The ten Startup Actions and five Daily Actions constitute a success methodology called *Weight Success Method™*. Doing these actions is the essential process to creating weight success forever — or living most or all of the rest of your days in your desired healthy-weight range <u>and</u> deriving benefits, enjoyment, and fulfillment from it.

Lastly, when you seek more in-depth information or an answer to a question, find it in the Backup Resource section (Chapters 2–27).

Weight Success is: Living most or all of one's days in one's desired healthy-weight range <u>and</u> deriving benefits, enjoyment, and fulfillment from it. The easiest way to create Weight Success is the **Weight Success Method** — first do the ten Startup Actions and then do the five Daily Actions each day for the rest of your life. By doing this, Weight Success Forever will be <u>YOURS</u>. So ... *read on.*

Part 1-C: Ten STARTUP Actions of the Method

The actions of the Weight Success Method come in two groups: (1) STARTUP Actions and (2) DAILY Actions. This is the FIRST group. Doing these 10 Startup Actions is the start of your Weight Success Journey.

DOING THE upcoming ten startup actions lays the foundation for succeeding at lifelong healthy-weight living. It helps you install Success Drivers into your weight success journey. You do these ten actions at the beginning. But bear in mind, to create maximal success in your weight success pursuit you must retain the result of these actions, or keep acting upon the decisions made in these actions, throughout your weight success journey — meaning, each day for the rest of your life.

> Note: For more information on success drivers, go to Ch. **19** at page 117.

The WEIGHT SUCCESS METHOD begins with these ten Startup Actions:

Action 1: **FAILURE CAUSE** (p. 14)

Action 2: **WEIGHT RANGE** (p. 14)

Action 3: **WEIGHT SUCCESS BENEFITS** (p. 15)

Action 4: **MANDATORY FEATURE** (p. 15)

Action 5: **MINDSET** (p. 15)

Action 6: **EATING APPROACH** (p. 17)

Action 7: **DIETARY PROGRAM** (p. 19)

Action 8: **REMINDER** (p. 20)

Action 9: **SCALE** (p. 20)

Action 10: **THE KEY** (p. 20)

Startup Action **1:** FAILURE CAUSE
Recognize the *real* cause of overweightness.

There's only one real cause of our overweightness. It's *overperformance* of a certain three-action process, the process of:

1 – Opening our mouth;

2 – Inserting a piece of metabolizable calorie-containing food into our mouth; and

3 – Swallowing the piece of food.

We call it the *Open–Insert–Swallow* process — or **O-I-S** process, for short.

Overperformance of this process is the <u>real</u> cause of overeating and weight gain. And, it's the only cause. This process is how we consume more metabolizable calories than what our body is metabolizing, or "burning up," per day, which in turn is what causes us to gain weight. Lastly, recognize that this process is *totally controllable* by each of us.

So ...

Even though much of society refuses to admit it, weight gain and overweightness is created by our actions and, therefore, is controllable by each of us.

OVERPERFORMANCE OF

☺-I-S

The REAL Cause of Overweightness

> **Definition:** *Overeating* is the act of consuming more calories than what our body is metabolizing, or "burning up," per day. ~ (<u>This</u> is how weight gain happens.)

Startup Action **2:** WEIGHT RANGE
Identify a desired healthy-weight *range.*

Instead of using a single pound or kilogram number as your weight target or goal, use a weight *range.* And, make the range wide enough that it's possible — with a reasonable effort — to get *within* the range on most or all of your days. By using a weight range as your goal you have opportunity to be a weight management *success* all or most of the time. This weight range becomes the essence of your Healthy-weight Goal — a.k.a. weight goal or achievement goal.

So …

For starters, set your ideal weight range span to be six, seven, or eight pounds or, if you weigh in kilos, three or four kilograms. Then, view every number in your healthy-weight range as being a *healthy weight* for you. Which means, whenever your body weight is in your healthy-weight range you're living at your healthy weight, a situation we call *healthy-weight living.* For example, if your weight range were 158–164 pounds, then each day your weight is between 158.0 to 164.9 pounds you would be "at your healthy weight."

> **For more**, go to Ch. **6** at page 56. Reading this is recommended.

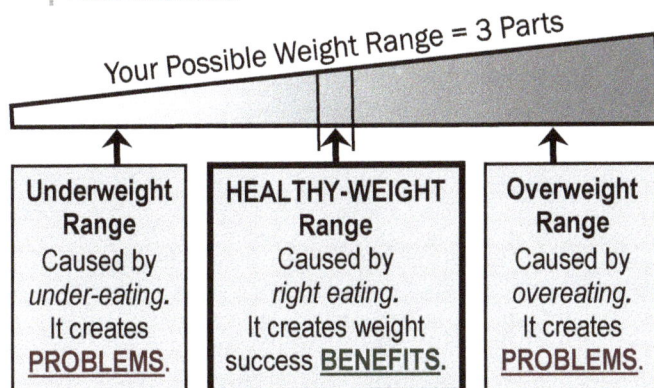

Your Possible Weight Range = 3 Parts

Underweight Range	HEALTHY-WEIGHT Range	Overweight Range
Caused by *under-eating.* It creates PROBLEMS.	Caused by *right eating.* It creates weight success BENEFITS.	Caused by *overeating.* It creates PROBLEMS.

Startup Action **3**: BENEFITS

Identify your weight success *benefits.*

Having a good reason for doing something builds our motivation to do it and increases our resoluteness to press on when a setback occurs. As regards the pursuit of weight success, the "good reason" we have for doing it is the benefits we gain from living in our healthy-weight range. We call these benefits *weight success benefits.*

> **For more** on weight success benefits go to Ch. **7** at page 60. Reading this is recommended.

So …

Identify your weight success benefits. Then reflect on these benefits *each day.* By doing this it moti-

vates your mind to pursue activities that lead to realizing these benefits, which includes the activity of creating healthy-weight living success. Here's an infographic.

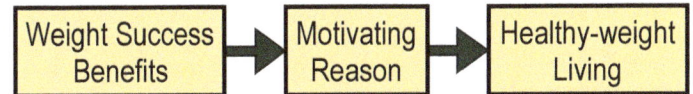

Weight Success Benefits → Motivating Reason → Healthy-weight Living

---

Startup Action **4**: MANDATORY FEATURE

Decide that healthy-weight living is a *mandatory* feature of your life.

Mandatory feature means: <u>non</u>-optional, <u>will</u>-do, <u>must</u>-have aspect of your existence. Most people who fail to create healthy-weight living have also failed to make the firm decision that living in their healthy-weight range is a mandatory feature of their life. When living in your healthy-weight range *isn't* a mandatory, must-have aspect of your life, you tend to get discouraged or quit whenever a setback arises.

So …

Decide right now that living in your healthy-weight range is — and will continue to be — a *mandatory* feature of your existence. Then, hold this decision in mind for the rest of your life.

Startup Action **5**: MINDSET

Adopt a *weight success mindset.*

Our dominant views and beliefs — a.k.a. assumptions — shape our life. They do this by triggering thoughts, feelings, and actions that work to create actual situations that correspond to the imagined situations depicted within our views and beliefs. In doing so, our beliefs affect every aspect of our existence, *including* that aspect called eating and weight management.

Sadly, as pertains to weight management many people hold self-defeating views and beliefs. They believe — or assume — that either (a) they can't succeed at living their desired weight or (b) if they do succeed at it it will involve hardship and suffering. This results in them never even trying to live their desired weight or, if they do try, eventually quitting because they find it to be "hard."

> SIDE NOTE: At this point I must make an admission. I believe *anyone* can (a) succeed at living most or all of their days at their healthy weight and (b) do it easily and enjoyably. I further believe, based on personal experience, that the quickest way to make this happen is by doing the Weight Success Method described in this chapter.

So ...

Realizing the huge impact of our beliefs on our life, what should we be doing? We should be holding views and beliefs that promote creation of the situations we want to have happen — including the situations of (a) controlling our weight and living in our healthy-weight range and (b) doing it *easily.*

As pertains to creating lifelong healthy-weight living, there's a particular mindset — which we call *weight success mindset* — that consists of seven key views and beliefs. Holding this mindset opens the door to the easiest way to create weight control and healthy-weight living. For ease of expression, I'll describe it like a person would express it.

My weight success mindset includes these views and beliefs:

1. Living in my healthy-weight range requires doing Weight Success Actions *every day.*

2. Living in my healthy-weight range is a <u>mandatory</u> feature of my existence — so, living outside that range is a <u>non-option</u>.

3. Living in my healthy-weight range provides me many great benefits.

4. I possess the power to make it happen — that is, I possess the power to (a) direct my eating, (b) direct my thoughts and feelings as pertains to eating, (c) live in my healthy-weight range *and* do it easily, and (d) surmount any fat-promoting factor I might encounter.

5. For me, right eating is more enjoyable and rewarding than wrong eating.

6. For me, correct calorie consumption is more important and rewarding than maximization of eating pleasure.

7. I view every challenge and setback in my weight success journey as a stepping stone to greater personal progress and future healthy-weight living, and not as a millstone holding me back from future success.

Holding a mindset of the above seven elements maximizes your effectiveness at achieving weight control and healthy-weight living. Here's why. Your mind — including your subconscious mind — creates thoughts and feelings that align with your major beliefs. Which is to say, your mind seldom operates in contradiction to your major views and beliefs, or outside the boundaries defined by those views and beliefs. So you should make sure all your eating- and weight-related mindset elements are ones that promote right eating and living in your healthy-weight range, and that none of them promote wrong eating or living outside your healthy-weight range. The above seven elements have maximal impact on creating the types of thoughts and feelings that promote right eating and healthy-weight living. So, they should be part of your "eating and weight management mindset."

Now here's a main point: <u>Doing the Weight Success Method assists you with installing these mindset elements into your mind</u>.

So, ask yourself this question: *How do I want my weight success journey to be?* Do I want it to be tough? (It can be that.) Or, do I want it to be easy? (It can be that, too.) So decide now how you *want* it to be and *believe* it will be:

Hard   *Easy* ✓

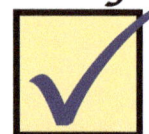

In short, weight management is either: (a) depressing drudgery or (b) uplifting journey. *You* determine, in large part, which it will be by the desires and the beliefs you hold in your mind. So, hold the desire and the belief that it will be *easy* ... or, at least, way easier than you ever imagined it could be. In short, succeeding at creating healthy-weight living depends, to a large extent, on you *believing*

and *acting as-if* you possess the power to make it happen.

How Believing and Acting As-if Work

Here's why believing and acting as-if are important. The act of *believing* that your mind is *in the process* of performing certain actions is one of the most powerful tools there is for succeeding at healthy-weight living (and other pursuits, as well). So, each day hold the belief that your mind — including your subconscious mind — is acting on what you want it to be doing. This includes holding the belief that your mind is pursuing the healthy-weight living goal you want it to be pursuing.

Also ... Act As-if

Along with believing, act as-if. That is, conduct your thinking, feelings, and actions in accordance with the belief that your mind — including subconscious mind — is right then in the process of listening to and taking action on everything you're telling it. When you do this it motivates your mind to create the types of thoughts and feelings you desire to have, which in this case are thoughts and feelings that steer you toward right eating and healthy-weight living.

But, what should you do if you find it hard to muster the belief that your mind is acting on what you're telling it? Again, the answer is: Act as-if. To do this, *you totally pretend you believe.* That is, you role-play that your mind — including subconscious mind — is right then in the process of doing what you're telling it to do. And, in doing this role-play you hold in mind the thoughts and feelings that would be present within your mind if your mind was, in fact, right then doing what you're telling it to do.

Perhaps all this seems a bit odd. But do it anyhow — it works. It triggers your mind to produce the thoughts and feelings you desire to have — in this case, thoughts and feelings that guide you to lifelong healthy-weight living.

Acting as-if is one of the most powerful tools there is for making healthy-weight living happen. So, hold in mind the assumption that you have the

wherewithal to easily make healthy-weight living happen, then conduct your thinking, feelings, and actions in accordance with that assumption.

> **Definition of Acting As-if:** *Acting as-if* is the act of holding in mind an assumption that a particular situation presently exists or is in the process of coming about, and then conducting one's thinking, feelings, and actions in accordance with that assumption.

Your thoughts and feelings determine your eating actions, your eating actions determine your weight. You <u>do</u> have the power to create and hold healthy-weight-promoting thoughts and feelings each day.

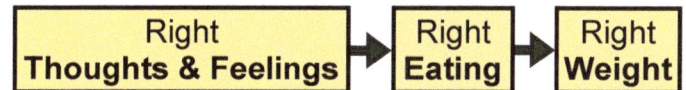

Right Thoughts & Feelings	→	Right Eating	→	Right Weight

Startup Action **6:** EATING APPROACH
Adopt the *Right Eating* approach to eating.

There are two main approaches to eating: (1) *pleasure* priority approach and (2) *healthy-weight* priority approach. Each exerts a powerful impact: one negatively, the other positively.

With the **PLEASURE priority approach** the main goal is *eating pleasure maximization*. Unfortunately, this leads to over-performing the Open–Insert–Swallow process. Which, in turn, results in overeating and weight gain. As such, the pleasure priority approach makes weight control *very* hard to do. This is a main factor causing people to struggle with creating healthy-weight living.

> **Definition of Overeating:** *Overeating* is the act of consuming a greater number of calories than what your body is metabolizing, or "burning up," per day.

But with the **HEALTHY-WEIGHT priority approach** the main goal is: eating an amount of calories that leads to healthy-weight living — otherwise called *healthy-weight calorie consump-*

tion. This approach results in performing the Open–Insert–Swallow process to a proper extent. As such, it leads to non-overeating and living in one's desired weight range, as depicted here.

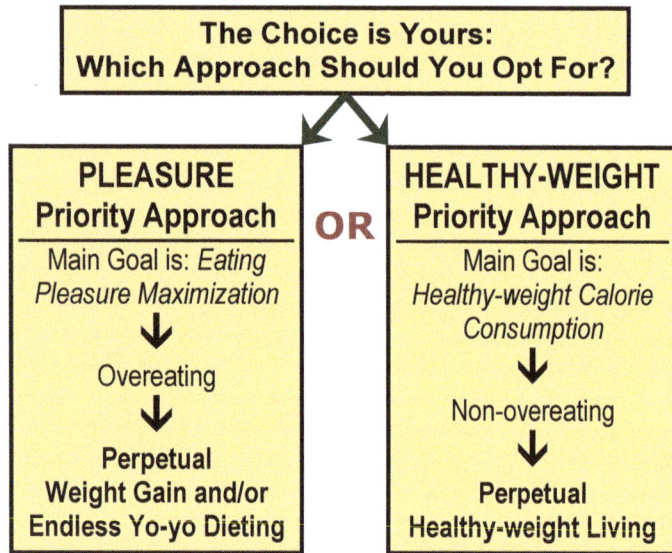

```
┌────────────────────────────────────────┐
│          The Choice is Yours:           │
│  Which Approach Should You Opt For?     │
└────────────────────────────────────────┘
        ↙                    ↘
┌──────────────────┐  ┌──────────────────┐
│   PLEASURE       │  │  HEALTHY-WEIGHT   │
│ Priority Approach│OR│ Priority Approach │
│                  │  │                   │
│ Main Goal is: Eating│ │ Main Goal is:    │
│ Pleasure Maximization│ Healthy-weight Calorie│
│        ↓         │  │   Consumption     │
│   Overeating     │  │        ↓          │
│        ↓         │  │  Non-overeating   │
│   Perpetual      │  │        ↓          │
│ Weight Gain and/or│ │    Perpetual      │
│ Endless Yo-yo Dieting│ Healthy-weight Living│
└──────────────────┘  └──────────────────┘
```

Regrettably, most persons opt for the pleasure priority approach. This dooms them to regular overeating and weight gain which, in turn, makes it nearly impossible for them to succeed at living their life in their desired healthy-weight range.

So ...

Avoid the pleasure priority approach to eating and embrace the healthy-weight priority approach.

Now, at this point you might be thinking: "Yes, healthy-weight calorie consumption looks like the smart option, but pleasure maximization is the *fun* option, so that's for me." That's how most people view it, which is why most people are endlessly gaining weight. But they're mistaken about the healthy-weight priority approach. It can be enjoyable and gratifying too, when applied a certain way. That "certain way" I call *right eating.*

Right Eating – Way to Healthy-weight Living

With **Right Eating** there are three priorities:

Priority #1 — Healthy-weight calorie consumption (top priority)

Priority #2 — Proper nutrition

Priority #3 — Eating enjoyment.

Each priority has a purpose. The purpose of priority #1 is healthy-weight living, or living your

life in your healthy-weight range. The purpose of priority #2 is having an optimally healthy body. The purpose of priority #3 is eating enjoyment derived while pursuing priorities #1 and #2. So, right eating promotes healthy-weight living, optimally healthy body, and eating enjoyment.

Also, each priority is achieved a certain way. You achieve priority #1 by eating a certain *amount* of food — specifically, an amount that results in healthy-weight calorie consumption. I call this amount **right amount.**

You achieve priority #2 by eating certain *types* of food — that is, types that promote good health. I call these types of food *right types,* or **right foods.**

You achieve priority #3 by performing priorities #1 and #2 with a certain enjoyment-creating approach — specifically, an approach that results in savoring and appreciating the flavors of right foods in right amounts. I call this *right eating enjoyment* or, simply, **right enjoyment.**

So here's my one-sentence definition of right eating. **Right Eating** is: Eating right foods in right amounts, and in a way that creates right eating enjoyment. Here's an infographic for it.

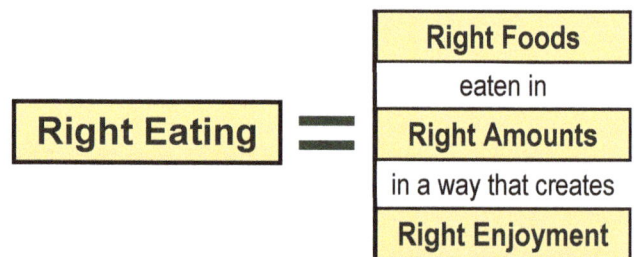

```
┌──────────────┐   ┌──────────────────┐
│              │   │   Right Foods     │
│              │   ├──────────────────┤
│              │ = │    eaten in       │
│ Right Eating │   ├──────────────────┤
│              │   │   Right Amounts   │
│              │   ├──────────────────┤
│              │   │ in a way that creates│
│              │   ├──────────────────┤
│              │   │  Right Enjoyment  │
└──────────────┘   └──────────────────┘
```

At this point you might be thinking, "Okay, sounds good, but how do I create right eating enjoyment?" Here are four guidelines for it.

> **Definition:** A *healthy-weight-promoting food* is a food that promotes creation of healthy-weight living.

Guidelines for Creating Right Eating Enjoyment

1. Create lower-calorie, *healthy-weight-promoting foods* that are <u>tasty</u> and <u>satisfying</u>.

2. Prepare *healthy-weight-promoting foods* that are easy to consume in right amounts and also <u>more satisfying</u>.

3. Eat *healthy-weight-promoting foods* in a way that maximizes <u>eating pleasure</u> derived from these foods.

4. Condition your mind to enjoy *healthy-weight-promoting foods* and to not enjoy overweight-promoting foods. This might sound hard to do, but actually it's fairly easy once you get into it.

> **Note:** For more on this subject, go to Ch. **12** at page 82.

Conclusion. Keep in mind the concept of Right Eating. It's a key concept to avoiding overeating and achieving easier healthy-weight living. And remember, of the three factors that constitute right eating, *healthy-weight calorie consumption* is the top priority. That's because the <u>real</u> cause of overweightness is overperformance of the Open–Insert–Swallow process.

OVERPERFORMANCE OF

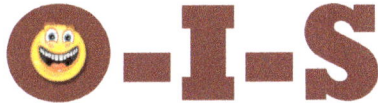

O-I-S

is how overeating and overweightness come about.

Startup Action **7**: DIETARY PROGRAM

Adopt a dietary program that fits YOU.

Almost every successful weight management pursuit involves a preferred dietary program. I define *preferred dietary program* as a set of eating guidelines and eating practices you prefer to follow and which, when followed, cause you to realize good health and healthy-weight living. When you don't have a dietary program that you're applying it increases the chances of you eventually straying "off course" and ending up gaining back the weight you once lost. Another name for preferred dietary program is preferred eating strategy.

Virtually any bona fide dietary program will work when it's *fully* applied. But most people never apply a program fully. Why? Because they're pursuing a program that doesn't fit their personal preferences, needs, and lifestyle. This results in them finding the program to be hard to do, so they quit.

So ...

Find the program that best fits your personal preferences, needs, and lifestyle. This is a key to dietary program success because the program that best fits you is the one you're most apt to apply fully. In short: full application = works fully; partial application = works partially or not at all. And, the program you're most apt to apply fully is the one that best fits you and your situation.

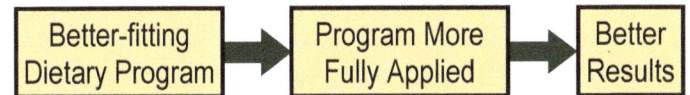

Better-fitting Dietary Program	→	Program More Fully Applied	→	Better Results

If you don't yet have a preferred dietary program you have a choice. It can be one of the bona fide established programs already on the market *or* it can be a program of your own design. Go whichever way will produce the best results for you.

> Your **preferred dietary program** is a set of eating guidelines and eating practices you prefer to follow and which, when followed, cause you to realize good health and healthy-weight living.
> For a preferred dietary program you have two choices:

Do one of the established bona fide dietary programs on the market.	OR	Do a dietary program of your own design (but make sure it's healthy).

If you're thinking about traveling the design-it-yourself road, be sure to apply the basic principles of nutrition so you avoid inadvertently adopting a harmful eating practice.

> **Note:** For info and ideas on creating a self-designed program, go to Ch. **11** at page 74.

A dietary program can be a straight-forward plan — such as eating a certain number of calories per day. Or, it can be a detailed program involving eating certain specific foods in certain amounts. Or, it can be any other nutritionally sound program involving a certain focus, procedures, or guidelines.

So, your objective should be either to find or to design the dietary program that *best fits you.* Hold this thought in mind: Somewhere in the world is a dietary program with "your name on it." If you desire to have it and believe you can get it, you'll eventually find it or create it.

Also, bear in mind you can change your dietary program any time you find a better one. So it's not required that you obtain the "perfect dietary program" before beginning weight management. You can start with an "acceptable" or "best available" program and then later, when you discover a better program, you can switch.

To conclude, it goes without saying that whatever dietary program you follow should be one that doesn't harm your health or create a potential medical problem. And, it could be a good idea to consult with your physician before adopting any new dietary program or making a major change in eating practices.

Startup Action **8**: REMINDER

Install a *failproof* reminder mechanism.

A main factor causing many people to fail at creating healthy-weight living is the act of *forgetting* to apply their weight management program.

So …

Set up a reminder mechanism that will remind you each day to apply the Weight Success Method. Make reminder messages to yourself. Then place these messages where you'll see them every day. Possibilities include: (a) in your bedroom, (b) on the refrigerator, (c) in your wallet or purse, (d) in your car, (e) on your computer, and (f) on your exercise equipment. Plus, put digital messages on your computer screen, smartphone, and other devices. Do whatever it takes to create a *failproof* reminder system. Here's a sample message.

Weight Success Method
Do it every day. Takes less than **8** minutes.
1 – Weighing
2 – Reinforcement or Correction
3 – Benefits Directive
4 – Goal Statement
5 – Guided Eating
(plus Daily Exercise Activity when possible)

Note: For more on this, go to *Setting Up a Failproof Reminder System*, in Ch. **27**, page 160.

Startup Action **9**: SCALE

Obtain a *good* scale.

The biggest irony in the world of weight control is this. The dreaded bathroom scale, which most folks despise and ignore, is the very thing that has the power to set them free. Here's why. When properly used, as described in Daily Action 1 of the Weight Success Method (p. 22), it delivers timely feedback that enables a person to take control of their weight management destiny.

So …

If you don't already have one, get a consistently accurate scale. Then make your scale a favorite tool and a friend.

> **Note:** For more on scales, go to Ch. **8** at page 62. Reading this is recommended.

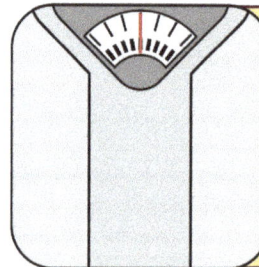

SECRET: Properly used, any good bathroom scale is the most powerful tool on the planet for creating healthy-weight living. Sadly, this fact is one of our "world's best-kept secrets."

Startup Action **10**: THE KEY

Commit to doing *Weight Success Actions* <u>every</u> day.

Never forget: The #1 reason why we fail at creating healthy-weight living is we fail to do Weight Success Actions every day.

So …

Apply the success methodology we call *Weight Success Method.* The five Daily Actions in the Method are some of the most powerful Weight Success Actions a person can do. Doing the Method installs and maintains success drivers in your weight success journey which, in turn, results in making most or all of your days be a Weight Success Day. Summed up, all this results in the Weight Success Dynamic shown next.

WEIGHT SUCCESS DYNAMIC

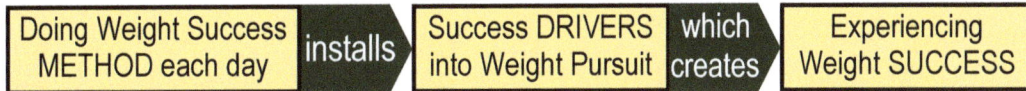

Doing Weight Success METHOD each day	installs	Success DRIVERS into Weight Pursuit	which creates	Experiencing Weight SUCCESS

WEIGHT SUCCESS = Living most or all of one's days in one's desired healthy-weight range <u>and</u> deriving benefits, enjoyment, and fulfillment from it. ~ For description of benefits, enjoyment, and fulfillment created by weight success, read Ch. **7** (p. 60), Ch. **17** (p. 103), Ch. **22** (p. 137), and Ch. **24** (p. 148). ~ A person who's in process of creating weight success we call a *Weight Winner.*

REMEMBER: The key to succeeding at healthy-weight living is: Do Weight Success Actions <u>every day</u>. The 10 Startup Actions are your launch pad in this process. They help install Success Drivers into your weight success pursuit.

KNOW THIS AND NEVER FORGET IT. You possess the capability to create healthy-weight living for life, and also the capability to create it **EASILY.** The five Daily Actions are your next step. They help further install and maintain Success Drivers in your weight success pursuit.

Part 1-D: Five DAILY Actions of the Method

The actions of the Weight Success Method come in two groups: (1) STARTUP Actions and (2) DAILY Actions. This is the SECOND group. Doing these five Daily Actions helps install and maintain Success Drivers in your Weight Success Journey.

AFTER COMPLETING the ten Startup Actions you begin the five Daily Actions. In doing so, bear in mind three things about these five actions.

1. They're *easy* to do.

2. In total, they typically take *less than* eight minutes of dedicated time per day.

3. They can be *combined* with any bona fide dietary program of your choice, including one of your own design.

   Side note: They're also highly effective for reversing Pandemic Fat Buildup.

The five DAILY ACTIONS of the Weight Success Method are:

Action 1: **WEIGHING** (p. 22)

Action 2A: **REINFORCEMENT** (p. 23)
           — OR —
Action 2B: **CORRECTION** (p. 26)

Action 3: **BENEFITS DIRECTIVE** (p. 28)

Action 4: **GOAL STATEMENT** (p. 34)

Action 5: **GUIDED EATING** (p. 35)

By doing these five Daily Actions each day (and also having done the ten Startup Actions) you go a long way toward installing and maintaining success drivers in your weight success pursuit. This results in you realizing the desired outcome, or goal, of the pursuit. The following pages tell how to do these five Daily Actions.

WEIGHT SUCCESS
——— is the GOAL ———

WEIGHT SUCCESS METHOD™
——— is the MEANS ———

Goal+Means+Action=WEIGHT SUCCESS™

Daily Action 1: WEIGHING

Correctly weigh yourself each day (and weigh only once a day).

This action typically takes *less than* 30 seconds.

WHY You Do It

Correct daily weighing is the *#1 most important* action for creating healthy-weight living. It's because of three outcomes. First, weighing each day creates *daily focus* on healthy-weight living. Second, it provides *timely feedback* on your prior day's healthy-weight efforts. Third, it enables you to give *immediate positive response* to your daily weight situation. There are two positive responses. When your daily weighing shows a <u>desired</u> weight you respond with reinforcement (Daily Action 2A). When the weighing shows an <u>undesired</u> weight you respond with immediate corrective action (Daily Action 2B). These three outcomes — daily focus, timely feedback, and immediate positive response — make correct daily weighing the #1 most important action in your weight success journey.

HOW to Do It

Create *accurate* weight readings. Your daily weight reading can vary slightly from weighing to weighing due to variables unrelated to fat gain or loss. We call these variables ***extraneous variables.*** Possible extraneous variables include: (a) when you last ate, (b) amount of water retention by your body, (c) amount of urine in your bladder, (d) amount of clothes you have on, (e) type of floor the scale is on, (f) location of the scale on the floor, (g) where you stand on the scale, and (h) where you distribute your body weight on your feet. You should strive to minimize the effect of these variables. To do that apply these eight rules.

Eight Rules for Correct Daily Weighing

Apply these eight rules every time.

1. **Use a good scale.** If possible, use one that's consistently accurate. Use the *same* scale for each weighing.

2. **Weigh at the *same time,*** or within the *same hour,* each day (and only once a day). The best time usually is in the morning prior to breakfast. Call it your Daily Weighing Hour. As an example, my daily weighing hour is 7:00 to 8:00 a.m.

3. **Avoid eating before weighing.** If you must eat soon, eat after the weighing.

4. **Empty your bladder before weighing.**

5. **Weigh yourself with nothing on,** or else with the same weight of clothing every time. (You'll likely find that weighing naked is the easiest way.)

6. **Position the scale on the same spot on the floor.**

7. **Stand on the same spot on the scale.**

8. **Use the same weight distribution on your feet.** It doesn't matter what the weight distribution is as long as it's the same with each weighing.

In short, weigh yourself in a way that accurately measures fat change (or non-change) from day to day. For this, weigh yourself at the *same time,* or in the same hour, and in the *same way* each day. The object is, make the extraneous variables be the same with each weighing. The best time for weighing is most likely in the morning before breakfast. Make it one of the first actions of each day.

Plus, when the final weight reading comes up on the scale, *SAY* that weight number to yourself.

Note on Scales. With many scales if you weigh yourself twice in a row it will give you two slightly different readings. If your scale is one of these, weigh yourself twice in a row at each weigh-in and then go with the *average* of the two numbers. But, if your scale is a consistently accurate one, weigh yourself just once.

Note: For more on scales and weighing, go to Ch. **8** at page 62.

SUMMING UP This Daily Action 1

Weigh every day, the same time, the same way, using the Eight Rules for Correct Daily Weighing each time. ~ Do this, and also the other four daily actions of the Weight Success Method, and lifelong healthy-weight living will be *yours.*

REMEMBER: The secret to succeeding at lifelong healthy-weight living is: Do Weight Success Actions <u>every</u> day. You accomplish this by doing the Weight Success Method, which typically takes <u>less than</u> **8** minutes of dedicated time per day. This causes vital *success drivers* to be installed and maintained in your weight success pursuit.

> Do the **Five Daily Actions** <u>every</u> day . . . and **Lifelong Weight Success** will be <u>Yours</u>.

Daily Action 2A: REINFORCEMENT

Each time your daily weight reading is a <u>desired</u> reading, respond with self-reinforcement.

This action typically takes *less than* 40 seconds.

Desired weight readings exist in two forms: (a) readings that come during weight maintenance pursuit and (b) readings that come during weight reduction pursuit. When in weight <u>maintenance</u> pursuit — or striving to maintain a certain weight — any reading that's within your healthy-weight range we call a *desired* weight reading. When in weight <u>reduction</u> pursuit — or striving to lose weight — any reading that's lower than the prior day's weight reading we call a *desired* weight reading.

Each day that you get a desired weight reading you follow up by delivering self-reinforcement to your mind — especially subconscious mind.

WHY You Do It

When your mind receives reinforcement — that is, an enjoyable or desirable response — for a particular action it performed, it motivates your subconscious mind to repeat that action. In this instance, the action for which your subconscious mind is receiving reinforcement is the act of creating thoughts and feelings that guide you to getting desired weight readings. Because of this dynamic, this Daily Action 2A increases the likelihood of having future desired weight readings.

HOW to Do It

One of the most powerful forms of reinforcement is sincere appreciation and praise. So, each day after your daily weighing, when you've discovered once again that you're living another day in your healthy-weight range, give your mind — that is, your self — praise and appreciation. Tell it you're super happy over the desired weight reading, and that you want it to keep up the good work. And, when delivering this self-communication, do it with exuberance and joy. In short, use your daily weighing each morning as a springboard for creating daily pride, happiness, and inspiration. It's a great way to start a day. I've been doing it for years. It never gets stale.

Recommended Message

To make it easy for you, following is a message I suggest you use for your self-reinforcement (the shaded italic paragraph in the next column). I call it the *Thank You, Keep It Up* message. For the blank line, insert one of these two phrases, whichever applies:

> *continue living in my healthy-weight range*
> — OR —
> *lose more weight.*

Insert the first phrase when you're in weight maintenance pursuit, the second one when in weight reduction pursuit.

You deliver the message by speaking either in regular-volume voice or in a whisper — your choice.

Thank you, thank you, thank you, subconscious mind! Thank you for guiding me to

_____.

*I really, truly appreciate you doing this. Keep it up. Keep on creating daily __thoughts__ and __feelings__ that guide me to consuming the **types** of food and the **amount** of food that results in me living each day of the rest of my life in my healthy-weight range. I __very much__ want you to do this. And, I believe __one hundred percent__ that you __will__ do it. Great work, subconscious mind! Keep it up. Thank you, thank you, thank you!*

The above Thank-you, Keep It Up message includes the phrase "subconscious mind." It's there to ensure that your subconscious mind focuses on what you're saying, so that it will "hear" the message and then *do it.*

A main driver of successful healthy-weight living is having your whole mind — that is, both conscious __and__ subconscious mind — involved each day in the pursuit of healthy-weight living.

> **Note:** For more discussion of Whole Mind Involvement, go to the *Success Driver 19* section in Ch. **19** at page 121.

One of the most effective ways of getting one's subconscious mind involved is direct communication — that is, directly communicating requests, directives, depiction statements, and thank-you messages to it. (This we do in Daily Actions 2A–5.)

For maximal impact, I suggest you address your subconscious mind by a name. It can be any name you like. You can use a person-type name, such as, for example, your first name. And, your subconscious mind will respond to that name as long as it knows you're speaking to it. Also, naming your subconscious mind "Subconscious Mind" is okay, too. Or, if you like, you can use a nickname such as, for example, "Sub-mind" or "Subby Mind" or "Subby." For what it's worth, I use the nickname Subby. Seems like a corny name, I know, but I've used it for years and my subconscious mind has readily responded to it.

To create maximal impact from saying your Thank-you, Keep It Up message, apply the following six actions when delivering it.

Six Actions for an Effective Thank You, Keep It Up Message

To maximize the effect of your Thank You, Keep It Up message, do these six actions when delivering it.

1. Use a **name**: Address your subconscious mind by *a name* — again, the name I use is "Subby," but the name "Subconscious Mind" and other names will work, too.

2. Be **specific**: Describe the *specific* desired action your subconscious mind has performed.

3. Express **appreciation**: Deliver *thanks and appreciation* for having performed the desired action.

4. Request **continuance**: Tell your subconscious mind to *continue performing* the desired action.

5. Express **desire**: Express the continuance request with *strong desire,* or emotional intensity.

6. Express **belief**: Express *firm belief* and also *act as-if* your subconscious mind is right then in the process of doing what you're requesting.

NOTE: The prior Thank You, Keep It Up message (p. **24**) incorporates all six actions — check it out.

The wording for the Thank You, Keep It Up message can vary slightly from weighing to weighing, as you might ad lib. But it mainly embodies the prior italic paragraph on page **24**. TIP: Make a copy of it and keep it where you can easily refer to it.

Deliver the Thank You, Keep It Up message in a way that creates maximum positive impact on your mind. So as you say it, generate a feeling of happiness and joy, joy over having gotten a desired weight reading for yet another day — which means

you're either in your healthy-weight range or moving toward it. The more joy you experience and express, the more it motivates your mind — in particular, your subconscious mind — to continue creating desired weight readings.

Also, when delivering the message — and during the rest of your day — *hold the belief* that your mind is right then, at that very moment, *in the process* of performing the actions described in the message. This enhances the impact.

> **For more information on believing and acting as-if**, go to the *How Believing and Acting As-if Work* section in Startup Action 5 (p. **17**). Reading this is recommended.

The prior example Thank You, Keep It Up message (p. 24) takes only about 30 seconds to deliver. Yet it's powerful. When reinforcing your subconscious mind there's no such thing as too much thanks and appreciation. So it's okay to include more praise and thanks than what's in the example message. Heap it on — with exuberance.

ADDITIONAL REINFORCEMENT. For more reinforcement for daily good performance, check out the *Mind Motivator 6: Goal Reminders* section in Ch. **13** at page 94.

An example of a strong visual reminder is the bulletin board note on page 8. It's recommended that you post visual reminders of your healthy-weight goal and of your ongoing realization of that goal. Then view these reminders throughout each day, and especially when doing this Daily Action 2A.

OPTIONAL PRAYER. If you're one who likes prayer, here's one you might use after each weighing.

I thank you, God, for making me to be,
and for the opportunity to become the finest person I'm
*   capable of being,*
and for the opportunity to live in my healthy-weight range,
and for the opportunity to do it easily.
I thank you very, very much.

It's a pithy expression of gratitude. It's also thought-provoking. I've been saying it for years right after delivering the Thank You, Keep It Up message. I find it motivating and uplifting.

SUMMING UP This Daily Action 2A

After each desired weight reading, thank and rein-force your mind — including your subconscious mind — and tell it to keep up the good work. When doing this, include the Thank You, Keep It Up message (p. **24**). Deliver the message using the Six Actions for an Effective Thank You, Keep It Up Message. ~ Do this Daily Action 2A each time you get a desired weight reading, and also do the other four daily actions of the Weight Success Method, and healthy-weight living will be *yours.*

REMEMBER: The secret to succeeding at lifelong healthy-weight living is: Do Weight Success Actions <u>every</u> day. You accomplish this by doing the Weight Success Method, which typically takes <u>less than</u> **8** minutes of dedicated time per day. This causes vital *success drivers* to be installed and maintained in your weight success pursuit.

> Do the **Five Daily Actions**
> <u>every</u> day . . .
> and **Lifelong Weight Success**
> will be <u>Yours</u>.

> ### Daily Action **2B**: CORRECTION
> **Whenever your daily weight reading is an <u>undesired</u> reading, respond with immediate corrective action that very day.**

So, what's an undesired weight reading?

When in weight <u>maintenance</u> pursuit, any daily weight reading that's outside, or above, your healthy-weight range we call an *undesired* weight reading. And, when in weight <u>reduction</u> pursuit, any daily weight reading that's higher than the prior day's weight reading we call an *undesired* weight reading.

Each time you get an undesired weight reading you should initiate corrective action.

WHY You Do It

Taking immediate corrective action fixes the undesired weight problem within 24 to 48 hours. This puts you instantly back on track to lifelong healthy-weight living and ensures that a small problem doesn't grow into a big one. In short, it *ensures* that your healthy-weight pursuit *never fails.*

The procedure for taking immediate corrective action varies between the two types of weight management pursuits. So, first I describe how to do it in weight maintenance pursuit, and then in weight reduction pursuit.

How to Take Corrective Action When in Weight *MAINTENANCE* Pursuit

To correct, or reverse, an undesired weight reading when in weight maintenance pursuit — or when striving to maintain a certain weight — do these two actions.

FIRST, avoid negative reaction. That is, don't get involved in second-guessing, self-doubt, self-pity, self-blame, guilt, or discouragement. Instead, declare the day to be a *Weight Correction Day.* View this Weight Correction Day as an exciting opportunity to build your personal strength and healthy-weight management expertise. This is *very* important.

SECOND, enact immediate corrective eating action. For the next 24 or 48 hours eat in a way that corrects the undesired situation in that time. To do this, go into *under-eating* mode. That is, consume fewer calories than what your body will be expending. You can do this with either total fasting or semi-fasting. With total fasting you eat nothing for that period. With semi-fasting you eat just a small amount.

> **Note:** If engaging in under-eating could create a problem or be harmful to you, find out from your doctor what a safe minimal number of daily calories is for you. Then consume that daily amount for the duration of your under-eating period. As always,

before adopting any new dietary program or major change in eating practices you should consult with your physician.

If you opt for semi-fasting do this. Pick a "calorie target" — like, say, for example, 1000 calories for the day. And then consume only that many calories. Does this seem like it would be hard to do? Well, it's not. Just make the decision to do it and then do it. If you feel that this would be difficult, or might be a burden on you, bear this point in mind.

Correcting a weight-gain situation after it has become big is about a *hundred* times harder than correcting it when it's small, or first crops up. So, eagerly correct the problem *now.* In doing this, don't view a weight correction day as a hardship; instead, view it as an opportunity — an opportunity to save yourself a massive amount of future hardship by expending a miniscule amount of effort and "suffering" today, or for just 24 hours. So, *never* procrastinate on fixing an undesired weight reading. Always do it *that very day.* Typically, going into under-eating mode will bring your body weight back into your healthy-weight range in just 24 to 48 hours.

> Special Note: When needed, do the *setback-reversal process* described in Ch. **10** at page 68.

Reminder: When your daily weight reading shows a <u>desired</u> weight, you do Action **2A** and not 2B. When it shows an <u>undesired</u> weight you do Action **2B** and not 2A.

Staving Off Hunger Pangs. If you find yourself being nagged by hunger pangs while doing this Action 2B, apply one or more of these three tactics.

Tactic 1: Drink Water. When you feel a hunger pang drink some water. This fills your stomach, which reduces the hunger pang.

Tactic 2: Deliver a Mini-directive. Before drinking the water, deliver this directive to your subconscious mind: "Subconscious mind, after I finish drinking this water, reduce my hunger pang for the next two hours. I *know* you can do it. I *want* you to do it. I believe one hundred percent that you *will* do it. And, I thank you for doing it."

Tactic 3: Say the Goal Statement. Silently say this healthy-weight goal statement throughout the day, especially whenever you feel a hunger pang.

"I <u>am</u> the person of my healthy weight.
I am healthy, happy, and doing great."
In short, whenever a hunger pang arises, focus your mind on your healthy-weight goal.

How to Take Corrective Action When in Weight *REDUCTION* Pursuit

To respond appropriately to an undesired weight reading when in weight reduction pursuit — or while striving to lose weight — do these four, or possibly five, actions.

ACTION 1: *Be Real.* ✒ Realize that an undesired weight reading can occur from extraneous variables (which are listed in Daily Action 1, page **22**). So, bear in mind that this particular undesired reading might be a result of that. If it is, then the variable that caused today's "weight gain reading" will likely cause a "weight loss reading" tomorrow or the day after, when the variable is working in reverse. Also, make sure you're applying the Eight Rules for Correct Daily Weighing every day (which are described in Daily Action 1).

ACTION 2: *Avoid Negative Reaction.* ✒ Avoid second-guessing, self-doubt, self-pity, self-blame, guilt, and discouragement. All these are counterproductive. Instead view the undesired weight reading as an opportunity to improve your weight management expertise. This is *very* important.

ACTION 3: *Do Your Full Dietary Program.* ✒ Make sure you're following your weight-loss regimen, or preferred dietary program, completely. If you haven't been, recommit yourself to doing so, then start doing it that very day. <u>Also</u>, make sure you're doing all five daily actions of the Weight Success Method <u>every day</u>.

ACTION 4: *Reverse the Setback.* ✒ If you've gotten an undesired, or weight gain, weight reading <u>three</u> days in a row, do the *setback-reversal process* described in Ch. **10** (p. 68) and also read Ch. **14** (p. 96).

ACTION 5: *If the Above Actions #1–4 Aren't Working, Consider a Change of Dietary Program.* ✒

If you've done the above four actions completely and are still getting too many undesired weight readings, give serious consideration to replacing your present dietary program with another one, one that better fits you and your situation. More on dietary programs is in Startup Action 7 (p. **19**).

In short, if your weight reduction pursuit is involving too many undesired weight readings it means one or both of two things: (a) you're not fully doing your preferred dietary program and/or (b) you're using the wrong dietary program and you need to switch to one that's better suited to your situation, needs, and preferences. Whichever is the cause, don't procrastinate on putting the corrective action into effect right away. If you have the *right* dietary program for you and you're imple-menting it *fully* each day, you *will* lose weight.

SUMMING UP This Daily Action 2B

Whenever you get an undesired weight reading while pursuing weight *maintenance*, (a) hold a positive outlook and (b) take immediate corrective action that very day — that is, immediately bring your weight back into your healthy-weight range, typically within 24 hours. ~ Whenever you get too many undesired weight readings while pursuing weight *reduction,* make sure that (a) you're apply-ing the optimal preferred dietary program for you and (b) you're implementing that program fully each day. ~ Do this Daily Action 2B when it's called for, and lifelong healthy-weight living will be *yours.*

REMEMBER: The secret to succeed-ing at lifelong healthy-weight living is: Do Weight Success Actions every day. You accomplish this by doing the Weight Success Method, which typically takes <u>less than</u> 8 minutes of dedicated time per day. This causes vital *success drivers* to be installed and maintained in your weight success pursuit.

> Do the **Five Daily Actions**
> <u>every</u> day . . .
> and **Lifelong Weight Success**
> will be <u>Yours</u>.

Daily Action **3**: BENEFITS DIRECTIVE

Each day, read your Weight Success Benefits Directive, then visualize one of the benefits as an accomplished fact.

This action typically takes *less than* three minutes.

A copy of the Weight Success Benefits Directive is at the end of this Daily Action 3 section, pages **32–33**.

WHY You Do It

Delivering your Weight Success Benefits Directive to your self does three powerful things. First, it describes for your mind — mainly, your subcon-scious mind — the exact mindset and actions that it should focus on bringing about for creating lifelong healthy-weight living. Second, it instructs your subconscious mind in what it should be doing each time you say your Healthy-weight Goal Statement (Daily Action 4). And, third, it reminds you of your weight success benefits. The result: Delivering the Directive motivates your subconscious mind to each day create the types of thoughts and feelings that lead you to creating lifelong healthy-weight living.

HOW to Set Up the Directive

In the Directive, fill in these blank lines: (a) healthy-weight range, (b) preferred dietary program, and (c) weight success benefits. You'll find the Directive on pages 32–33 and also in the Toolkit at: correllconcepts.com/toolkit.pdf

> **Note:** For more on setting up the Directive, go to Ch. **9** at page 65. Reading this is recommended.

HOW to Deliver the Directive

When delivering the Directive each day do these four things.

First, do the actions described in the instructions section at the top of the first page.

Second, read the Directive aloud. (Reading aloud is best, but when you can't do that, whisper it to yourself.)

Third, after reading it, pick out one of the more exciting weight success benefits and visualize yourself enjoying it. Visualize for at least 30 seconds.

Fourth, when delivering the Directive — and throughout the rest of your day — *hold the belief* that your subconscious mind is right then, at that very moment, *in the process* of performing the actions described in the Directive. For more information on this, go to the *How Believing and Acting As-if Work* section in Startup Action 5 (p. **17**).

How to Get Copies of the Directive

Make several copies of the Weight Success Benefits Directive (p. 32–33) for your personal use, and place the copies in spots where it'll be convenient (like, perhaps, a copy in your suitcase).

Also, there's an extra copy at the end of this book (p. **185**), in case you'd like to cut it out.

Plus, another way to get copies is go to the free online Toolkit at:

correllconcepts.com/toolkit.pdf

There you'll find a PDF document of the Benefits Directive formatted for printing on 8.5×11-inch paper. If you like, you can print it out two-sided and, thereby, have the entire Directive on a single sheet.

Also, if you'd like to have the Directive in a format that might be handy for keeping on a digital device — computer, tablet, or smartphone — copy or upload this to your digital device:

correllconcepts.com/dir-dig2.pdf

How to Deliver the Directive for Maximal Effect

For extra impact, consider applying creative delivery techniques when reading the Weight Success Benefits Directive. Doing this can cause your mind — especially your subconscious mind — to pay extra attention to what you're telling it to do. Here are five examples to consider.

First, emphasize the key words. You can do this by speaking slightly louder, or slower, or more forcefully. These key words are printed in *italic,* underline, or **bold.**

Second, repeat (reread) a particular phrase or sentence for emphasis. So, what parts should you be focusing on? Reread whichever actions of the five directive actions you feel are most relevant at the time. If you happen to be in a period of progress slowdown, it likely means some action called for by the Directive is not being fully performed by your subconscious mind. So, emphasize to your mind that you definitely want it to be doing this action.

Third, read the entire Directive slowly and deliberately. This will require one or two extra minutes. But it can pay dividends. It can cause your subconscious mind to pay special attention to the five actions prescribed in the Directive. To do this, pause for a few seconds after each action or paragraph. During the pause, reflect on the meaning or main message of the action.

Fourth, ad lib whenever you see fit. Insert spontaneous additional instructions to your subconscious mind to emphasize key points or actions.

Fifth, deliver the Directive in a different place or position. For example, if you've been delivering the Directive sitting down, do it standing. Or, deliver it while pacing, like you're delivering a speech. Include arm movement and gesticulation of main points. This can be a powerful form of delivery. It can enhance your emotional impact. Experiment and find out what works best for you. Or, just change delivery style from time to time for variety.

Also, if there's a word in the directive and you'd like to delete it, just draw a line through it. If you'd like to replace it with a different word, write in the new word above the word that has the line through it.

> **Note:** For more instructions on the Directive, go to Ch. **9** at page 65. Reading this is recommended.

SUMMING UP This Daily Action 3

Each day deliver the Weight Success Benefits Directive (which starts on page 32). Deliver it to your subconscious mind, and also visualize one of your weight success benefits. During the day, believe and act as-if your subconscious mind is in the process of performing every instruction you give it. ~ Do this Daily Action 3, and also the other four daily actions of the Weight Success Method, and lifelong healthy-weight living will be *yours.*

REMEMBER: The secret to succeeding at lifelong healthy-weight living is: Do Weight Success Actions <u>every</u> day. You accomplish this by doing the Weight Success Method, which typically takes <u>less than</u> **8** minutes of dedicated time per day. This causes vital *success drivers* to be installed and maintained in your weight success pursuit.

Do the **Five Daily Actions** <u>every</u> day . . .
and **Lifelong Weight Success** will be <u>Yours</u>.

WEIGHT SUCCESS
—— is the GOAL ——

WEIGHT SUCCESS METHOD™
—— is the MEANS ——

Goal+Means+<u>Action</u>=WEIGHT SUCCESS™

WEIGHT SUCCESS = Living most or all of one's days in one's desired healthy-weight range AND deriving benefits, enjoyment, and fulfillment from it.

Coming up next is the Weight Success Benefits Directive. The Directive consists of two pages. The easiest way to read and comprehend it is to start the Directive on an even-numbered page, so that both pages of the Directive are visible at the same time. Thus, this extra page has been inserted here to make the Weight Success Benefits Directive begin on an even-numbered page (specifically, page 32).

Weight Success Benefits Directive

INSTRUCTIONS: Use this Directive for Daily Action 3. ● Where there's a dotted line (...........), say the name you use when speaking of or to your subconscious mind. ● Read this directive aloud <u>and</u> say it with some emotional intensity. (Reading aloud is best, but when you can't do that, whisper it to yourself.) When reading it, ***strongly desire*** for the actions it describes to be realized. And, ***hold the belief*** and act as-if what's described in this statement is *in the process of happening.* After reading the list of weight success benefits, for at least 30 seconds ***visualize*** at least one of the benefits as an accomplished fact. As you go through the day, *continue* believing and acting as-if what's described in this directive is in the process of happening. ● For set-up, insert your healthy-weight range and preferred dietary program into the blanks. For the "pounds–kilos" phrase, draw a line through the word that doesn't apply. List your weight success benefits on the lines at the end. Hint: Use pencil, not pen. Or, type it up and tape it in. (For more, see Ch. **9** at page 65.)

*   *   *

........................., today and *every* day for the rest of my life, do these five very important actions.

1 – Guide me to *easily* living in my **healthy-weight range,** which right now is
_____ to _____ pounds–kilos.

2 – Guide me to *fully* doing my **preferred dietary program**, which right now is the
_____ program.

3 – When I say my Healthy-weight Goal Statement while eating, automatically create thoughts and feelings that guide me to Right Eating, that guide me to eating the ***types*** of food and the ***amount*** of food that results in me living in my healthy-weight range.

4 – Whenever I make a decision to stop eating, make the urge to eat *immediately* begin to fade away for that eating session. And, if anytime I happen to accidentally overeat, create an uncomfortable bloated feeling that lasts for a short time.

5 – Whenever I say my Healthy-weight Goal Statement, bring to mind a thought of at least one of my weight success benefits. And, then, create within me a *happy, positive feeling.*

The Weight Success Benefits I gain from living in my healthy-weight range include:
1. A greater chance of *living healthier longer* — or greater chance of living free of debilitating accidents, illnesses, diseases, and bodily malfunction.

_____

_____

_____

_____

_____

_____

_____

_____

_____
_____
_____
_____
_____
_____
_____
_____
_____
_____
_____
_____
_____
_____
_____
_____
_____

I thank you, God, for the opportunity to live my life this way.

......................., please do *everything you can* to assist me in creating lifelong healthy-weight living in a positive, pleasurable way. This benefits me *greatly.* I realize you're now doing it, and I thank you for it.

Living in my healthy-weight range is a *mandatory,* <u>must</u>-have feature of my existence. I am doing it *now* and for the rest of my life — and doing it *easily* <u>and</u> *enjoyably.* Yes! Yes! YES!

*   *   *

NOTE: After delivering the directive, close your eyes and say your Healthy-weight Goal Statement <u>three</u> times. Do it with intensity. ~ Plus, each day allow yourself to get a *good feeling* from making your weight losses stick and from having realized healthy-weight living. You deserve it. It's a **substantial** praiseworthy achievement.

> The **Weight Success Benefits Directive** is an important message for your mind, especially your subconscious mind. Deliver it like it is and your subconscious mind will act accordingly.

Daily Action **4**: GOAL STATEMENT

Each day, say your Healthy-weight Goal Statement at least 25 times.

This action typically takes *less than* 120 seconds.

To do it you need a healthy-weight goal statement. The one I recommend (and have been personally using since 2008) is this:

> *I am the person of my healthy weight.*
> *I am healthy, happy, and doing great.*

As previously explained, every weight in your healthy-weight range is considered to be a *healthy weight* for you.

WHY You Do It

Saying your Goal Statement each day focuses your mind — in particular, your subconscious mind — on the desired ultimate outcome of your healthy-weight pursuit. This triggers your subconscious mind to create daily thoughts and feelings that guide you toward right eating and living your life in your healthy-weight range.

HOW to Do It

Each day say your Healthy-weight Goal Statement at least 25 times. (Note: 25 times is a minimum, not a maximum. You can say it more than 25 times, if you like.) Does saying it 25 times a day seem like it would be time-consuming? It's not. You're able to say your Goal Statement *three times* in 12 to 15 seconds, which is 12 to 15 times a minute. Which means, saying it 25 times per day uses *less than* 120 seconds per day. So there's no reason why you can't do this Daily Action 4 every day.

Plus, the Goal Statement need not be said all at once. You can divide it into several sessions. Or, if you like, you can spread it throughout the day.

Plus, you can say it aloud, either in full voice or in a whisper. Or, you can say it silently to yourself — your choice. So, you can do this Action 4 *any time, any place.* Also, you can vary the *way* you say the statement from time to time. Sometimes do it more rapidly, other times more slowly. And, for

variety put emphasis on different words at different times.

Plus, you can fit them into "free time." Each of your days contains numerous "free time" periods where statement iterations can be fit in. These periods are when you're doing something but also can be thinking about something else at the same time. Examples include when you're lying in bed, dressing, showering, driving, walking from here to there, taking a break, eating, using the bathroom, exercising, and watching TV. So, each day holds opportunities where you can fit in five or ten iterations of your Healthy-weight Goal Statement. Because you're doing this while also doing something else, you can consider the time involved to be non-dedicated time, or free time. In short, there are so many opportunities for free-time statement iteration you can, if you wish, easily fit 40, 50, or even 100 or more into a day without any special time allotment.

Plus, here's an easy way to keep tract of your goal statement iterations: Count them in units of five using one of your hands. After each iteration move one of your fingers (either in or out). After moving all five fingers, say the total number to that point. So, after counting the first five say "Five" (either aloud or silently), after the second five say "Ten," after the third five "Fifteen," and so on.

Even though you can say your Goal Statement any time you want, some particularly good times to say it are (a) when you awaken in the morning, (b) whenever you feel an urge to eat, (c) *while you're eating*, (d) before you go to sleep at night, and (e) whenever you wake up in the night. Saying it at these times can have extra-powerful impact.

Finally, whenever you're saying your Healthy-weight Goal Statement — either aloud or silently in your mind — *hold the belief* that your mind is right then in the process of transforming you into the person described in the Statement — that is, "the person of your healthy weight" and one that's "healthy, happy, and doing great." Also, *act as-if,* or totally pretend, you're that person. Believing and acting as-if motivate your mind — in particular, your subconscious mind — to create the types of thoughts and feelings that steer you toward lifelong healthy-weight living. For more on this, go to the *How Believing and Acting As-if Work* section in Startup Action 5 (p. **17**).

> **Note:** Also, consider applying optional backup depiction statements. For this, go to the *Motivator 2* section in Ch. **13** at page 90.

SUMMING UP This Daily Action 4

Each day say your Healthy-weight Goal Statement at least **25** times. You can say it any way you like (including silently to yourself) and also any time you like. But always say it at least once *before each eating session.* ~ Do this Daily Action 4, and also the other four daily actions of the Weight Success Method, and lifelong healthy-weight living will be *yours.*

REMEMBER: The secret to succeeding at lifelong healthy-weight living is: Do Weight Success Actions <u>every</u> day. You accomplish this by doing the Weight Success Method, which typically takes <u>less than</u> 8 minutes of dedicated time per day. This causes vital *success drivers* to be installed and maintained in your weight success pursuit.

Do the **Five Daily Actions**
<u>every</u> day . . .
and **Lifelong Weight Success**
will be <u>Yours.</u>

Daily Action **5:** GUIDED EATING

Each time you eat, apply the Guided Eating Process.

This action typically takes *less than* 15 to 20 seconds of <u>non</u>-dedicated time per meal.

In any given eating session we pursue eating in one of two modes: (1) unguided or (2) guided.

Unguided Eating. Eating activity that's not guided by the eater — meaning, it's done automatically and without conscious deliberation — we call *unguided eating.* So, with unguided eating we don't guide our eating actions. Instead, the food items around us do that. These food items are visual cues. The cues trigger a certain behavior. This certain behavior consists of performing a series of eating actions that results in consuming the cues. We mostly perform this behavior automatically, or with minimal deliberation or conscious direction. (Note: Other names for unguided eating are automatic eating, undirected eating, and non-controlled eating.)

So, unguided eating is a 3-action process. First, we confront food items, which are cues. Second, the food cues trigger an automatic-eating response. Third, we engage in undirected or automatic eating until the cues disappear from being eaten. During this time we aren't thinking about what we're doing. As a result, we're not guiding our eating activity. For most persons nearly all eating is unguided. This is why many folks engage in frequent overeating — and, thereby, fail at creating healthy-weight living. So we should replace unguided eating with guided eating.

> **Note:** For more on unguided eating, go to Ch. **21** at page 132.

Guided Eating. In guided eating *we* guide the eating process. Meaning, instead of the food items determining what and how much we eat, *we* do it. This might sound hard to do, but it's not. You can easily create guided eating any time you want. To do this, apply a certain 3-action process which we call **Guided Eating Process.** (Other names for guided eating are directed eating and controlled eating.) Guided eating is a *major* key to replacing overweight living with healthy-weight living for life.

> **Note:** In this book the word *eating* encompasses drinking. And the word *food* encompasses beverages. So wherever you read the terms *eating* and *food* know that it includes drinking and beverages.

WHY You Do It

Whenever you're not guiding your eating activity, your eating activity is <u>un</u>controlled. This is why unguided eating leads to overeating. Doing this Daily Action 5 *reduces* the amount of unguided eating and *increases* the amount of guided eating. Which makes for *non*-overeating meals. This, in turn, leads you to weight success.

HOW to Do It

To create guided eating in any particular meal or eating session, apply this guided eating process: **C**ommunicate, **B**elieve, **A**ppreciate. It's your key to easy guided eating.

> TIP: To easily recall the three steps of the upcoming Guided Eating Process (**C**ommunicate, **B**elieve, **A**ppreciate), think of **C-B-A**. Which is <u>A-B-C in reverse</u>.

The C-B-A Guided Eating Process

Each time you eat perform these three steps.

1. **Communicate.** When you begin eating, deliver *guided-eating self-talk* to your self.
2. **Believe.** As you eat, *hold the belief* and also act as-if your subconscious mind is right then, at that very moment, in the process of performing the actions described in your guided-eating self-talk. Which means, be on the lookout for a stop-eating signal.
3. **Appreciate.** When a stop-eating signal comes, *thank* your subconscious mind for sending the signal and then <u>act on it</u> — that is, *stop eating.*

Doing this process takes no extra time. It's done on non-dedicated time, or while you're eating. Here's fuller explanation of how to do the three C-B-A steps.

Step 1: COMMUNICATE

Whenever you start eating, deliver guided-eating self-talk to your self. *Guided-eating self-talk* is any message delivered to your self while eating, for the purpose of causing your subconscious mind to assist with guiding you away from overeating and toward non-overeating. You can deliver self-talk either by whispering to yourself or by speaking

silently in your mind. Do it whichever way works best for you at the time. To deliver guided-eating self-talk, do these two actions:

1 – Say your Healthy-weight Goal Statement;
2 – Describe how you want the eating session to turn out.

I'll explain these two actions.

ACTION 1: Silently say your Healthy-weight Goal Statement <u>three</u> times when you start eating. This takes only about 15 seconds. The Statement is:

> I <u>am</u> the person of my healthy weight.
> I am healthy, happy, and doing great.

ACTION 2: Silently tell your subconscious mind how you want the upcoming eating session to turn out. For this, use one or both of the following two guided-eating statements, *or* something like them. Either way, the object is to describe how you want the eating session to be.

Sample Guided-eating Self-talk Statement #1
This food is filling me up, filling me up, <u>filling me up</u>. I might not be able to eat it all.

Sample Guided-eating Self-talk Statement #2
This food is very, very, <u>very</u> satisfying. By the time I finish eating it I'll be <u>fully</u> satisfied and have <u>no</u> desire to eat any more this meal.

Now, both these statements refer to whatever amount of food constitutes a right amount for that meal. Typically it's the food that's on your plate or in hand, not everything on the table or in the refrigerator. Or, it's the amount of food prescribed by your preferred dietary program.

Also, if you like you can combine the two self-talk statements, like this:

> *This food is filling me up, filling me up, <u>filling me up</u>. I might not be able to eat it all. It's also very, very, <u>very</u> satisfying. By the time I finish eating it I'll be <u>fully</u> satisfied and have <u>no</u> desire to eat any more this meal.*

Doing this triggers your subconscious mind to cause you to feel both filled up and fully sated with eating pleasure without overeating.

Note: the above statements are given as samples. If you so choose you can deviate from them or add to them. In short, ad lib whenever you feel like it. Also, to reiterate, you deliver guided-eating self-talk either by whispering or by speaking silently in your mind.

> For more on communicating to your subconscious mind, go to the "Six Actions for an Effective Thank You, Keep It Up Message" (p. **25**).

Step 2: BELIEVE

As you eat, hold the belief and also act as-if your subconscious mind is right then, at the present moment, in the process of performing the actions described in your guided-eating self-talk. Which means, as you're eating be on the lookout for a stop-eating signal. That is, expect that your mind will be creating a stop-eating signal at the point you should cease eating. (Note: It likely will include the full-stomach feeling.) Coming up is a list of seven possible stop-eating signals.

> For more on believing and acting as-if, go to the *How Believing and Acting As-if Work* section in Startup Action 5 (p. **17**).

Step 3: APPRECIATE

When a stop-eating signal comes, thank your subconscious mind for sending the signal and then act on it — that is, stop eating. How do you thank your subconscious mind? It's easy — like this:

> *"Subconscious mind, I thank you very much for sending the stop-eating signal. I really appreciate it."*

And, how do you act on the signal? Immediately after getting just a slight full-stomach feeling, or any other form of stop-eating signal, stop eating. Do *not* eat "just a few more bites." Do *not* decide to "finish off" what's on your plate or in your hand. Instead, stop eating right then. And, if there's any leftover food, immediately discard it or push it out of reach or put it into the refrigerator for eating the next day.

It might seem like this would be hard to do. That's because most of us have, at one time or another, acquired an eat-it-all, fill-'er-up habit. But

overcoming this habit is easier than you might imagine. To do so, immediately follow the stop-eating signal when it comes. When you do this the urge to continue eating *immediately begins to fade away.* Which means, within about 30 to 60 seconds after you stop eating you no longer have an urge to continue eating.

And don't forget, after the signal comes, express appreciation and thanks to your subconscious mind for sending it. Conveying this thanks motivates your mind to keep assisting by sending further stop-eating signals when needed. Note: You can convey thanks by speaking either aloud, such as in a whisper, or silently in your mind — your choice.

When you do this Step 3 you get a bonus. You get a great feeling from having turned a potential overeating situation into a non-overeating victory. And, believe me, this feeling is way more gratifying than any feeling you get from continuing to eat.

At this point you might be thinking, "What happens if one ignores the stop-eating signal?" When you fail to follow a stop-eating signal — that is, when you continue eating or proceed into overeating — your mind retracts the signal. As a result, the feeling or thought that constituted the signal fades away. And, in its place, the "old" urge and habit to pursue overeating usually reappears.

What's more, if you repeatedly ignore the stop-eating signals your subconscious mind sends, it will eventually stop sending stop-eating signals. So, whenever you get a Stop-eating Signal, **act on it.**

Some Common Stop-eating Signals

Here's a list of seven common signals your subconscious mind might use for telling you to stop eating or to refrain from eating.

1. The full-stomach feeling. This typically involves a feeling of pressure or tightening at the top of your stomach, or where your stomach joins your throat. Even just a slight full-stomach feeling is a stop-eating signal. This feeling can come even when your stomach isn't completely full. The full-stomach feeling is likely the most common, or #1, stop-eating signal.

2. A reduced urge to eat or to continue eating. Even just a slightly-reduced urge is a stop-eating signal.

3. The food you're eating or thinking of eating suddenly loses its appeal or begins to "lose its taste." Even just a slight reduction in the food's appeal or taste is a stop-eating signal.

4. A feeling or suspicion that if you eat a certain food or a certain amount of food it will give you a bloated or overly-full feeling. Even just a slight feeling that this might happen is a stop-eating, or don't-eat-it, signal.

5. A thought of something you haven't yet done but that needs doing.

6. A thought of something you need to say to someone.

7. An urge to pursue some other activity, with this other activity being a non-eating activity. Even just a slight urge to pursue another activity is a stop-eating signal.

A stop-eating or don't-eat-it signal typically involves one or both of two types of actions: deactivating and diverting. The first three actions in the above list are *deactivating* actions. The last four are *diverting* actions. Also, it's possible your subconscious mind might devise a stop-eating signal not on this list! So be on the alert for some new form of stop-eating signal your mind might devise.

How to Trigger a Stop-eating or Don't-eat-it Signal. The key to having your subconscious mind send a stop-eating signal before the point of overeating is this. Make sure you're applying Step 2 — the Believing or "B" step (p. **37**) — of the Guided Eating Process. This puts you on the lookout for the signal. Which, in turn, causes your subconscious mind to send it. But, if you like you can do more. Try this handy technique. Pause your eating for a few seconds and then whisper or silently say to yourself: *Subconscious mind, have I eaten enough? If so, send me the full-stomach feeling this very moment.*

Then focus on your stomach. If you sense just the slightest feeling of "change" or pressure or fullness in your stomach or where your stomach

joins your throat, that's a stop-eating signal. So stop eating right then. When you do this — that is, follow the signal — the urge to continue eating *immediately begins to fade away.*

Conversely, if your subconscious mind doesn't send you a stop-eating signal when you ask "Have I eaten enough?" it could mean that you haven't overeaten at that time. Or, if you complete a meal and never get a stop-eating signal it might mean that your subconscious mind has concluded that eating that amount of food at that time will lead you to having an overeating-free day.

During-eating Self-talk — *Powerful!*

Now and then you might find yourself in a situation that appears like it could lead to overeating — like, for example, a super-strong eating urge or an extra-tempting meal. For this you can apply extra guided-eating self-talk. We call it *during-eating self-talk.* Here's how to do it.

First, make sure you do the self-talk prescribed for Step 1 of the Guided Eating Process (p. **36**). *Then, include additional self-talk as you're eating.* Every couple minutes or so, silently describe to yourself the way that eating session is, or should be, turning out. If you like, you can silently repeat the initial two Guided-eating Self-talk Statements (p. **36**). Every time you deliver this self-talk, hold the belief and act as-if your subconscious mind is right then in the process of bringing about the situation depicted in the self-talk message. For more on believing and acting as-if, go to the *How Believing and Acting As-if Work* section in Startup Action 5 (p. **17**).

This tactic might seem gimmicky, but it's powerful. During-eating self-talk is your never-fail SWAT team for neutralizing mealtime overeating and turning any eating session into an overeating-free victory. Use it anytime you need to stifle overeating.

Snack-time Procrastination

The prior-described during-eating self-talk tactic works for defeating overeating during extra-tempting meals. But now and then you might have need to defeat overeating that arises from eating too much between meals, called over-snacking.

When you're grappling with over-snacking you might apply the *procrastinate tactic.* That is, don't decide to not snack; instead just postpone the decision. Tell yourself you'll take up the matter in a little while, perhaps *after* completing some activity. In doing this you avoid the snacking self-argument. You don't become involved with the question "Should I snack, or should I not?" So, you don't end up enflaming the snacking urge by making a don't-snack decision. Instead, you sidestep it by postponing the decision. When you do this the snacking urge dissipates as soon as you start pursuing the other activity. Usually that's the only time you'll need to deal with the snacking urge for that portion of the day. But, what do you do if some time later the snacking urge reappears? You do

what all good procrastinators do: You procrastinate again.

SUMMING UP This Daily Action 5

Each time you eat do guided eating with the C-B-A process: **(1)** **C**OMMUNICATE guided-eating self-talk to your self — including to your subconscious mind, **(2)** **B**ELIEVE and act as-if your mind is in the process of doing what you're describing, and when a stop-eating signal comes, **(3)** **A**PPRECIATE the signal, thank your subconscious mind for it, and *immediately stop eating.* When you do this the urge to continue eating immediately begins to fade away. ~ Do this Daily Action 5, plus the other four Daily Actions, and lifelong healthy-weight living will be *yours.*

> **Note:** For deeper insight into *why* the Weight Success Method works, read Ch. **18** (p. 109) and Ch. **22** (p. 137).

We conclude this part with this summation.

The Weight Success Secret is this:
To succeed at lifelong healthy-weight living, **do Weight Success Actions <u>every</u> day.** By doing a certain amount of Weight Success Actions every day it causes you to *succeed* at creating lifelong healthy-weight living — a.k.a. Weight Success Forever. (And, conversely, by <u>not</u> doing Weight Success Actions every day it likely results in you failing at creating healthy-weight living.)

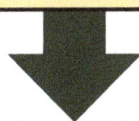

The most powerful Weight Success Actions are the ten STARTUP actions and the five DAILY actions of the **Weight Success Method.** So, first do the ten *Startup* Actions. Then, thereafter do the five *Daily* Actions **every day.** The five Daily Actions include: Weighing, Reinforcement or Correction, Benefits Directive, Goal Statement, and Guided Eating.

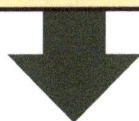

The next most powerful Weight Success Actions are certain optional actions described in Backup Resource Chapters **6–16, 21,** and **27.**

Part 1-E: Model Day with the Method

The Weight Success Method might look complex, but actually it's *simple and easy.* And, it typically takes *less than* 8 minutes of dedicated time per day.

TO ENSURE clarity I'm now going to provide an example: a fictional day that involves the five daily actions. This model day is presented in first-person singular, or as if it were happening to <u>me</u>. We'll assume I'm in weight maintenance mode, which I have been for a number of years now.

In this model day the first thing I do when I wake up in the morning is say my Healthy-weight Goal Statement three times. Shortly after that I weigh myself, in the buff. I apply the Eight Rules for Correct Daily Weighing (p. **23**). This is Daily Action 1. It takes only about 20 seconds.

When my daily weight reading is a desired reading, which it almost always is, I immediately deliver positive reinforcement to my subconscious mind. This includes the Thank You, Keep It Up message (p. **24**). While delivering this self-rein-forcement, and afterward as well, I'm *holding the belief* and *acting as-if* my subconscious mind is right then listening to what I'm saying and is in the process of performing the actions described in the message. This is Daily Action 2A. It takes only about 30 to 40 seconds.

But if my daily weight reading happens to be an undesired reading, I skip Action 2A and do Action 2B instead. For this action I take immediate correc-tive action. For the next 24 to 48 hours I do under-eating, or consume far less calories than what I'm expending. This typically corrects the undesired situation in 24 hours. Doing this requires no extra dedicated time to do.

So, the weight reading I get in Daily Action 1 determines the following action that I do. When I get a desired reading I do Action 2A and not Action 2B. When I get an undesired reading I do Action 2B and not Action 2A. (For clarity, I note that I very seldom need to do Action 2B any more.)

Shortly after completing Daily Actions 1 and 2A, I deliver the Weight Success Benefits Directive (p. **32**) to my mind. The Directive instructs my

subconscious mind to perform certain actions that assist me with realizing right eating and healthy-weight living. Throughout the day I'm holding the belief and acting as-if it's performing these actions. This is Daily Action 3. It takes only about two to three minutes to do.

Also throughout the day I say my Healthy-weight Goal Statement at least 25 times. Often I end up saying it more than that. Some of the times I say it speaking aloud, and sometimes in a whis-per, and some of the times I say it speaking silent-ly, or in my mind. I often say it during the "free time" periods in my day, or when I'm doing some-thing else at the same time. So I'm using non-dedicated time. When I say it I'm holding the belief and acting as-if my mind — in particular, my subconscious mind — is right then in the process of creating the types of thoughts and feelings that steer me toward being the person described in the Goal Statement. This is Daily Action 4. It takes less than 120 seconds of <u>non</u>-dedicated time per day.

When I eat I usually apply the 3-step Guided Eating Process — **C**ommunicate, **B**elieve, **A**ppreci-ate (p. **36**), called C-B-A for short. This helps me turn the session into guided eating, which steers me away from overeating. Also, I'm diligent about applying the Process during the last meal of the day, which usually is supper. I do this because the last meal is often the *make-it-or-break-it time;* it determines whether the day turns out to be a non-overeating day or an overeating day. This is Daily Action 5. It takes only about 15 to 20 seconds of <u>non</u>-dedicated time per meal to do.

After I go to bed at night I silently say my Healthy-weight Goal Statement at least three times before falling asleep. If I wake up in the night, such as for going to the bathroom, I silently say it at least three times as I'm going back to sleep.

CONCLUDING NOTE: The total time consumed by all five daily actions is *less than* eight minutes of dedicated time for the 24-hour day. To me, this is a miniscule investment for gaining years of non-overweight living and the weight success benefits that come with it.

Five Big Points

Enact these five powerful tips.

1 – Never stop. After achieving your desired weight or going into maintenance mode, do not do what many dieters do. Do not decide to "take a break" or to "coast for a while." If you take a break you'll likely gain back all the weight you lost. Instead, continue doing the Weight Success Method for life. Remember, it typically takes less than eight minutes of dedicated time per day.

2 – Routinize and habituate. Make doing the five Daily Actions a *routine* in your life. As much as possible, do each of the Actions the same time and place every day. In short, make doing them a *habit.*

3 – Feel good about it. Each day allow yourself to get a *good feeling* from living yet another day in your healthy-weight range. You deserve it. It's a substantial praiseworthy accomplishment.

4 – It has worked for the author for *over ten years* — it'll work for you, too. The writer of this book has been using and refining the Weight Success Method since 2007. He's been doing it because it works, and works easily. With it, you too can maintain your weight in your healthy-weight range the rest of your life *and* you can do it easily.

5 – Pursue it for what it is: a *daily success-creation process.* Remember this. To succeed at lifelong healthy-weight living, do Weight Success Actions *every day.* Any action that contributes to creating weight success qualifies as a Weight Success Action. Five very powerful Weight Success Actions are the five Daily Actions of the Weight Success Method. Doing these five actions typically takes *less than* **8** minutes of dedicated time per day. The result is it causes success drivers to be installed and maintained in your weight success pursuit, which, in turn, results in you realizing lifelong weight success — a.k.a. Weight Success Forever.

So, What's the Next Step?

Your next step in weight management decision-making could be one of the most impacting decisions of your life. If you make the decision to do nothing it'll likely result in ongoing weight gain and yo-yo dieting. But, if you decide to do the actions of the Weight Success Method, it'll almost certainly result in you living the rest of your life in your healthy-weight range, and doing so more easily and enjoyably than you ever thought possible. Put simply, it comes down to this.

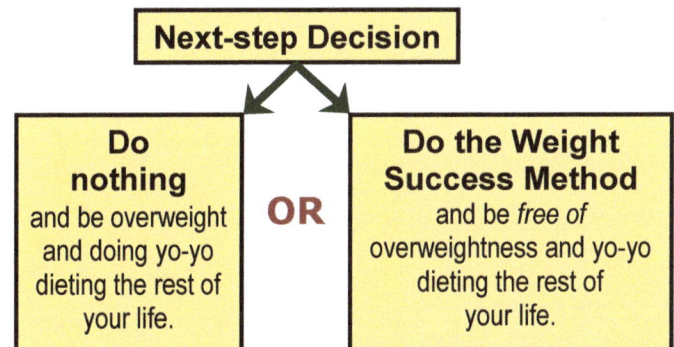

Next-step Decision

Do nothing and be overweight and doing yo-yo dieting the rest of your life.	**OR**	**Do the Weight Success Method** and be *free of* overweightness and yo-yo dieting the rest of your life.

~ Important Recommendation ~

At least once each month, take a few minutes to read (or perhaps reread) a portion of this book. By reading new material you'll acquire new insights. By rereading "old" material you'll also capture new insights. The more insights you have, the more *effective* you'll be in your weight success journey. And, also, the more *fulfillment* you'll derive.

THE BACKUP RESOURCE CHAPTERS (2–27)

FOR YOUR easy reference, here's a list of the additional chapters, which are available as an optional Backup Resource.

NOTE: For virtually any unusual weight management problem or challenge you need to surmount, it's likely that the information you need for doing this is contained in either (a) Chapter 1 or (b) one of the above Backup Resource Chapters 2–27.

CHAPTER 2: Lifelong Weight Success Empowerment

**The essential elements of the Weight Success Method are depicted in Chapter 1.
Now here's additional information you might find worth knowing.**

A *SUCCESS METHODOLOGY* is an action plan that pertains to a certain pursuit and consists of specific actions that, when performed by a person, cause a maximal number of success drivers to be included in that pursuit, thereby resulting in easiest possible creation of the desired situation or outcome associated with the pursuit. As stated in Chapter 1, the particular success methodology we're talking about is the **Weight Success Method.**

> For an explanation of success drivers, see Ch. **19** at page 117.

A success methodology comprises two types of actions: (1) STARTUP actions and (2) DAILY actions.

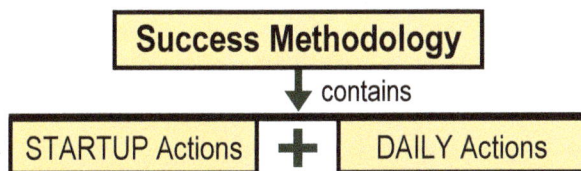

As the term is used here, a *startup action* is an action that's performed at the startup of a particular pursuit. Each startup action installs at least one vital success driver into the pursuit. As pertains to the pursuit of healthy-weight living, there are ten startup actions

A *daily action* is an action that's performed every day for the duration of a particular pursuit. Each daily action installs into that pursuit one or more vital success drivers. In some pursuits, such as the pursuit of weight success, for example, the duration of the pursuit is "the rest of one's life." As pertains to the Weight Success Method, there are five daily actions.

Two Types of DAILY Actions

For maximal effect a success methodology should include two types of daily actions: (1) goal-realization actions and (2) mind-motivation actions.

A *goal-realization action* is a daily action that leads to attainment or realization of the desired situation or goal associated with a certain pursuit.

As regards your weight success pursuit, the actions involved in performing your preferred dietary program (described in Startup Action 7, page 19) are the main goal-realization actions of your weight success journey.

A *mind-motivation action* is a daily action that motivates a person to perform goal-realization actions. Why are mind-motivation actions included in a success methodology? It's because many success pursuits are derailed not because a person doesn't know the actions needed for realizing a particular goal but, rather, because they fail to keep their mind focused and motivated on performing these goal-realization actions each day. In short, mind-motivation actions keep a person focused on performing goal-realization actions.

So, to recap, in your weight success journey the main *goal-realization actions* are those actions involved in performing your chosen dietary program, as described in Startup Action 7 (p. 19), and the main *mind-motivation actions* are the five Daily Actions of the Weight Success Method.

Five Pointers for Maximizing Success on Your Upcoming Weight Success Journey

While on your weight success journey keep the following five pointers in mind. By doing so you will maximize your effectiveness and success.

Success Pointer 1 — *Focus on Daily Progress Action.* Realize that success in any major pursuit derives from small progress actions performed day after day. (Another term for *progress action* is "step in the right direction.") Further, realize that small daily progress actions can be performed at any chosen time on any given day. Still further, realize that, distilled to its essence, your weight success journey constitutes an endless series of daily progress actions — or "steps in the right direction" — performed day after day for a lifetime. Finally, realize that performing these progress actions can be simple, easy, and enjoyable.

Success Pointer 2 — *Hold a Can-do, Will-do Mindset.* Hold the view and belief — a.k.a. assumption — that you can and will achieve lifelong healthy-weight living. And, also hold and act on the assumption that you'll achieve it *easily,* or at least more easily than you likely ever imagined.

Success Pointer 3 — *Keep in Mind that the Easiest Road to Healthy-weight Living is the Weight Success Method.* Realize that this is because the Weight Success Method is the easiest way to bring success drivers into your weight success pursuit which, in turn, enables creating the desired outcome of the pursuit.

Success Pointer 4 — *Take Advantage of All Available Resources.* The Backup Resource section of this book (Chapters 2–27) holds a plethora of optional backup resources. More than likely, whenever you have a question or seek more in-depth information or come upon a special problem, the insight and information you need and seek exists within Chapters 2–27. To find it, review the Table of Contents (p. **4**) *and/or* go to the Index (p. **175**) *and/or* check out the Glossary (p. **168**).

Success Pointer 5 — *Adapt, Improvise, Enhance.* As of the start of writing weight management books I've spent more than twelve years creating, personally testing, modifying, refining, editing, and writing the success methodology I call Weight Success Method. As a result, the ten Startup Actions and the five Daily Actions that constitute this Method are exact procedures. I urge you to put these procedures to the test by applying them specifically and fully. I do this because I'm convinced that if you fully apply these procedures you'll reap rewarding results.

But, very few things in this world are perfectly perfect. No matter how good and complete something is there's usually some way — if only a small way — that it can be modified to be better or more effective. This is especially the case when dealing with a human-applied methodology created for worldwide individual use. This happens because each of the several billion members of humankind is, in at least some small way, unique unto itself.

So in addition to my urging you to exactly, fully apply the prescribed actions of the Weight Success Method I *also* urge you to be open and eager to adapting, improvising, and enhancing any of those actions to your personal situation, should you see a way of doing so. This could maximize the impact of the Method in your weight success journey.

I believe you'll find the Weight Success Method to be the beginning of one of the most rewarding accomplishments of your life: the noble, noteworthy accomplishment known in this book as *weight success* — a.k.a. living most or all of the rest of your days in your desired healthy-weight range and deriving benefits, enjoyment, and fulfillment from it.

WEIGHT SUCCESS DYNAMIC

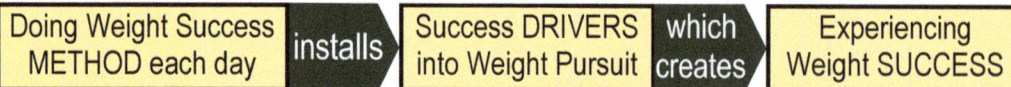

Doing Weight Success METHOD each day **installs** Success DRIVERS into Weight Pursuit **which creates** Experiencing Weight SUCCESS

Lifelong Weight Success Empowerment

You've learned of the Weight Success Dynamic in Chapter 1. We depicted it in infographic form, as shown above. This dynamic consists of three factors connected by two impact bridges, one of the bridges being indicated by the word "installs" and the other by "which creates." But it also can be expressed in text, like this.

Doing the Weight Success Method each day installs success drivers into one's weight success pursuit which, in turn, results in experiencing weight success.

As previously stated, we define weight success as: Living most or all of one's days in one's desired healthy-weight range and deriving benefits, enjoyment, and fulfillment from it. Now a question arises: How long will the Weight Success Dynamic continue? This is a vital question, because for every 10 persons who lose weight about 9 of them are gaining it back, or going from "weight success" to "weight failure."

The answer to that question is this: The Weight Success Dynamic can continue *for the rest of your life* ... and will do so with just a reasonable amount of diligence by you. Why does this happen? It's because there's a third impact bridge in the Weight Success Dynamic. It's depicted by the blue line in the infographic below.

This blue line extends from the Success block to the Method block and includes the words "which promotes continuation of." This bridge exists because of *positive reinforcement.* It works like this.

Upon achieving weight success via doing the Weight Success Method a person comes into a wonderful situation. They're now living most or all of their days in their desired healthy-weight range and deriving benefits, enjoyment, and fulfillment from it.

The "benefits, enjoyment, and fulfillment" part of weight success is *positive reinforcement* that promotes continuation of doing the Weight Success Method.

Summed up, weight success acts as positive reinforcement that motivates continuation of doing the Weight Success Method or, put another way, weight success increases the likelihood of a person continuing to do the Method each day. This "continuation-promoting effect" of positive reinforcement works to propel the Weight Success Dynamic for life. So, we now relabel the Dynamic to include the word *Lifelong* in the name, as shown in the infographic below.

Now here's the vital final point: This Lifelong Weight Success Dynamic enables a person to develop an ability, or power, to create weight success for life. We call this ability **Weight Success Empowerment.** (It's depicted by the green portion in the infographic.) Now this is what you need to know: I believe virtually anyone can acquire weight success empowerment by *continually doing the Weight Success Method.*

LIFELONG WEIGHT SUCCESS DYNAMIC

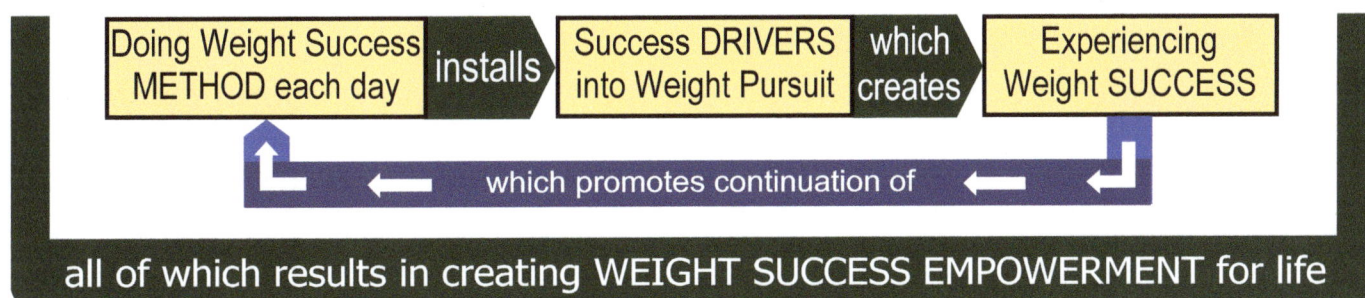

Doing Weight Success METHOD each day	installs	Success DRIVERS into Weight Pursuit	which creates	Experiencing Weight SUCCESS

← which promotes continuation of ←

all of which results in creating WEIGHT SUCCESS EMPOWERMENT for life

WEIGHT SUCCESS = Living most or all of one's days in one's desired healthy-weight range <u>and</u> deriving benefits, enjoyment, and fulfillment from it. ~ For description of benefits, enjoyment, and fulfillment created by weight success, read Ch. **7** (p. 60), Ch. **17** (p. 103), Ch. **22** (p. 137), and Ch. **24** (p. 148). ~ A person who's in process of creating weight success we call a *Weight Winner.*

CHAPTER 3: Why We've Been Struggling with Weight Control

Weight control — a.k.a. weight management — is the act of regulating one's amount of body fat for maintaining one's weight in a certain weight range.

FOR THIS CHAPTER, I propose and then answer one of the most vexing questions of our time: Why have we, as a society, been struggling with weight control? To answer this question I present five key concepts. Three have already been introduced in Chapter 1; two are new here. These concepts enable us to understand why achieving weight control has been such a widespread struggle in our modern world. Here they are.

1 – Primary Purpose of Eating
2 – Cause of Fat Gain
3 – Factors that Promote Overperformance of the O-I-S Process and Fat Gain
4 – New-situation Creation
5 – To Achieve Weight <u>Control</u>, Pursue Weight <u>Success</u>

We'll now examine each concept.

KEY CONCEPT 1:
Primary Purpose of Eating

Eating is a pleasurable experience. As such, humankind — or at least modern humankind — has come to assume that the primary purpose of eating is to derive maximal eating pleasure.

But this assumption is dangerous and destructive. How so? It's because when we assume that the primary purpose of eating is to derive maximal eating pleasure it causes an undesired outcome; it causes us to engage in *overeating,* which results in continual weight gain, which results in continual overweight living.

So, what is, or should be, the primary purpose of eating? The primary purpose of eating should be: To consume the *types* of food and the *amount* of food that contributes to (a) creating optimal health and (b) living in one's healthy-weight range.

Once we are accomplishing the primary purpose of eating on a daily basis, then we add in a secondary purpose of eating: Deriving eating pleas-

ure in conjunction with accomplishing the primary purpose. For easy reference we call this right eating. So, *right eating* is: Eating right foods in right amounts and in a way that creates right eating enjoyment. Right eating is the roadway to lifelong healthy-weight living.

> More information on this subject can be found in "Startup Action 6: Eating Approach," page 17.

KEY CONCEPT 2:
Cause of Fat Gain

One of the biggest impediments to weight control in modern society is that we've become confused over what is the *cause* of fat gain. So here's the nitty-gritty on it (previously explained in Startup Action 1, page 14).

Fat gain is caused by one — and only one — thing: overeating. We define *overeating* as: Consuming more calories than what one's body is metabolizing, or "burning up," per day.

Or, put another way, the cause of fat gain is *overperformance* of a certain three-action process, the process of:

1 – Opening our mouth;
2 – Inserting a piece of metabolizable calorie-containing food into our mouth; and
3 – Swallowing the piece of food.

We call it the *Open–Insert–Swallow* process — or **O-I-S** process for short. Overperformance, or over-repetition, of this process is the <u>real</u> cause of overeating and weight gain. And, it's the only cause. This process is how we consume more metabolizable calories than what our body is metabolizing, or "burning up," per day, which in turn causes us to gain fat and to struggle with achieving weight control. And, finally, it's important to note that this O–I–S process is totally controllable by each of us.

So, what about all the "zillion" other factors that researchers and writers of the past thirty years have been "discovering" and calling the "cause" of weight gain and overweight living?

KEY CONCEPT 3:
Factors that Promote Overperformance of the O-I-S Process and Fat Gain

Even though there is only one cause of fat gain, which is overeating — a.k.a. overperformance of the Open–Insert–Swallow process — there's a slew of factors that promote fat gain. Or, put another way, there are dozens, maybe hundreds, of factors that promote or facilitate doing overeating and deriving fat gain from it. For simplicity I call these factors fat-promoting factors. I define *fat-promoting factors* as: Factors that promote overeating or fat gain, or make it easier for a person to overeat and gain weight.

> A list of fat-promoting factors can be found in a "Fat-promoting Factors" discussion on page **126.**

But, in my opinion, of all the many fat-promoting factors five of them stand out as being most powerful in promoting overeating and in making us struggle with weight control. They are:

1 – Hunger pangs;
2 – Eating pleasure;
3 – Non-satiability of eating pleasure;
4 – Endless opportunity to experience instant eating pleasure; and
5 – Habit of unguided eating.

I refer to them as the "Big Five" of fat-promoting factors. I also call them Weight-control Inhibiting Factors, a term I'll be using in this discussion.

Weight-control Inhibiting Factor 1:
Hunger Pangs

The first major factor that has been promoting overeating and inhibiting our efforts to achieve weight control is that when we're involved in undereating we experience hunger — a.k.a. hunger pangs. This experience is distinctly annoying or even painful, so we strive to avoid it. But undereating is necessary for weight reduction. And, brief

periods of temporary weight reduction are necessary for most people to achieve ongoing weight control — a.k.a. lifelong healthy-weight living. So, refusal to experience any form of hunger pang, even briefly, has been deterring our achievement of weight control.

Why do we experience hunger pangs? Most likely it's an aspect of our human species that has arisen through evolutionary process. By motivating us to obtain and consume food to nullify the hunger pang, this aspect results in us acquiring the physical sustenance we need to survive and reproduce, which results in continuation of our species.

Weight-control Inhibiting Factor 2:
Eating Pleasure

The second major factor that has been promoting overeating and inhibiting our efforts to achieve weight control is that eating is a distinctly pleasurable experience for us. Most people enjoy this pleasure a lot. But when the desire to experience this pleasure becomes priority #1 it triggers overeating. And, this has been deterring our achievement of weight control.

Why do we experience eating pleasure? Again, most likely it's an aspect of our species that has arisen through evolutionary process. By us deriving pleasure from eating, it motivates us to create eating occasions, which results in us acquiring the physical sustenance we need to survive and reproduce, which results in continuation of our species.

So, the act of eating produces two simultaneous desired results. First, it causes an immediate reduction in pain (by removing any hunger pang) and, second, it provides an immediate jolt of pleasure (in the form of eating pleasure). As such, hunger pangs and eating pleasure are flipsides of a same "eating stimulus coin." Together, they work as an evolutionarily created double-whammy that moves us to constantly seek out or create eating occasions.

Weight-control Inhibiting Factor 3:
Non-satiability of Eating Pleasure

The third major factor that has been promoting overeating and inhibiting our efforts to achieve weight control is that we seldom tire of experiencing eating pleasure.

Many types of pleasures can become boring to us, or somehow decline in strength, or diminish in appeal. But not so with food. Eating pleasure seems to be non-satiable. We seem to never tire of it or lose interest in experiencing it every day. Indeed, it seems to work "in reverse," the more we experience of it, the more we seem to want it. This non-satiability of eating pleasure triggers overeating, which has been deterring our achievement of weight control.

Why does this situation exist? Again, perhaps it's an evolutionarily created aspect of our species that serves to perpetuate the species. Or, perhaps it's an evolutionarily created aspect "run amok."

Weight-control Inhibiting Factor 4:
Endless Opportunity to Experience Instant Eating Pleasure

The fourth major factor that has been promoting overeating and inhibiting our efforts to achieve weight control is that in modern society there is endless opportunity to experience instant eating pleasure. Meaning, it's because readily consumable food is everywhere. So most persons, or those not living in severe poverty, have the easy opportunity to eat any time, any place.

Having universal abundance of instantly consumable food is a huge blessing, but it also can be a trap. In prior centuries eating required special preparation and work. So eating was confined to a few (such as three) distinct eating sessions per day. And, each eating session had boundaries, a beginning and an ending.

But with readily consumable food everywhere, the natural boundaries of eating have tended to fade away. No longer is work required for eating and no longer are there beginning and ending points. Instead, eating has morphed into an effort-less process that tends to flow through every day without major interruption or lengthy breaks. As a result, this situation of having universal abundance of instantly consumable food promotes overeating, which has been deterring our achievement of weight control.

Each of weight-control inhibiting factors 1, 2, and 3 is, in itself, a powerful force for promoting overeating and weight gain and, thereby, it's a powerful factor deterring weight control. But, when factors 1–3 are joined by this factor 4, overeating and weight gain become supercharged, and weight control becomes a daunting challenge. This is the predicament that modern society is in today.

Weight-control Inhibiting Factor 5:
Habit of Unguided Eating

The fifth major factor that has been promoting overeating and inhibiting our efforts to achieve weight control is that the activity of unguided eating has become a deeply ingrained habit with most humans. This habit results in overeating, and this, in turn, has been deterring our achievement of weight control.

> **Definition for review:** *Unguided eating* is eating that's not guided by the eater; it's eating that's done automatically and without conscious deliberation.

Why do we have this habit? It's because the activity of unguided eating is an activity that starts shortly after birth and is then repeated numerous times every day thereafter, resulting in *thousands* of repetitions every year. This constant daily repetition of unguided eating makes it become a strong, deeply ingrained habit that promotes daily overeating.

> For more on unguided eating, see "Daily Action 5: Guided Eating" in Ch. **1** at page 35. ~ For more on habits, see Ch. **21** at page 132.

Summation of the "Big Five" Weight-control Inhibiting Factors

We now provide a summary.

Weight control is the act of regulating one's amount of body fat for maintaining one's weight in a certain desired weight range. Many factors —

a.k.a. fat-promoting factors — can affect the degree of difficulty in achieving weight control. But, in my opinion, five factors have been having an outsized impact on inhibiting the achievement of weight control within modern society. I call them the "Big Five" Weight-control Inhibiting Factors, or WCIF for short. In summary, they work like this.

WCIF #1: *Hunger Pangs.* This factor deters weight reduction by making undereating to be a pain-producing experience.

WCIF #2: *Eating Pleasure.* This factor promotes weight gain by making eating, including overeating, to be a pleasure-producing experience.

WCIF #3: *Non-satiability of Eating Pleasure.* This factor promotes weight gain by making eating, including overeating, to be a pleasure-producing experience we never tire of.

WCIF #4: *Endless Opportunity to Experience Instant Eating Pleasure.* This factor promotes weight gain by making eating, including overeating, to be an easy, instantaneous pleasure-producing experience that can be had any time of every day.

WCIF #5: *Habit of Unguided Eating.* This factor promotes weight gain by making eating, including overeating, to be a habitual unguided activity that happens automatically, or without deliberate conscious thought, every day.

> **Definitions for review:** *Under-eating* is consuming fewer calories than what your body is metabolizing, or "burning up," per day. ~ *Overeating* is consuming more calories than what your body is metabolizing, or "burning up," per day.

This brings us to the fourth key concept.

KEY CONCEPT 4:
New-situation Creation

"Life-enhancing situation" is a key term in this discussion. I define *life-enhancing situation* as: a new situation that's an improvement over a present situation. The story of humankind is a story of an endless pursuit of creating life-enhancing situations.

There are two main ways we create life-enhancing situations. The first way is we eradicate

a particular factor that's causing a problem at the present time. I call this *causal-factor eradication.* The second way is we create a desired *new* situation that, when actualized, automatically replaces a non-desired present situation. I call this *new-situation creation.* Here's how these two approaches work.

WAY #1: Causal-factor Eradication

Causal-factor eradication involves four actions.

First, we identify a problem or malady we'd like to eliminate.

Second, we identify the cause of the malady — a.k.a. causal factor.

Third, we identify, obtain, or create an antidote that, when applied, will eradicate the causal factor.

Fourth, we apply the antidote and, thereby, eliminate or nullify the causal factor, which results in eliminating the problem or malady.

Causal-factor eradication can be best illustrated using the field of medicine. This approach is how we free our self from a medical problem. First, we identify a particular sickness, illness, ailment, or malady we'd like to be free of. Second, we identify the causal factor that's creating the malady. Third, we obtain or create an antidote that, when applied, will eradicate the causal factor. Fourth, we apply the antidote, which results in curing or mitigating the sickness, thereby creating a life-enhancing situation. The antidote typically involves some sort of injection, pill, medication, surgery, or activity that reduces, eliminates, or overrides the illness-causing factor.

WAY # 2: New-situation Creation

The second main way we create life enhancement is we create a desired *new* situation that, when actualized, automatically replaces a non-desired present situation. For this to work, the desired new situation and the non-desired present situation must be mutually exclusive. That is, only one of the situations can exist at a time. For example, right eating and overeating are mutually exclusive situations; the presence of one rules out, or nullifies, the presence of the other.

The new-situation creation approach to creating a life-enhancing situation involves four actions.

First, we identify or envision the desired new situation we want to create or have actualized.

Second, we identify the factors required for succeeding at creating the desired new situation. We call these factors success-creation drivers, or success drivers for short.

> **Definition for review:** A *success driver* is a condition or activity that, when present, increases the likelihood of a person succeeding at a certain pursuit — or, more specifically, increases the likelihood of a person performing actions that contribute to creating a certain desired situation or outcome associated with the pursuit. ~ (More information on success drivers can be found in Ch. **19** at page 117.)

Third, we obtain or formulate a methodology — a.k.a. success methodology — that, when enacted, will bring success drivers into the pursuit of creating the desired new situation.

> **Definition for review:** A *success methodology* is an action plan that pertains to a certain pursuit and consists of specific actions that, when performed by a person, cause a maximal number of success drivers to be included in that pursuit, thereby resulting in easiest possible creation of the desired situation or outcome associated with the pursuit.

Fourth, we do the success methodology — that is, we perform the actions described in the action plan. By doing this we actualize the desired new situation. And, because the desired new situation and the non-desired present situation are mutually exclusive, the desired new situation replaces the non-desired present situation, thereby resulting in life enhancement.

Although most people haven't realized it, the above two approaches to creating life enhancement — the causal-factor eradication approach and the new-situation creation approach — have been used for years, and each has played a key role in humankind's quest and creation of ongoing life enhancement. But, the results achieved from these two approaches can vary depending on the situation.

What's the Best Approach for Weight Control Success?

Some life-enhancing situations are most easily achieved via applying the causal-factor eradication approach. Other situations are most easily achieved via the new-situation creation approach. Now here is a sixth Weight-control Inhibiting Factor (in addition to the five previously described). As a society, we've been focusing on the least-effective approach to creating weight control. We've been trying to achieve weight control via application of the causal-factor eradication approach to creating life enhancement. But this endeavor has been less-than-fully effective. Indeed, it has been a dismal failure.

Why has that been the case? It's because the primary causal factor that's been creating the problem of fat gain and overweight living is not a condition or a thing. Rather, it's a *human activity* — specifically, it's the activity of daily overperforming the three-action process of opening our mouth, inserting food into our mouth, and swallowing the food. Now here's the rub. When human activity is a causal factor of a particular problem, that causal factor can be especially hard to eradicate. The reason for this is, in order for us humans to eradicate this causal factor we first must acknowledge that *we* — that is, our *controllable actions* — are the *cause* of the problem.

But, individually and as a society, we resist doing that. We do so because acknowledging that we — or our controllable actions — are the *cause* of the weight-gain problem is distressing and embarrassing to us. So, for the past 20 or so years, instead of acknowledging and addressing the *actual* causal factor of fat gain and overweight living — which is the act of consuming more calories than what our body is metabolizing per day — we've been diverting our attention to discovering and identifying sideline fat-promoting factors — which are factors that promote overeating and fat gain but *aren't the actual cause of it*. As a result, we've been acting as-if these sideline fat-promoting factors are what's causing our weight gain and weight control failure when, in fact, they are not.

Definition for review. A *fat-promoting factor* is a factor that promotes overeating or fat gain, or makes it easier for a person to overeat and gain weight (but isn't the cause of overeating or fat gain). There's a long list of fat-promoting factors (one depiction of the list is provided on page **126**) and also the five biggest of them are described in the "Summation of Big Five Weight-control Inhibiting Factors" section (p. **48**).

So, the end-result is we've identified "zillions" of fat-promoting factors and not one is the actual cause of weight gain and overweight living. As a result, we still haven't solved the overweightness problem. Indeed, the problem has actually grown. Which brings us to the question "What should we be doing now?"

One of the keys to achieving weight control success is: *Apply the new-situation creation approach to life enhancement.* Doing this involves these four actions.

ACTION ONE: *Identify and envision the new situation that we desire to create, or to actualize.* As pertains to the pursuit of weight control, the desired new situation we seek to realize is lifelong weight success — a.k.a. weight success forever.

> **Definition review.** *Weight success* is: Living most or all of one's days in one's desired healthy-weight range and deriving benefits, enjoyment, and fulfillment from it.

ACTION TWO: *Identify the factors required for succeeding at creating the desired new situation of lifelong healthy-weight living.* We've already identified nineteen of these factors in Chapter 1 (p. **9**). For easy reference we call these factors success drivers.

> **Definition review.** A *success driver* is a condition or activity that, when present, increases the likelihood of a person succeeding at a certain pursuit — or, more specifically, increases the likelihood of a person performing actions that contribute to creating a certain desired situation or outcome associated with the pursuit.

ACTION THREE: *Obtain or formulate a methodology — a.k.a. success methodology — that, when enacted, brings success drivers into our pursuit of creating the desired new situation of lifelong weight success.*

> **Definition review.** A *success methodology* is an action plan that pertains to a certain pursuit and consists of specific actions that, when performed by a person, cause a maximal number of success drivers to be included in that pursuit, thereby resulting in easiest possible creation of the desired situation or outcome associated with the pursuit.

As pertains to the pursuit of weight control and weight success, the most effective methodology we know is the *Weight Success Method,* described in Chapter 1.

ACTION FOUR: *Do the actions specified in the success methodology.* Which means, as pertains to the pursuit of weight control we do the actions described in the Weight Success Method. This method comprises two sets of actions: (a) startup actions and (b) daily actions. By doing these actions we actualize, or bring about, the desired new situation of lifelong healthy-weight living. And, because healthy-weight living and non-healthy-weight living — a.k.a. overweight living — are mutually exclusive, the desired new situation of healthy-weight living automatically replaces the "old" non-desired situation of non-healthy-weight living. Further, by continuing to do the daily actions specified in the Weight Success Method for the rest of our life we continue living in our healthy-weight range the rest of our life. Or, in other words, we succeed at creating lifelong weight success.

This Action Four of the weight control process can be distilled to an essence that's expressed in a single sentence, which is this: To succeed at lifelong healthy-weight living, do Weight Success Actions <u>every day</u>. For easy reference we've dubbed this activity **Weight Success Secret** (and described it in Chapter 1 on page 12).

> **Definition review.** A *Weight Success Action* is an action that contributes to creating weight success. Or, more specifically, it's an action that promotes living most or all of one's days in one's desired healthy-weight range <u>and</u> deriving benefits, enjoyment, and fulfillment from it. Examples of Weight Success Actions include the ten Startup Actions, the five Daily Actions, the actions described in the Weight Success Benefits Directive, and any of the actions prescribed in Chapters 2–27.

KEY CONCEPT 5:
To Achieve Weight Control, Pursue Weight Success

We begin this section with our initial definition. *Weight control* is the act of regulating one's amount of body fat for maintaining one's weight in a certain weight range. Individually and as a society, we've been struggling mightily to achieve weight control. But as a society we've been failing.

Now the time has come to disclose a little secret. The easiest, most effective way to achieve weight control is to aim *beyond* weight control. That is, strive to achieve *more* than weight control; strive to achieve weight *success.*

As defined throughout Chapter 1, **weight success** is: Living most or all of one's days in one's desired healthy-weight range <u>and</u> deriving benefits, enjoyment, and fulfillment from it. When one is pursuing weight *success,* achieving weight *control* happens automatically. That's because weight control is no longer merely a "daily grinding must-do struggle." Instead, it becomes an exciting progress action, or uplifting daily step, in a greater quest, the quest of succeeding at creating lifelong healthy-weight living <u>and</u> deriving daily benefits, enjoyment, and fulfillment from it.

So, how does one put oneself on the road to lifelong weight success? I realize you already know the answer: Do the success methodology known as *Weight Success Method.* Doing the Weight Success Method automatically activates a certain cause-effect chain that we call Lifelong Weight Success Dynamic (depicted on page 45). And, once this dynamic is operating a person acquires the ability, or power, to create weight success for life. We call this power *weight success empowerment.* A main purpose of this book is to enable and inspire you to acquire the ability of weight success empowerment, thereby enabling you to live most or all of the rest of your days in your desired healthy-weight range <u>and</u> derive benefits, enjoyment, and fulfillment from it — a situation also known in this book as Weight Success Forever.

WEIGHT SUCCESS FOREVER
The 4 Steps to Creating It

1 – Read Chapter **1** of this book.

2 – Do the ten STARTUP Actions.

3 – Start the five DAILY Actions.

4 – Keep doing <u>all five</u> Daily Actions <u>every</u> day ... forever.*

* Typically takes less than 8 minutes of dedicated time per day.

CHAPTER 4: Attributes of an Ideal Weight Management Program

Weight control — a.k.a. weight management — is the act of regulating one's amount of body fat for maintaining one's weight in a certain weight range.

IF SOMEONE were to ask me what the attributes should be for an ideal weight management program, I would give them this list of sixteen.

1 – It includes **SUCCESS DRIVERS:** By applying the program one automatically includes most or all of the 19 success drivers in their weight success pursuit and, thereby, overcomes a main reason why many people fail at creating lifelong healthy-weight living — that reason being: Failure to do Weight Success Actions every day.

2 – Is **EASY:** No hard work or deep thought needed. Involves simple daily actions anyone can do in a few minutes per day.

3 – Is **ECONOMICAL:** Fits the budget of ordinary persons.

4 – Is **SAFE:** Doesn't require possibly-risky weird foods or procedures.

5 – Is **HEALTHY:** No radical less-than-fully-healthy eating regimen required. You pursue a dietary program that's healthiest for you.

6 – Is **FLEXIBLE:** No excessive time demands. Can be configured to fit one's daily schedule.

7 – Is **FOCUSED:** Is built on core concepts anyone can remember. Not a collection of cutesy topics with no connecting message.

8 – Is **COMBINABLE:** There's no requirement to adhere to a single dietary approach. Can be combined with almost any bona fide dietary program of one's choice, including a program of one's own design.

9 – Is **CUSTOMIZABLE:** Doesn't take a "you must do it only this way" approach. Includes all the tools needed for instant, easy startup, but they're all customizable, should one want to tweak any.

10 – Is **ENJOYABLE:** No pain, stress, or inconvenience. Involves activities most persons find enjoyable and gratifying. (For more on this, go to Ch. **17**, page 103.)

11 – Is **DUAL-FUNCTION:** Is specially designed to create (a) change achievement that's needed for achieving weight reduction <u>and</u> (b) maintenance achievement that's needed for achieving lifelong healthy-weight living. (For more on this, read Ch. **23,** page 146.)

12 – Is **PROVEN:** Has been proved to work, preferably through verification by scientific methodology. But, lacking that, has been proved to work by the creator of the program.

13 – Is **SETBACK APPLICABLE:** Contains a specific procedure for converting any problem or setback into a progress action. (For more on this, read Ch. **10,** page 68.)

14 – Is **LIFE JOURNEY ENHANCING:** Use of the program expands the basic elements of human flourishing: (1) positive emotions, (2) engagement (a.k.a. flow), (3) positive relationships, (4) meaning, and (5) accomplishment. (For more on this, read Ch. **22**, page 137.)

15 – Is **MINDSET ENHANCING:** Helps a person to build a healthy-weight-promoting mindset (as described in Startup Action 5, page 15).

16 – Allows for optional **ADVANCED DEVELOPMENT:** Provides a way for those seeking more in-depth knowledge and procedures to get it. Chapters 2–27 are for this purpose. For examples, see Ch. **13** (p. 90) and Ch. **24** (p. 148).

So, which weight management programs come closest to matching this ideal description? I don't know about every program out there. But it's my judgement that the Weight Success Method hits all 16 of the above descriptors. So, the Weight Success Method might not be the only ideal program, but if there are multiple ideal programs, the Weight Success Method is surely one of them.

Of all the attributes of the **Weight Success Method,** the most unique and most powerful is: It results in you doing Weight Success Actions <u>every day</u>.

It Comes Down to This

THE EASIEST WAY TO DO
WEIGHT SUCCESS ACTIONS
EVERY DAY IS DO THE
WEIGHT SUCCESS METHOD.

DOING THE METHOD PUTS
SUCCESS DRIVERS
INTO YOUR
WEIGHT SUCCESS PURSUIT,
WHICH CAUSES YOU TO DO
WEIGHT SUCCESS ACTIONS
EVERY DAY,
WHICH RESULTS IN YOU
SUCCEEDING AT CREATING
HEALTHY-WEIGHT LIVING
<u>FOR LIFE</u>.

Do the **Five Daily Actions** <u>every</u> day . . .
and **Lifelong Weight Success** will be <u>Yours</u>.

Typically takes <u>less than</u> **8** minutes of dedicated time per day.

CHAPTER 5: Two Main Processes in Weight Management

Weight management comes down to two things: (1) a PROBLEM and (2) a SOLUTION.

WHEN THE world of weight control — a.k.a. weight management — is distilled to its essence it amounts to two main processes. The first process is the dynamic that causes weight gain. We'll label it Problem Process — a.k.a. *overweight* creation process. The second process is the dynamic that causes weight control or the healthy-weight condition. We'll label it Solution Process — a.k.a. *healthy-weight* creation process. These two processes look like this.

1–The PROBLEM Process
(a.k.a. OVERWEIGHT Creation Process)

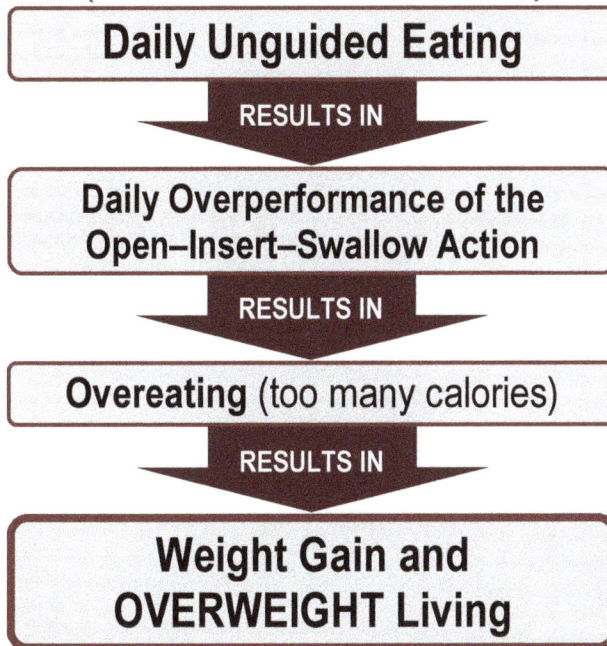

Daily Unguided Eating

RESULTS IN

Daily Overperformance of the Open–Insert–Swallow Action

RESULTS IN

Overeating (too many calories)

RESULTS IN

Weight Gain and OVERWEIGHT Living

2–The SOLUTION Process
(a.k.a. HEALTHY-WEIGHT Creation Process)

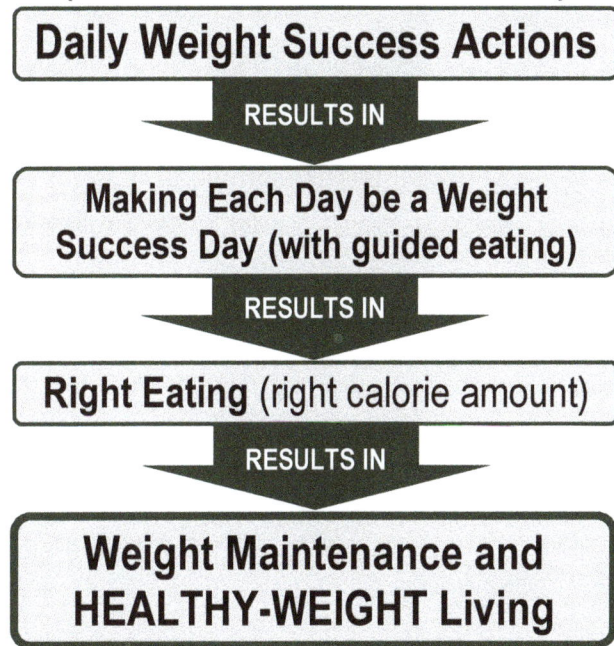

Daily Weight Success Actions

RESULTS IN

Making Each Day be a Weight Success Day (with guided eating)

RESULTS IN

Right Eating (right calorie amount)

RESULTS IN

Weight Maintenance and HEALTHY-WEIGHT Living

With the thousands of hours and millions of dollars that we've spent in the past 50 years on researching the "zillions" of fat-promoting factors in our world we've adopted the assumption that the cause and cure of overweightness is *COMPLEX*. But in actuality, it's *SIMPLE*. Once society realizes this truth, overweightness will <u>decline</u> and healthy-weight living will <u>ascend</u>.

CHAPTER 6: Healthy-weight Range in Detail

A key factor in creating healthy-weight living is: Identify an achievable healthy-weight *range*.

SOCIETY HAS long overlooked this crucial point: A main cause of our failure to achieve weight management success is we've been defining weight management success in terms of a single number (pound or kilogram). A pound number is a weight target that's just 16 ounces wide. Using a single pound number as one's daily weight target is like having a football goalpost that's 16-inches wide and then defining field goal kicker success in terms of kicking the ball through this ultra-narrow goalpost on every kick. It's so narrow of a target the kicker will miss it on most days. So, for most days the kicker is a *failure*. It's no wonder the pursuit of weight management has been one of the most discouraging endeavors of modern life.

What's the solution? Define weight management success in terms of a weight *range*. By having a weight range as the target it creates the opportunity to be a weight management success every day. I call this range your *healthy-weight range*. I define it as: the weight range that maximizes the likelihood of you living in optimal health. So, your entire healthy-weight range is regarded as being a healthy weight for you. Which means, whenever your body weight is in your healthy-weight range, you're a "weight management *success* who's living at their *healthy weight."*

Guidelines for Your Healthy-weight Range

There's no one perfect method for setting one's healthy-weight range. But here are some helpful guidelines. Use these and also include your own good judgement. Plus, it could be a good idea to factor in the opinion of a health professional, such as your doctor.

Start by Ascertaining Your Ideal Weight

For the past 150 years the medical profession has created formulas for calculating ideal body weight. These formulas go by various names, typically the name of the inventor. It appears that, at the present time, the most widely accepted formula is the **Robinson formula,** created in 1983.

On the Internet you can find automatic ideal weight calculators based on this formula. You enter your age, gender, and height and it shows an ideal weight number. Here's the URL for one such calculator:

calculator.net/ideal-weight-calculator.html

You'll note that this site also shows the ideal weight derived from some of the other formulas. And you'll further note that all these weights differ from one another. Which tells us that ideal weight calculation isn't an exact science. But, again, the Robinson formula appears to be the one most widely recognized — at the time this book was written — so I suggest going with that one.

If Needed, Modify the Ideal Weight Number to Fit Your Situation

Now here's a major point. If in your opinion the ideal weight number produced by the calculator doesn't fit your situation or won't produce the most effective weight management outcome for you, *adopt whatever ideal weight number you believe will produce the most effective weight management outcome on your weight success journey.* Make sure it's a weight number that's healthy for you. Again, you might find it helpful to factor in the opinion of a physician.

Here are two factors that might warrant changing the ideal weight number produced by the calculator: (a) frame size and (b) muscle mass.

Frame Size. Your frame size — a.k.a. skeletal size or bone size — could be a reason for deviating from the ideal weight number produced by the calculator. The term "frame size" pertains to the width of your bones. Researchers apply three categories to it: small, medium, large — a.k.a. narrow, normal, wide. The weight calculator's number is based on a medium, or normal, frame size. So, generally speaking, if you have a large or wide frame size — sometimes called "big boned" or "large boned" — it might be a good idea to adjust your ideal weight number upward. How much? There's no exact amount, but 10 pounds or more might be called for.

Conversely, if you have a narrow frame size, it might be a good idea to adjust your ideal weight number downward.

So how does one determine whether their frame size is narrow, medium, or wide? There are two ways. One is: measure the circumference of your wrist at the narrowest point. The other is: measure the width of your elbow at the widest point. There's a specific method for doing each. If you're interested in exact instruction, go to the Internet and do a search for "ideal weight based on frame."

Muscle Mass. In addition to being based on normal frame size, the ideal weight calculator is also based on normal muscle size. Which means, if you happen to be genetically endowed with larger than normal muscle size, or if you're a bodybuilder that has acquired extra-large muscles, it might be a good idea to adjust the calculator's ideal weight number upward. How much? That depends on how much larger your muscles are from normal. If you're a bodybuilder with very large muscles, the upward adjustment could be considerable.

Determine How Large Your Healthy-weight Range Span Will Be

So, what should be the size, or span, of your healthy-weight range? I'll begin with this general guideline.

If you weigh in pounds, consider having your healthy-weight range span be either six, seven, or eight pounds.

If you weigh in kilograms, consider having it be either three or four kilos.

But, if you believe an eight pound or a four kilo healthy-weight range is too small for your situation, feel free to expand it slightly to, say, a nine, ten, or eleven pound (or a five kilo) range. Also, if you're a woman who undergoes considerable premenstrual water retention you might find it handy to use a slightly expanded healthy-weight range. That way, you have ample opportunity to maintain your body weight within your healthy-weight range during the premenstrual period.

In short, consider setting the span of your healthy-weight range to be _about five percent_ of your ideal weight number. But, if you have good reason to make it slightly larger or smaller than that, do so.

I'll explain how the "five percent guideline" works. Assume that a person has a 160 pound ideal weight number. Five percent of 160 is eight ($0.05 \times 160 = 8$). So this suggests a healthy-weight range span of eight pounds. Which means, the person would use this 8-pound span number as a starting point and, if necessary, increase or decrease the span from that point to create a healthy-weight range that, in their opinion, will produce the most effective weight management outcome on their weight management journey.

Determine the Upper and Lower Numbers of the Range

So how does one go about setting the high end and low end numbers of their healthy-weight range? There are three ways. Pick the one you believe will work best for you.

WAY #1: *Make Your Ideal Weight the Center Point of the Range.* ✒ For this, have your ideal weight number be near the center of the range, and then build above and below it.

To illustrate, let's assume your ideal weight number is 168 pounds. And, let's further assume you want to have a 7-pound healthy-weight range. To create a 7-pound range around this number you could go three pounds down and three pounds up from 168. This results in a healthy-weight range of 165 to 171 pounds. Which means, any weight within this range (or between 165.0 to 171.9) is considered to be a *healthy weight* for you. So, whenever your body weight is 165, 166, 167, 168, 169, 170, or 171 pounds (or between 165.0–171.9 lbs.) you're living at your healthy weight.

And what about kilograms? If your ideal weight number happened to be 76 kilos and you wanted a

3-kilo healthy-weight range, you could go one kilo down and one kilo up from 76, thereby creating a healthy-weight range of 75 to 77 kilos. So, any weight between 75.0–77.9 kilos would be considered to be a healthy weight for you.

WAY #2: *Make Your Ideal Weight Number the Lower Limit of the Range.* ❧ For this, have your ideal weight number be the bottom point of the range, and then build upward from there.

To illustrate, let's assume once again your ideal weight number is 168 pounds. And, let's further assume you want to have a 7-pound healthy-weight range. To create a healthy-weight range with this number at the bottom you would go six pounds up from 168. This results in a healthy-weight range of 168 to 174 pounds. Which means, any weight within this range (or between 168.0 to 174.9) is considered to be a *healthy weight* for you. So, whenever your body weight is 168, 169, 170, 171, 172, 173, or 174 pounds (or between 168.0–174.9 lbs.) you're living at your healthy weight.

And what about kilograms? If your ideal weight number happened to be 76 kilos and you wanted a 3-kilo healthy-weight range with your ideal weight at the bottom, you would go two kilos up from 76, thereby creating a healthy-weight range of 76 to 78 kilos. So, any weight between 76.0–78.9 kilos would be considered to be a healthy weight for you.

WAY #3: *Make Your Ideal Weight Number the Upper Limit of the Range.* ❧ For this, have your ideal weight number be the top point of the range, and then build downward from there. The procedure for this is the same as for doing Way #2 (above), except in the opposite direction.

So, which of these three ways is best for you? I suggest you use whichever one you believe will produce the most effective weight management outcome for you.

Your Ideal Weight and Healthy-weight Range Can Change Over Time

Evolving conditions can warrant a change in ideal weight number and healthy-weight range. For example, if you're growing taller your ideal weight

and healthy-weight range will likely move upward. And, if your muscle mass is shrinking, as happens to most persons after about age 35 or 40, your ideal weight and weight range will likely move downward. Also, as you grow older your ideal weight goes down. So, as your age, height, and amount of muscle mass changes, you should adjust your healthy-weight range accordingly. And, you should reflect this in your Weight Success Benefits Directive by changing your healthy-weight range numbers.

Closing Comment and Warning

In setting your ideal weight number, bear this point in mind: Good health is always more important than "good looks." Meaning, don't be tempted into pursuing a super-low, or ultra-thin, ideal weight number just because you, or friends or family, think you look "good" or "sexy" at that weight. Conversely, don't be seduced into keeping your body weight in the overweight range just because you, or friends or family, think you look "good" or "strong" or "healthy" at that weight. Living overweight increases the likelihood of incurring any of numerous debilitating conditions. Ditto for living underweight. In short, there's nothing good-looking, healthy, or sexy about being the victim of some debilitating illness caused by living overweight or underweight.

Also, you'll likely discover that most people don't know what constitutes healthy body weight. What they view as an ideal or healthy weight is about 25 pounds higher than an actual ideal body weight. Which means, if you rely on what other people think is the "right weight" for you, you'll likely end up being about 25 pounds *overweight*, or 25 pounds beyond your ideal or healthiest weight.

Why do most people carry this distorted view? It's because, in our world correct weight is the *exception*, overweightness is the *rule*. We're removed from the womb by overweight doctors and nurses. We grow up playing with overweight friends. We're raised by overweight parents. We're taught by overweight teachers, coaches, and role models. The result: We automatically view the overweight body as being the norm and view the correct weight body as an underweight "ab-norm."

To illustrate, here's a story. Shortly after starting the Weight Success Method in 2007 I moved my weight down some pounds, to live in what I figured was my healthy-weight range. This change prompted a family member to occasionally tell me "you're too skinny," "you need to put on some pounds," and so on. Finally, I decided action was in order. I did some Internet research to find out exactly what my ideal weight number was. As it turned out, depending on how it was calculated I was either right at my ideal weight or *slightly above* it. I typed up my findings and gave copies to family members. The comments on my body weight came no more.

It's about Living in the Right Range

View it this way. You have an overall possible body weight range that consists of three parts: underweight range, healthy-weight range, overweight range. Make sure you live your life in the one that produces greatest health benefit. As an infographic it looks like this.

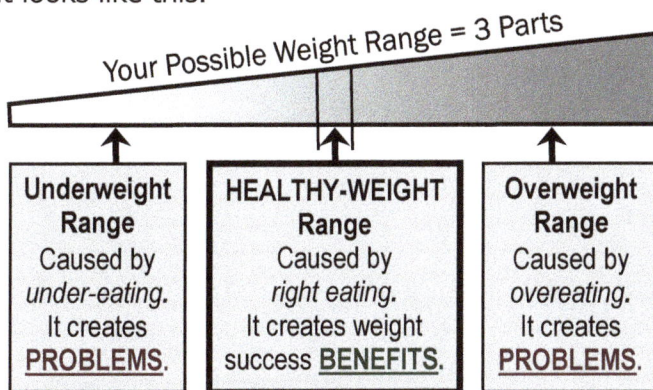

Your Possible Weight Range = 3 Parts

Underweight Range	HEALTHY-WEIGHT Range	Overweight Range
Caused by *under-eating*. It creates PROBLEMS.	Caused by *right eating*. It creates weight success BENEFITS.	Caused by *overeating*. It creates PROBLEMS.

☺

Did You Know ...

Research indicates that when we're living <u>non</u>-overweight, or at our ideal weight, the likelihood of us living FREE OF a major affliction is *much greater* than when we're living overweight. Here's a list of the bad situations that <u>non</u>-overweight living helps a person to <u>avoid</u>: high blood pressure · high blood cholesterol · congestive heart failure · heart attack · blood clots in legs and lungs · stroke · gout · Alzheimer's disease · osteoarthritis · type 2 diabetes · colon cancer · breast cancer · uterine cancer (women) · prostate cancer (men) · liver cirrhosis · gallstones and gall bladder disorders · sleeping disorders such as sleep apnea and excessive snoring · joint and lower back problems · infertility · incontinence · menstrual problems and pregnancy issues · and psychological disorders such as depression and lowered self-esteem.

If you happen to be one who easily gains weight (and most people are), achieving the goal of living out your life in your healthy-weight range is a **commendable, noteworthy accomplishment.** It's an accomplishment you should appreciate, and derive a good feeling from, **every single day.**

CHAPTER 7: Weight Success Benefits in Detail

Once you fully identify and then daily visualize the benefits of healthy-weight living and weight success, self-motivation becomes *easier.*

TO MAXIMIZE the likelihood of creating lifelong heathy-weight living, you must clearly identify your weight success benefits. Then reflect on these benefits each day. By doing this it motivates your mind to pursue activities that result in realizing these benefits, which includes the activity of creating lifelong healthy-weight living. Here's how to identify your weight success benefits.

Create a list of the good things that will come your way from living in your healthy-weight range. We call these good things *weight success benefits.* To make your benefits listing job easy I've included this list of 20 possible benefits. Of course, *you should ignore those that don't apply to you.* Plus you should add in any benefit that does apply but isn't on the list. Your final list can include both general benefits and specific. Use whatever wording carries the most meaning for you.

20 Possible Benefits from Living in Your Healthy-weight Range

1. I have a greater chance of *living healthier longer* — or greater chance of living free of debilitating accidents, illnesses, diseases, and bodily malfunction.
2. I experience greater eating pleasure.
3. I feel better.
4. I look better.
5. I move better.
6. I have greater agility.
7. I have greater energy and stamina.
8. I experience greater happiness, including a daily good feeling from creating lifelong healthy-weight living.
9. I have a stronger self-image and enhanced self-esteem.
10. I have better overall health and fewer annoying ailments.
11. My clothes fit better and feel more comfortable.
12. I'm no longer constantly growing out of clothes.
13. I can do more [of a particular fun thing or things].
14. I eliminate [a particular illness or affliction].
15. I improve [a particular relationship].
16. I overcome [a particular problem].
17. I can better engage in [a particular activity or pursuit].
18. I have a greater chance of avoiding debilitating physical accidents, such as broken bones from falling.
19. I have a greater chance of living longer.
20. I will be more active in my latter years.

Write down your list of weight success benefits in the Benefits section of the Weight Success Benefits Directive. Note: Don't assume that the prior list of 20 benefits includes every possible weight success benefit. There may be additional benefits not on this list, which you might want to include.

REPEAT: Write It Down!

Either (a) *write down* or (b) *type up and print out* your list of weight success benefits. Then insert this list into your Weight Success Benefits Directive, which you use in Daily Action 3.

Be Sure to Include Benefit #1

You can include whatever benefits you want in your weight success benefits list. But I suggest you be sure to include Benefit #1 (shown in prior list). That benefit is: a greater chance of living healthier longer — or greater chance of living free of debilitating accidents, illnesses, diseases, and bodily malfunction.

Perhaps you're wondering why Benefit #1 is Number One. It's because as a person ages the chance of contracting a debilitating affliction increases substantially. Research shows that when you're living <u>non</u>-overweight the likelihood of you living FREE OF a major affliction is much greater than when you're living overweight. Here's a list of the bad situations that <u>non</u>-overweight living helps a person to <u>avoid</u>: high blood pressure • high blood cholesterol • congestive heart failure • heart attack • blood clots in legs and lungs • stroke • gout • Alzheimer's disease • osteoarthritis • type 2 diabetes • colon cancer • breast cancer • uterine cancer (women) • prostate cancer (men) • liver cirrhosis • gallstones and gall bladder disorders • sleeping disorders such as sleep apnea and excessive snoring • joint and lower back problems • infertility • incontinence • menstrual problems and pregnancy issues • and psychological disorders such as depression and lowered self-esteem.

Increasing the likelihood of living FREE OF those conditions is a high priority to many folks, which is why "a greater chance of living healthier longer" is the #1 weight success benefit.

TO CONCLUDE, each day read your weight success benefits list and visualize at least one of the benefits as an accomplished fact. Generate a good feeling from the visualization. This motivates your mind — especially your subconscious mind — to create thoughts and feelings that guide you toward creation of that benefit, which will involve creation of healthy-weight living.

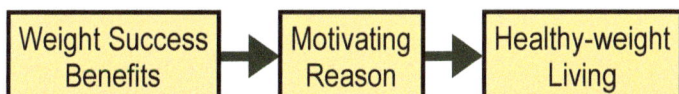

| Weight Success Benefits | → | Motivating Reason | → | Healthy-weight Living |

A Final Big Reason

Here's one more reason for living your life in your healthy-weight range. Many of us express how much we love and care for our children, grandchildren, and other family members. But I suggest, also include this action: *Live the rest of your life in your healthy-weight range.* Doing so is one of the truest love expressions of all, in two ways.

First, by living the rest of your life in your healthy-weight range you provide family members with an inspiring role model to emulate — a role model of healthy-weight living. The result: at least some will follow your example, which will cause them to live a healthier, happier, more fulfilling life.

Second, by living in your healthy-weight range you greatly *reduce* the chance of you contracting a debilitating condition as a result of extended overweight living. This, in turn, reduces the likelihood of your children or other family members having to bear the crushing responsibility of looking after you for years while you're living out your life in an incapacitated state.

Indeed, living the rest of your life in your healthy-weight range is one of the most loving, caring, thoughtful things you can do for those who are nearest and dearest to you. So, engaging in healthy-weight living isn't merely an act of self-development and personal achievement. It goes way beyond that.

> Do the **Five Daily Actions**
> <u>every</u> day . . .
> and **Lifelong Weight Success**
> will be <u>Yours</u>.

Healthy-weight living provides a plethora of benefits — way more than most persons imagine it to be. Perhaps the greatest benefit of all is having a greater chance of
living healthier longer.

CHAPTER 8: Weighing and Scale Info

A consistently accurate bathroom scale, *properly* used each day, is the most powerful tool on the planet for creating healthy-weight living.

YOU MIGHT find this hard to believe, but it's true. Correct daily weighing (Daily Action 1) combined with a certain right response (Daily Action 2A or 2B) is the core element to creating lifelong healthy-weight living. So, you need a scale that delivers a consistently accurate weight reading every time. If you already have such a scale, great. But, if you don't have a consistently accurate scale it would likely be a good idea to get one.

Contrary to what you might assume, many bathroom scales do *not* produce a consistently accurate weight reading. Meaning, if you step on the scale two times in a row you'll get two different readings — sometimes as much as two or three pounds (or a kilo) apart. This type of scale doesn't best serve our purpose.

Also contrary to what you might assume, there seems to be no correlation between a bathroom scale's accuracy and its stylishness, size, type, or price. Meaning, a fancy stylish scale will deliver an inaccurate or inconsistent reading as often as a plain-looking scale — a big scale will deliver an inaccurate or inconsistent reading as often as a smaller scale — a digital (electronic sensor) scale will deliver an inaccurate or inconsistent reading as often as a mechanical (spring) scale — and an expensive bathroom scale will deliver an inaccurate or inconsistent reading as often as a lower-priced scale.

If you don't believe it, do as I did. Go to the scale section of a well-stocked bathroom supplies store — like, for example, Bed Bath & Beyond — and conduct a test. Weigh yourself on the various sample test models. With each one, stand on it three times in a row. I predict you'll find the inconsistency to be eye-opening.

Finally, as a result of your testing, get the best-performing scale your budget will allow. By "best-performing scale" I mean the scale that comes closest to delivering a *consistently accurate* weight reading for you.

Eventually, I did some Internet research and ended up buying a type of scale used in most doctors' offices. Such a scale typically comes in two types: (a) a high-end digital scale and (b) a balance beam, or weigh beam, scale. The weigh beam scale is the traditional type of scale that has been used in doctors' offices for about the past century or so. It's the one that looks like a giant "T" and has a weigh bar with a sliding weight at the top of the "T", as depicted in this Microsoft clipart sketch.

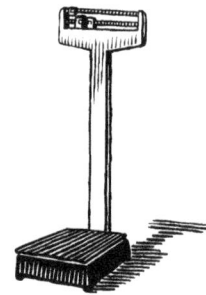

The digital scale, on the other hand, is more recent. It's slick looking and gives an instant reading. But it can be somewhat pricey. You might find that a "home version" of the weigh beam scale carries a more reasonable price tag.

My personal preference is the weigh beam, not just because of its lower price but because I like the way it works. I like sliding the weigh bar weight to the proper spot. Plus, it doesn't require batteries or electric cords. Plus, because of its tall height I see it many times each day, which makes it a reminder to do the five daily actions.

TIP 1: If you happen to get a weigh beam scale here's a handy suggestion. Each time after getting onto the scale or after sliding the weigh-bar weight, slightly raise your arms up and down a little bit. Do this just once. This "jiggles" the weigh beam, which causes it to instantly move to a new correct position. You might find that you do this "arm jiggle" movement several times during a weighing (each time after adjusting the weigh beam), in order to ascertain the final correct weight in that weighing.

TIP 2: After many years of using the weigh beam scale I wanted to achieve a more precise weighing, or smaller opening where the "needle" floats to indicate a weight reading. To do that, I cut a small piece of aluminum bar and bolted it to the scale to reduce the size of the opening. Here's a photo that illustrates.

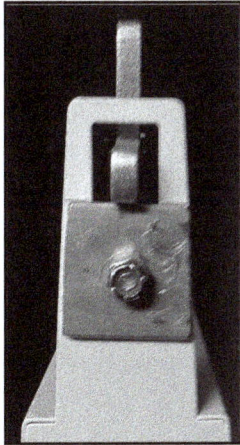

Moving on, several manufacturers make doctor's office scales. Some produce a broad line of both digital scales and weigh beam scales. The scale I personally use, for example, is the *Detecto physician weigh beam scale model 437* — website: detecto.com. It runs about $150 (in 2013). This might seem like a lot of money for a scale. But likely it will last a lifetime. So, what's the annualized cost? If, say, you use it for 20 years, the cost amounts to about $7.50 per year ($150 ÷ 20 = $7.50 per year), or just two cents a day. It's sold through various online sellers including through amazon.com. Also, should you happen to get this scale you might like to know that the company has an operating manual titled "Trouble Shooting Guide for Detecto Mechanical Physicians Balance Beam Scales." They will email it upon request.

Important Final Note on Scales

I've mentioned the above-cited specific scale model to provide possibly helpful info. This is <u>not</u> a product promotion or endorsement. There are a number of good scales that can do the job. I've opted for a balance beam scale because it fits my personal preferences. <u>But</u> you might find that a *digital* scale best fits *your* preferences. ***You should get the type and brand of scale that, in your opinion, will work best for YOU and YOUR SITUATION.***

Do the **Five Daily Actions** <u>every</u> day . . .
and **Lifelong Weight Success** will be <u>Yours</u>.

Typically takes <u>less than</u> **8** minutes of dedicated time per day.

– "2B or Not 2B" –
Two Opposite Approaches

There are two opposing approaches to solving the worldwide overweight problem. They work like this.

APPROACH #1: We continue doing those "cause of our overweightness" or "fat-promoting factors" studies that tell us we humans have no control over how much we eat and weigh. (For a listing of fat-promoting factors, go to "False Assumption 1" in Ch. **20** (p. 126).

APPROACH #2: Everyone go on a diet and take their weight down to their healthy-weight range; then weigh themselves each day and whenever their daily weight reading goes above their healthy-weight range they enact a Weight Correction Day of total fasting or semi-fasting and, so, bring their weight back into their healthy-weight range in 24–48 hours. (See Daily Action 2B, page 26).

The first approach will continue costing millions and solve nothing. The second would cost virtually nothing and solve the worldwide overweight problem in a year. Here's an infographic.

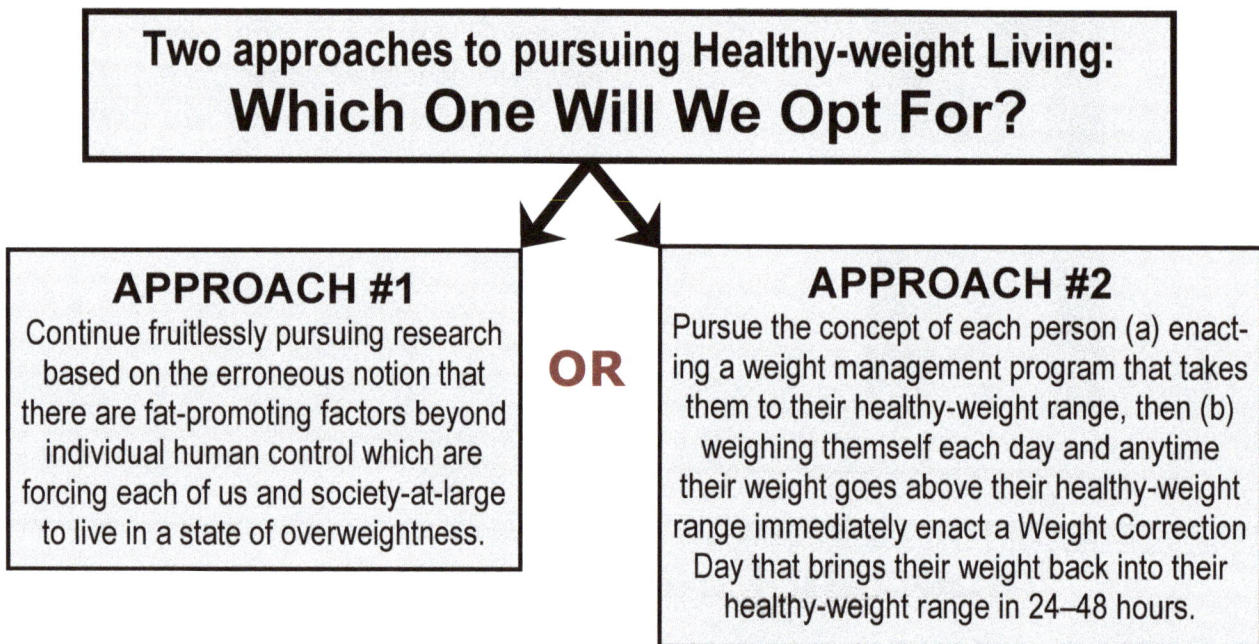

Two approaches to pursuing Healthy-weight Living:
Which One Will We Opt For?

APPROACH #1
Continue fruitlessly pursuing research based on the erroneous notion that there are fat-promoting factors beyond individual human control which are forcing each of us and society-at-large to live in a state of overweightness.

OR

APPROACH #2
Pursue the concept of each person (a) enacting a weight management program that takes them to their healthy-weight range, then (b) weighing themself each day and anytime their weight goes above their healthy-weight range immediately enact a Weight Correction Day that brings their weight back into their healthy-weight range in 24–48 hours.

There's a driving dynamic in the world of weight management and healthy-weight living — it's **Calorie Consumption.** It works like this — <u>remember it</u>.

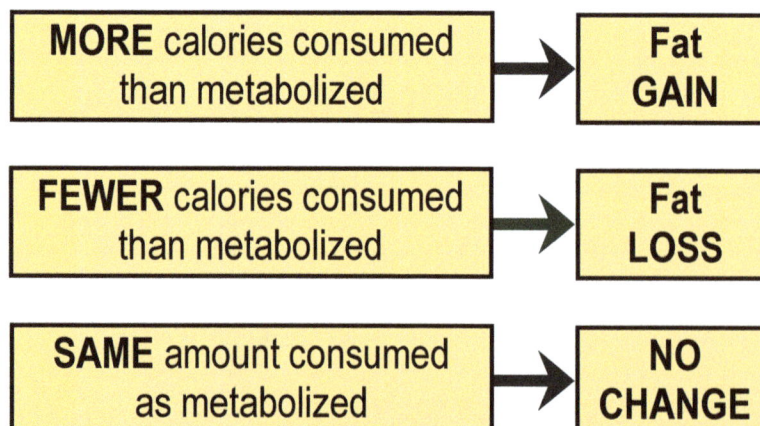

MORE calories consumed than metabolized	Fat **GAIN**
FEWER calories consumed than metabolized	Fat **LOSS**
SAME amount consumed as metabolized	**NO CHANGE**

CHAPTER 9: Detailed Instructions for Weight Success Benefits Directive

Apply these simple instructions for setting up and delivering the Weight Success Benefits Directive (p. 32) and you'll greatly magnify the positive impact of the Directive.

TO GET maximum results from your Weight Success Benefits Directive you need to do three things: (1) fill in the blank sections of the Directive, (2) enhance the Directive, if needed, and (3) deliver the Directive in a way that produces maximum effect. The next three sections tell how to do those three things.

1 – Filling in the Blanks

The Weight Success Benefits Directive contains three blank line (_____) sections. TIP: For filling in these blanks I suggest you use a pencil, not a pen. Here's how to do it.

Healthy-weight Range

In the first two blanks insert your desired healthy-weight range in either pounds or kilos. Your healthy-weight range should be a *bona fide* healthy-weight range for your gender, height, and age. For the "pounds–kilos" phrase draw a line through the word that doesn't apply. For explanation of how to set your healthy-weight range, go to the Healthy-weight Range in Detail chapter (p. **56**).

Preferred Dietary Program

In the next blank insert the name of your preferred dietary program. I define *preferred dietary program* as a set of eating guidelines and eating practices you prefer to follow and which, when followed, lead you to good health and healthy-weight living. Another name for preferred dietary program is preferred eating strategy.

So, if you're presently in weight reduction pursuit, then whatever eating program you're pursuing for your diet, weight loss, or weight reduction program is what you specify as your "preferred dietary program" in the Weight Success Benefits Directive. After you go into weight maintenance pursuit, you then specify the maintenance eating program you'll be following for staying in your healthy-weight range.

Your preferred dietary program can be any bona fide dietary program presently on the market <u>or</u> it can be a program of your own design. For more info on identifying a preferred dietary program, read Startup Action 7 (p. 19). If you think you might want to create a program of your own design, I suggest you first read the Author's Approach to Eating chapter (p. **74**).

Weight Success Benefits

In the last blank section — which consists of a set of lines — insert a listing of the benefits you'll derive from living in your healthy-weight range. For help in defining your weight success benefits, I suggest reading the Weight Success Benefits in Detail chapter (p. **60**).

The Weight Success Benefits Directive contains about 20 lines for listing weight success benefits. You're not required to fill every line. Some people have just three or four weight success benefits. Others have a dozen or more.

To install your list into the Directive you can either write it in or type it up and tape it in. If you write it in I suggest using a pencil.

As you already know, you'll be reading your Weight Success Benefits Directive each day. If your weight success benefits list is a lengthy one it will add an extra minute or so of reading time. But if it happens you'd like to keep reading time to a minimum, here's an optional tactic to consider. Divide your weight success benefits list into seven groups. Assign each group to a particular day of the week. Then, each day when reading the Directive, read the group of benefits assigned to that day, and overlook reading the other six groups on that day.

2 – Enhancing the Directive, If Needed

The Weight Success Benefits Directive isn't carved in granite; instead it's a changeable document. So, if there's something you'd like to delete, draw a line through it. If there's something you'd like to change, draw a line through it and write the new word or words above.

Reading the Directive the first few times might seem like work. But, after a few days it begins to become enjoyable, even fun. This especially occurs when results start happening, which is almost immediately.

3 – Seven Actions for Delivering the Directive for Maximum Effect

To maximize the results you get from the Weight Success Benefits Directive, apply these seven actions when delivering it. (Note: You can advantageously apply these actions to delivery of any mind directive, not just this directive.)

1 – Speak it. ✎ Speaking aloud is best, but when you can't do that, whisper it to yourself. As you whisper it make your tongue and lips move. (Note: You can convey directives to your mind by speaking silently in your mind. But, for the Weight Success Benefits Directive I recommend that you speak it aloud or at least whisper it.)

2 – Act as-if your mind is a *distinct being* that's listening to every instruction you're giving it. ✎ (For more about your mind, go to the Why the Weight Success Method Gets Your Whole Mind Involved chapter, page **109.**)

3 – Use some **emotional force**. ✎ That is, put some passion or emotional intensity into the delivery. Note: Happiness and excitement are forms of emotional intensity.

4 – Hold a **strong desire** for your mind to do every action described in the Directive. ✎ The stronger you desire for your mind to perform the actions described in the Directive, the more important these actions appear to your mind — including subconscious mind. And, the more impor-

tant these actions appear to your mind, the more diligently it strives to do them.

So, how do you strengthen your desire for your mind to do what's called for in the Weight Success Benefits Directive? You imagine how good you'll feel and how great your life will be from gaining the benefits of maintaining your weight in your healthy-weight range. These benefits, by the way, are the items you list in the Weight Success Benefits section of the Directive. The more vividly you imagine how good you'll feel from deriving these benefits, the more diligently your mind — especially your subconscious mind — will pursue actualization of the benefits.

5 – Hold the **belief** that your mind can and will perform the actions. ✎ Hold this belief not only while delivering the Directive but afterward, as well. This is vital. When you hold doubt, or halfway belief, that your mind will do the actions described in a request or directive it creates a problem. It causes your mind to ignore doing the actions. This happens because your mind seldom performs in contradiction to the belief system held in your mind. So, when you hold the belief "I can't do action X" or "my mind won't do action X" or "action X is impossible to do," your mind — including your subconscious mind — will respond accordingly. As a result, it likely won't perform the actions described in the Directive.

So, how do you replace disbelief with belief? You make-believe, or act as-if, you believe. That's right, you totally pretend you're holding the belief that you — or your mind — can and will perform the actions described in the Weight Success Benefits Directive. I realize this instruction might sound hokey. But do it anyhow; it works. For more on this, see the *How Believing and Acting As-if Work* section, in Startup Action 5 (p. 17).

6 – Visualize one or more of your weight success benefits as an accomplished fact. ✎ After reading the list of weight success benefits take 30 seconds to visualize, or imagine, yourself at that very moment enjoying having at least one of the exciting benefits.

7 – Apply **creative delivery techniques** for extra effect. ✍ Doing this can cause your mind to pay extra attention to what you're telling it to do. Here are some examples to consider.

FIRST, emphasize the key words. You can do this by speaking slightly louder, or slower, or more forcefully. These key words are printed in *italic,* underline, or **bold.**

SECOND, repeat (reread) a particular phrase or sentence for emphasis.

THIRD, read the entire Directive slowly and deliberately. This will require one or two extra minutes. But it can pay dividends. It can cause your subconscious mind to pay special attention to the instructions contained in the Directive. To do this, pause for a few seconds after each sentence.

During the pause, reflect on the meaning or main message of the sentence.

FOURTH, ad lib whenever you see fit. Insert spontaneous additional instructions to your subconscious mind to emphasize key points.

FIFTH, deliver the Directive in a different place or position. For example, if you've been delivering the Directive sitting down, do it standing. Or, deliver it while pacing, like you're delivering a speech. Include arm movement and gesticulation of main points. This can be a powerful form of delivery. It can enhance your emotional impact. Experiment and find out what works best for you. Or, just change delivery style from time to time for variety.

To sum up, the Weight Success Benefits Directive is an *important* message for your mind. Deliver it like it is and your mind — especially your subconscious mind — will act accordingly

---

Right-eating mindset creates right-eating actions which create right-weight living. Yes, mindset is the key.

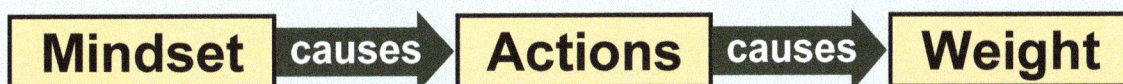

Mindset causes➤ **Actions** causes➤ **Weight**

Do the **Five Daily Actions** every day . . .
and **Lifelong Weight Success** will be Yours.

Typically takes less than **8** minutes of dedicated time per day.

CHAPTER 10: Setback Reversal Made Easier

In every endeavor, challenges and setbacks happen. Succeeding at an endeavor requires converting setbacks into progress actions. Those who do this, succeed. Those who don't, fail or quit.

WITH ALMOST every pursuit a person can accidentally deviate from the program now and then. So, on your weight success journey you might now and then forget to do what you want to be doing and, instead, accidentally engage in wrong eating. I call this a *misstep* — also known as accidental oversight. Here's an example. A special meal comes along and you become caught up in the moment and, thereby, overlook doing the Guided Eating Process (of Daily Action 5 of the Weight Success Method) and you end up accidentally overeating.

Here's another example of a misstep. An old overeating-causing habit or craving that you've shut down now temporarily reactivates during a certain meal or on a certain day. You unthinkingly respond to this temporarily reactivated habit or craving the wrong way — that is, by eating too much — and this results in overeating for the day.

Also, with every endeavor there are periods when progress seems to stop. For example, when striving to lose weight, weight loss might stop. Or, when living in your healthy-weight range, a jump in weight that takes you outside the range might occur. I call this a *progress lapse.*

In both these situations — misstep and progress lapse — you should apply the same response: *Immediately turn the setback into a progress action.* You can easily do this by applying a certain six actions plus an optional seventh action. I call it the *setback-reversal process.* It works like this.

Setback-reversal Process

To easily convert a progress lapse into a forward step, do these six actions (and perhaps an optional seventh action).

ACTION 1: Avoid a counterproductive response and adopt a productive one.

This is Action 1 because if you don't do this nothing else works, or works well. Examples of a counter-

productive response include second-guessing, self-doubt, self-pity, self-blame, guilt, and discouragement. These things never help and usually hurt. They make it harder to create a timely correction or reversal of the misstep or progress lapse. So, avoid every type of counterproductive response. Instead, adopt the attitude "What has happened is over; I'm now going to *learn* and *benefit* from it." In short, shun negative responses; embrace a positive one.

ACTION 2: Identify the cause.

The next step to creating a progress action out of a misstep or progress lapse is identify the cause. The cause of most missteps and progress lapses is a failure to remember to do what you needed to be doing. Or, in short, a failure to apply all five daily actions of the Weight Success Method each day.

ACTION 3: Identify the future corrective action.

For this step you identify the specific corrective action you'll be taking in the future to avert a repeat of the misstep or progress lapse. Basically, what you want to be doing next time is take the opposite action to whatever action caused the misstep.

For example, let's assume the misstep was caused by you forgetting to do the Guided Eating Process during a meal. In this case, next time a similar situation arises the corrective action would be for you to remember to do the Guided Eating Process during the meal.

ACTION 4: Deliver a misstep-reversal directive.

Deliver a mini directive to your self — or your mind — that orders it to apply the corrective action the next time you encounter the type of situation that resulted in the past misstep or progress lapse. Here's how it might go.

Subconscious mind, the next time I encounter [the situation that resulted in the misstep], you are to remind me to [take such-and-such corrective action]. I <u>strongly</u> <u>desire</u> for you to do this and I <u>firmly</u> <u>believe</u> you will do so. Working together, we <u>will</u> convert the past misstep into a progress action, and <u>will</u> avoid the misstep happening again. I greatly appreciate your help in this, and I thank you for it.

ACTION 5: Deliver your Healthy-weight Goal Statement 100 times.

Yes, you read it right. Say your Healthy-weight Goal Statement 100 times. You can either do this aloud, including in a whisper, or do it silently in your mind. Do it within 24 hours after the misstep. You need not do it all in one session. You can spread it out over the 24-hour period if you like.

Does repeating the Statement 100 times seem like a lot? Well, it's not. You're able to say it three times in 12 to 15 seconds. That's 12 to 15 times a minute. Which means, you can do it 100 times in less than eight minutes. If you prefer, you can break it up into two or more sessions. And, you can do them in bed when going to sleep and when you awaken in the morning, and during all the numerous "free time" periods in your day. For more, see the "How to Do It" section in Daily Action 4 (p. 34).

ACTION 6: Make certain you're doing all five Daily Actions, in entirety, each day.

My personal experience has been this. Whenever I've had a misstep or progress lapse — which, by the way, is very infrequently any more — it has occurred during a brief period when I had been "slacking off" on doing all five daily actions of the Weight Success Method each day.

Also, it has been my further experience that most of my progress lapses occurred on days when I had been involved in an "extra-tempting meal" situation and had forgotten to do Daily Action 5

(Guided Eating) during that meal. If it happens that this is the situation with your present misstep or progress lapse, do this. For the next seven days deliver this backup depiction statement to yourself at least 10 times each day.

I am right now in a guided-eating week.
I do guided eating every time I eat.

Again, say it at least 10 times each day for a week. If you need to refresh yourself on the Guided Eating Process, go to Daily Action 5 (p. 35).

OPTIONAL ACTION 7: Squelch recurring undesired weight readings.

Are you presently experiencing too many days of "undesired-weight readings," or too many recurring days of gaining weight or going over your healthy-weight range? If so, in addition to doing Actions 1–6 also do this Action 7. It involves three steps.

STEP 1: Check your healthy-weight commitment. Is living in your healthy-weight range a *mandatory*, <u>non</u>-optional, <u>will</u>-do, <u>must</u>-have aspect of your life? If it's not, make the firm decision — right now — that it will be for the rest of your life, and remember this decision *each day.*

STEP 2: Check your healthy-weight beliefs. Are you holding can-do, will-do beliefs as regards living in your healthy-weight range? Each day are you acting on the assumption that living in your healthy-weight range is, or can be, *easily* doable by you? If you're not doing this, or are finding it hard to do, read the *How Believing and Acting As-if Work* section in Startup Action 5 (p. 17). Then apply those instructions, including the part about each day *acting as-if* you possess the capability to easily live your life in your healthy-weight range. Also, when doing Daily Actions 3 and 4, be sure to believe and act as-if what they describe is actually happening.

STEP 3: Increase your right-eating *focus* and right-eating *communication*. No matter how many "undesired-weight days" you might be experiencing, no matter how much you might be struggling with overeating, no matter what fat-promoting factor you might be confronting, there's an amount of focus and communication that will reverse the situation. So your job is this: Ratchet up your right-eating focus and right-eating communication to the point it *overpowers* the situation that's making it hard for you to be free of frequently-recurring undesired weight readings. The rest of this chapter explains how to do this.

How to Increase Right-eating FOCUS and Right-eating COMMUNICATION

The first essential condition to overcoming a situation of recurring undesired weight readings is to ratchet up your right-eating resolve. The way to do this is: Make the resolute decision to immediately begin reversing the situation, *starting that day.* Then deliver a right-eating directive to your mind. Tell it how much you desire to be doing daily right eating and living your life in your healthy-weight range. Describe how doing this will greatly benefit you and your life. And, deliver this communication with vehemence. Lastly, increase your commitment to doing all five daily actions of the Weight Success Method, in entirety, *every day.*

The second essential condition to overcoming a situation of recurring undesired weight readings is to increase right-eating communication to your mind — including to your subconscious mind. You have three options for doing this, cleverly called Options 1, 2, and 3. Select the one you'd like to do.

Option #1 (p. 70) involves doing an expanded version of the five daily actions of the Weight Success Method. It's the simplest option of the three.

Option #2 (p. 71) involves adding a new mind motivator to the five daily actions. You have a choice of six new motivators. The Six More Mind Motivators chapter (p. 90) describes them. This option is a bit more complex than Option 1, but you might find it more powerful.

Option #3 (p. 71) — which I call *High-power Eat-right Solution* — involves a set of seven specific actions. It's an all-in, pedal-to-the-metal technique aimed at squelching creeping weight gain, or ending recurring overeating progress lapses. It's the most complex of the three options, but you'll likely find it the most powerful.

So, which option should you do? Do whichever one you think will work best. If you're not sure, you might start with Option #1. If it does the job, stick with it. If it doesn't, do Option #2. If #2 works — great. If it doesn't, do Option #3.

It's virtually certain at least one of these three options will result in you conquering whatever situation is causing your recurring overeating missteps or weight gain progress lapses. But always bear in mind, regardless of which option you choose, the key to success is: *Increase* the amount of right-eating focus and right-eating communication to the point it overwhelms, or conquers, the weight-gain-causing overeating. I call this the "Overeating-reversal Dynamic." Here's the infographic.

Overeating-reversal Works Like This

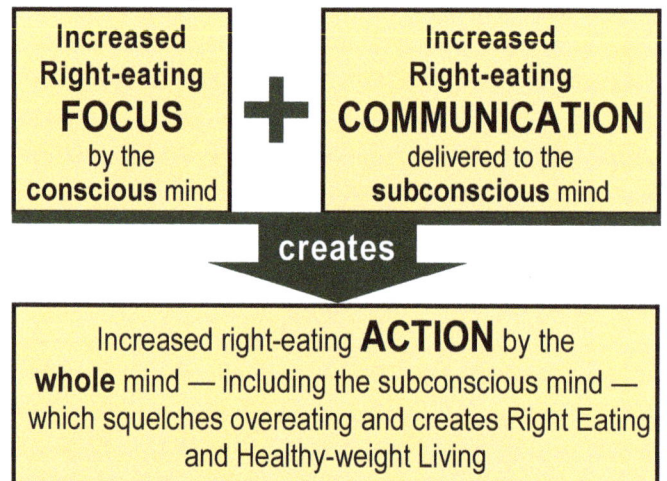

Increased Right-eating **FOCUS** by the **conscious** mind	**+**	Increased Right-eating **COMMUNICATION** delivered to the **subconscious** mind

creates ⬇

Increased right-eating **ACTION** by the **whole** mind — including the subconscious mind — which squelches overeating and creates Right Eating and Healthy-weight Living

Right-eating FOCUS = Time spent thinking about, talking about, pursuing, and enjoyably doing right eating and healthy-weight living.

Right-eating COMMUNICATION = Communication that tells your mind to steer you toward right eating and healthy-weight living.

> **Overeating-reversal OPTION #1:**
> **Expand the Five Daily Actions**

Setback reversal often boils down to doing the daily actions of the Weight Success Method with greater frequency and intensity. Here are some ways to do that. You can use just one way or you can use more than one — your choice.

In Daily Action 2A, increase the emotional intensity, or exuberance, you use when delivering the Thank You, Keep It Up message.

In Daily Action 3, enhance the delivery of your Weight Success Benefits Directive to increase its motivating impact on your mind. See the "Seven Actions for Delivering the Directive for Maximum Effect" section, page **66**, for ways you can enhance delivery.

In Daily Action 4, increase the number of times you say your Healthy-weight Goal Statement throughout the day. And, say it with increased passion. Also, make sure you say it *every* time you begin eating.

In Daily Action 5, increase the amount of guided-eating self-talk during eating sessions. This includes both the number of times you say your Healthy-weight Goal Statement and also the amount of ad lib self-talk. For more on this see the During-eating Self-talk section in Daily Action 5 (p. 38). Plus, make sure you're holding the belief and acting as-if your mind is right then in the process of doing what's described in your Weight Success Benefits Directive. And, when doing this be on the lookout for a stop-eating signal. (A listing of possible stop-eating signals is given in Daily Action 5, page 37.) Finally, when the stop-eating signal comes, follow it immediately and also thank your subconscious mind for sending it.

Overeating-reversal OPTION #2: Include Optional Mind Motivators

Would you like to test some additional ways of motivating your mind to assist with creating right eating and healthy-weight living? These techniques are powerful. Plus they can be fun.

Go to the Six More Mind Motivators chapter (p. **90**) and check out the optional six mind motivators. Choose the one that looks most promising and give it a try. If it works, do it each day along with the five daily actions. If it doesn't work, try another one of the six optional motivators. Note: You can do more than one a day, if you like. The more you do, the greater the impact.

Overeating-reversal OPTION #3: Do the High-power Eat-right Solution

You use this High-power Eat-right Solution along with the Weight Success Method, not in place of it. It's an all-in, super-powerful, pedal-to-the-metal fix for preventing recurring weight gain and also creeping weight gain. You can use it one or both of two ways.

Firstly, as previously explained, you can use it for this optional Action 7 of the setback-reversal process. Secondly, you can, if you like, use it whenever you confront a day that holds high potential for overeating. I'm talking about those days that contain extra-tempting food and a lot of it — like social events, picnics, parties, weddings, religious celebration days, Thanksgiving, and the like.

Now that you know *when* to use the Solution, here's *how* to do it. It involves seven actions.

ACTION 1: *Recognize the real cause of weight gain.* Bear in mind that weight gain comes from consuming more metabolizable calories than what your body is metabolizing, or "burning up," per day — called *overeating.*

Further, bear in mind that small daily amounts of overeating create small daily amounts of weight gain. So, to avoid creeping weight gain, avoid overeating even in small daily amounts. For more on this, go to Startup Action 1 (p. 14).

ACTION 2: *Realize that right eating is the fix for recurring weight gain.* Or, put another way, realize that to end recurring or creeping weight gain you must end daily overeating, even in small amounts, and install right eating in its place. *Right eating* is the act of eating right foods in right amounts and doing it in a way that creates right eating enjoyment (see Startup Action 6, page 18).

ACTION 3: *Define your daily maximum calorie allotment number.* For each day you're using this Solution, define the maximum number of daily calories you want to be consuming for that day. If it happens that your preferred dietary program specifies certain types of food you should be eating, then determine what amounts of these foods will equate with your daily maximum calorie allotment number.

Note: This number is not a wish-for number or a nice-to-attain number; it's a *firm, fixed, must-not-exceed* number. Consuming a little less than the daily calorie allotment number is okay, but consuming more is absolutely forbidden. So, do <u>not</u> exceed your daily calorie allotment number for the day.

To make it easier, you might divide the daily calorie allotment number into either meal calorie allotments or day-part calorie allotments. For example, if your daily calorie allotment is, say, 1000 calories, you might assign 200 calories to the breakfast meal, 200 calories to lunch, and 600 calories to dinner. Or, if you use the day-part approach, you might assign 200 calories to the 7 a.m. to noon part, 200 calories to the noon to 4:00 p.m. part, and 600 calories to the 4:00 to 7:00 p.m. part. Note: this amount and distribution of calories is an example, not a recommendation.

Then, every time you eat something, record what you ate and the number of calories consumed from that particular food. Keep a running total for the day, to ensure you don't go over your daily calorie allotment.

Or, if you like, for ultimate simplicity create an eating menu or plan covering the entire day. Specify the exact foods you're going to eat, the exact portion amount of each item, and the number of calories in each item. Set the portion amounts so the total number of calories equals your daily calorie allotment. Then eat exactly what the menu specifies, and no more.

ACTION 4: *Create and hold a weight success mindset.* ❧ Having such a mindset is vital to achieving sustained right eating and healthy-weight living. To create a weight success mindset hold these two assumptions in mind:

1. "Doing right eating and living in my healthy-weight range is a *mandatory* feature of my existence. It's a <u>non</u>-optional, <u>will</u>-do, <u>must</u>-have aspect of my life." For more on this, see Startup Action 4 (p. 15).

2. "Doing right eating and living in my healthy-weight range is *easily* doable." For more on

weight success mindset, see Startup Action 5 (p. 15).

ACTION 5: *The night before, do an upcoming-day description with right eating in it.* ❧ Before you go to sleep at night, probably while lying in bed, deliver an upcoming-day description to your subconscious mind. That is, describe to your subconscious mind how you want the next day to turn out. To illustrate, here's some sample wording.

Subconscious mind, tomorrow is going to be a <u>perfect</u> right-eating day. It will happen like this. I will consume my daily calorie allotment of _____ calories for the day, and no more. I'll find this to be <u>easy</u> to do. Each of my daily meals will make me feel like I'm <u>filled up</u>. I will have the full-stomach feeling after each one. And after each one I'll feel <u>fully satisfied</u> for the next _____ hours. And I'll be free of cravings and hunger pangs between meals. It will be a <u>great</u> right-eating day. It will be easy and fun to do, and I'll enjoy it immensely. Subconscious mind, please do whatever you can to positively assist me in making the day happen this way, and in making it be a pleasant, positive day. I believe 100% that you will do this. Thank you very, very much.

Note: This is sample wording, not a must-follow script. Use whatever wording best describes the way you want the day to turn out. And, if you have a nickname for your subconscious mind, you can use that name instead of the name "Subconscious Mind," if you so desire.

Also, if you like, you can repeat this description on the morning of that day. Doing it immediately after waking up, while still lying in bed, is a good time. For more on upcoming-day descriptions, go to "Motivator 3: Upcoming-day Description" (p. **92**) in the Six More Mind Motivators chapter.

ACTION 6: *Reiterate a right-eating backup depiction statement throughout the day.* ❧ Say the following backup depiction statement at least 25 times throughout the day.

I am right now in a right-eating day — a right-eating day in every single way.

Note: Saying it "at least 25 times" defines a minimum, not a maximum. For extra impact, if you so desire, say it more than 25 times — like say it 40, 50, or even 100 times during the day. For other backup depiction statements you might find helpful in creating right eating, go to "Motivator 2: Backup Depiction Statements" (p. **90**) in the Six More Mind Motivators chapter.

ACTION 7: *Do during-eating self-talk through-out each eating session.* For how-to instructions, see the During-eating Self-talk section in Daily Action 5 (p. 38).

OPTIONAL ACTION 8: *Ask God to disclose to you an insight, tactic, or opportunity you might use for ending creeping weight gain.* My experience has been that when I've requested insight from God on how I might solve a certain problem (of any kind) or accomplish a certain life-enhancing goal (of any kind), and I've requested it a certain way, I've received what I requested. If you'd like infor-mation on that process, go to the *Three Steps to Getting and Using Input from God* (p. **97**).

Concluding Thoughts

Setback reversal involves a choice between two "stones." Every adversity — challenge, misstep, progress lapse, discouragement — can be viewed either as a millstone pulling you down to failure or as a stepping stone that can lift you to further success. When you view the adversity as a millstone, that's what it becomes. When you view it as a stepping stone, that's what it becomes. So, adopt the Stepping Stone viewpoint for every adversity.

Also, keep in mind that the dividing line between winning and losing is a certain act: the act of converting setbacks into progress actions. So, convert each weight management setback into a progress action and you'll keep lost weight from returning and be a Weight Success Winner for life.

The Weight Success Secret is:
To succeed at healthy-weight living,
do Weight Success Actions every day.
— WHICH MEANS —
The way to overcome an extra-large weight management adversity (challenge, misstep, progress lapse) is:
INCREASE the number, type, duration, and/or intensity of Weight Success Actions you do each day.
~
For more on this subject, see Ch. **14** (p. 96) and Ch. **21** (p. 132).

CHAPTER 11: Author's Approach to Eating

This is an example of one person's self-designed dietary approach; it's not provided as a recommended universal program.

IN CASE YOU might find it handy to know, I'm now going to describe my personal approach to eating. But before doing this I must define a term and mention three points.

Definition. A key term used in the Weight Success Method is "preferred dietary program." I define *preferred dietary program* as a set of eating guidelines and eating practices I prefer to follow and which, when followed, cause me to realize good health and healthy-weight living. Another term I use is "preferred eating strategy." It's synonymous with preferred dietary program. Now to three points.

Point One. I'm not saying my eating strategy is the best program or approach for everyone. In my view there's no such thing as "one best dietary program for all."

Point Two. I'm not suggesting that because I use a self-designed program you should too. There are a number of established dietary programs on the market. So there's a good chance at least one of these programs would be a good fit for you.

Point Three. Whatever dietary program or strategy you might choose to go with — and regardless of whether it's a self-designed program or an established program — I suggest you do the five Daily Actions of the Weight Success Method at the same time.

Three Ways Eating Affects Me

Eating impacts my life three ways. Firstly, it affects my *weight.* That is, it either promotes me living at my desired weight <u>or</u> promotes me living at an undesired weight, or overweight. Secondly, it affects my *health.* That is, it either promotes a healthy body <u>or</u> promotes a non-healthy body. Thirdly, it affects the type of daily *pleasure* I experience. That is, I either derive pleasure from right eating <u>or</u> derive it from wrong eating.

So, my eating can impact my life either positively or negatively. The three negative effects are living overweight, poor health, and lack of right-eating pleasure. The three positive effects are living at my desired weight, good health, and experiencing right-eating pleasure. So, what are the factors that determine each of these effects?

Weight Effect. The weight effect derives mainly from the *amount* of food I eat. Meaning, when I eat the right amount of food it moves me toward living in my healthy-weight range. Conversely, when I eat too much food — or frequently engage in overeating — it moves me toward living outside my healthy-weight range, or being overweight.

Health Effect. The health effect derives mainly from the *types* of food I eat. Meaning, when I mostly eat right types of food in proper amounts it promotes me having a healthy body. Conversely, when I mostly eat wrong types of food in certain amounts it promotes me having a non-healthy body.

Pleasure Effect. The pleasure effect depends mainly on the *way* I prepare and eat foods. It also depends on what I *condition* my mind to like. When I prepare and eat foods the right way, and condition myself to like it, I experience right-eating pleasure, which promotes healthy eating. Conversely, when I don't do this I experience wrong-eating pleasure, which promotes non-healthy eating.

So, to sum up: I derive optimal weight, health, and pleasure from my eating by motivating myself to eat right foods in right amounts and by eating in a way that creates right eating enjoyment. Or, put another way, I derive optimal weight, health, and pleasure from applying right eating. The rest of this chapter describes how I do that. For easy identification I call this program the "John Correll Good Health Program."

My Three Eating Objectives

In light of the three ways eating affects me I have three objectives for eating.

Objective one is: Consume an amount of daily calories that results in me living in my healthy-weight range.

Objective two — which goes hand-in-hand with objective one — is: Maintain an optimally healthy body, or maximize the likelihood of living free of debilitating accidents, illnesses, diseases, and bodily malfunction.

Objective three is: Derive maximal pleasure from right eating and minimal pleasure from wrong eating.

Put another way, I strive to enact the three priorities of right eating, as described in Startup Action 6 (p. 17).

My Five Guiding Principles

In pursuing these three eating objectives I apply these five principles to my eating.

PRINCIPLE 1: *Whole Mind Involvement.* ❧ Here is a central principle of my approach to eating: My mind — including my subconscious mind — will create the types of thoughts and feelings that guide me toward right eating and away from wrong eating *provided that* (a) I focus each day on right eating and healthy-weight living, (b) I daily communicate to my subconscious mind that I want it to be steering me toward right eating, (c) I hold the belief that it's in the process of doing it, and (d) I express appreciation when right things happen. In briefest form the principle is this: My mind will steer me toward enjoyably living in my healthy-weight range *if* each day I motivate it to do so.

I discovered several years ago that the easiest, most effective way to apply this principle is do the five daily actions of the Weight Success Method. So, this method is the backbone of my eating strategy. Meaning, it's the vehicle by which I get myself to easily, enjoyably engage in right eating and refrain from wrong eating, or overeating, most of the time.

There are many approaches to enacting weight control. But my experience has led me to conclude that the Weight Success Method is the easiest, cheapest, safest, healthiest, most enjoyable one.

PRINCIPLE 2: *Maximize Pleasure While Minimizing Calories.* ❧ The second principle I apply to eating is this: Each day I strive to maximize the eating pleasure I derive from consuming my daily calorie allotment. My "daily calorie allotment" is the amount of daily calories that results in me living in my healthy-weight range. I've dubbed this principle the "secret to easier calorie control."

I discovered that when I derive only a minimal amount of eating pleasure from my daily calorie allotment I experience "eating-pleasure deprivation," which, in turn, tends to push me toward eating more than I should be eating. But, on the other hand, when I derive a maximal amount of eating pleasure from my daily calorie allotment I experience little or no eating-pleasure deprivation, which, in turn, makes it easier for me to eat a proper amount, or to avoid overeating.

Finally, I discovered that I could maximize the eating pleasure of my daily calorie allotment by applying eight basic eating actions. The Eight Actions for Easier Calorie Control chapter (p. **82**) describes these actions. Applying them on a daily basis is part of my approach to eating.

PRINCIPLE 3: *Moderation and Balance.* ❧ The third principle I apply to eating is this. Almost any "bad" food can be eaten without incurring weight gain or ill health *if* it's not eaten to excess. Conversely, almost any "good" food will incur a bad consequence *if* it's eaten to excess. So, achieving good health and weight control is not so much a matter of "always eat this and never eat that" but, rather, is a matter of *moderation and balance.*

So, I diligently strive to eat "good" foods in a healthful amount and refrain from eating "bad" foods to excess. And, as long as I'm doing this — that is, eating "good" foods in a healthful amount and refraining from eating "bad" foods to excess — I don't become angry or upset, or engage in self-criticism, after those occasional times when I happen to eat a small amount of a "bad" food.

PRINCIPLE 4: *Law of Predominant Activity.* ❧ The fourth principle I apply to eating is: When it comes to good health and weight control, what I do only now and then seldom makes a difference but, rather, what makes the difference is what I do *most of the time.* So, I don't hold the goal of "never ever do wrong eating" or "always and forever do right eating." Rather, my objective is to have right eating be my predominant type of eating. So, when now and then I might accidentally or deliberately happen to engage in a small amount of "wrong" eating I don't get angry or upset with myself, or engage in self-criticism.

PRINCIPLE 5: *Twelve-hour Non-eating Period Each Day.* ❧ The fifth principle I apply is: For most days I have a minimum 12-hour non-eating, or "fasting," period each 24-hour day. I do this by avoiding consuming food and beverage, other than water, between 7 p.m. and 7 a.m. In other words, I don't eat between supper and breakfast. Typically, I finish supper by 7 p.m. and start breakfast after 7 a.m.

To conclude, I discovered that applying these five principles makes weight management and eating control easier and more enjoyable.

The Times I Eat

Some research suggests that *when* we eat makes a difference. I suspect this might be true. Although I don't know if there's one universal eating schedule that's best for everyone. So here's the approach that has turned out best for *me.*

Years ago I would do after-dinner, or late-night, snacking. I no longer do that, as indicated by the above Principle 5. After-dinner eating produces unwanted outcomes for me, including weight gain. So, most days my daily eating occurs in the 12-hour period of 7:00 a.m. to 7:00 p.m.

Breakfast. I usually eat breakfast shortly after my daily morning weighing (Daily Action 1). So I do it around 7 or 8 a.m. It's typically a light meal consisting of oatmeal, tomato juice, and perhaps a small amount of fruit or a small bowl of cold cereal. Total calorie load amounts to around 400–500 calories.

Supper. I usually eat supper around 6 to 7 p.m. It can consist of about anything. But, much of the time it fits the general guidelines and eating practices described in the upcoming two sections. I have no set calorie target for supper. Instead, I use this meal as my *daily calorie adjuster.* It's when I ensure that I consume an amount of daily calories that will keep me in my healthy-weight range. It works like this.

If during-day calorie consumption has been less than usual <u>or</u> if during-day calorie expenditure has been greater than usual — like if I happened to take, say, a long bike ride — my supper meal would likely be slightly larger than usual. Conversely, if during-day calorie consumption has been greater than usual <u>or</u> during-day calorie expenditure has been minimal — like working on book-writing all day and doing no exercise — my supper meal would likely be slightly smaller than usual. So, for me, supper is the *pivotal* meal. It's when I ensure that my calorie intake for each day is an amount that will maintain me in my healthy-weight range. Or, put another way, it's when I ensure that each day turns out to be a right-eating day. Which means, supper for me is the "make it or break it time."

Lunch. So, when do I eat lunch? Answer: Any time I get the urge to do it. Meaning, I have no set time for lunch. I might eat it at 10:30 or at noon or at 2:00. I eat it when I'm feeling "hungry for lunch."

<u>Or</u>, I might eat no lunch and, instead, end up just doing a series of mini-snacks through the day, if that's what I feel like. I've found that, for me, sometimes it's easier to subvert hunger pangs and overeating by eating three, four, or five small meals — a.k.a. mini-snacks — throughout the day, or a mini-snack every couple hours, in place of eating one big lunch meal at noon.

Now, in mentioning this mini-snack approach I must impart a warning. Mini-snacking can be a slippery slope. It can easily, unknowingly transform into automatic eating that leads to *over*-snacking that results in excessive daily calorie consumption and weight gain. I speak from personal experience.

The reason is, when doing mini-snacking it's easy to overlook doing Daily Action 5 — the guided eating process. So, if you should decide to test out this mini-snack approach, make sure you're doing the guided eating process *every* time you're doing a mini-snack, no matter how small.

Lastly, I remind you that in describing my approach to eating I'm not suggesting that I think it's the best approach for you. The approach that works for me might or might not work for you. Only you can determine — by personal testing and perhaps physician advice — which eating approach or dietary strategy is best for you.

My Two General Eating Guidelines

Now we come to the question "What types of foods do I focus on eating?" Something that has bugged me for years is the confusing mish-mash of contradictory diets and dietary recommendations. In an attempt to escape this swamp I gravitate to those eating guidelines that have received either governmental endorsement or endorsement of a recognized professional association, such as, for example, the American Heart Association or American Medical Association.

For simplicity, or perhaps sanity, I've distilled this stuff into two eating guidelines. These two guidelines, in conjunction with Principles 1–5, are what I bear in mind when making food decisions.

Eating Guideline 1 – I strive to minimize excessive consumption of:
- high-sugar foods, which includes high-sugar beverages
- refined grains and foods made from it
- *trans* fat
- saturated fat
- nitrates and nitrites (i.e., cured or processed meats)
- red meat, especially fatty red meat
- fried foods.

Eating Guideline 2 – I strive to consume an ample, or government-recommended, amount of:
- fruits
- vegetables
- whole grain products

- low-fat and no-fat dairy products
- and occasionally include fish, nuts, and beans (meaning, legumes).

My Specific Eating Practices

Now we come to the specific eating practices I frequently apply. When I put the five principles and two guidelines together, and then translate it into specific actions, what has resulted is the following set of eating practices.

> **But here's an important side note.** My eating practices are not fixed. Instead, they evolve over time. Meaning, I modify, delete, and add actions as I see fit, for the purpose of producing optimal healthy-weight results and eating enjoyment. I also might modify them as government recommended eating guidelines evolve.

In year 2016, my eating practices generally included the following:

- I drink fat-free milk instead of whole milk most of the time.

- I eat fat-free or low-fat cheese instead of regular or "full-fat" cheese most of the time.

- I eat whole wheat bread instead of white bread much of the time.

- I use reduced-fat butter-type spread instead of regular butter much of the time.

- When I'm using or consuming oil I opt for olive oil most of the time, and when olive oil isn't available I tend to go with canola oil. I minimize solid or hydrogenated fats when I can.

- I opt for low-fat or fat-free salad dressing over regular or "full-fat" dressing most of the time. *Or,* I go with a "half-portion," or reduced amount, of regular dressing and "fortify" its flavor with a sprinkling of red wine vinegar or balsamic vinegar. Tastes great, by the way.

- I use stevia for my main sweetener in place of conventional sugar most of the time. Over the years I've tested a number of non-sugar sweeteners, and finally landed with stevia. For the first week or two of using stevia it seemed to have a "slightly different" sweet flavor to me. But after a couple weeks I ceased noticing the difference, with the result being that stevia and sugar now taste the same to me.

- I eat a bowl of oatmeal cereal almost every morning for breakfast. I go with traditional or "old-fashioned" oatmeal over the quick-cook or instant variety. I eat it with skim milk and add stevia for sweetener. Having oatmeal every morning is easy for me as I like cereal. I've been eating the traditional brands of whole-grain hot and cold cereals since I was about five. Occasionally, along with the oatmeal I include whole wheat toast or a small bowl of whole-grain cold cereal with skim milk and stevia.

- Along with oatmeal for breakfast I drink a small — approximately 5 ounce — glass of tomato juice. I opt for tomato juice over other juices — such as orange, apple, and grape juice — because tomato juice is relatively low in sugar and also lower in calories. I "spike" it with white vinegar in a ratio of 10:1 tomato juice to vinegar. It makes a zippy drink. Plus according to some research, high-acid food tends to diminish the blood glucose spike that can come from eating a glucose-creating food, such as a bowl of oatmeal.

- I drink a glass of water — about 6–8 ounces — with most meals. I'm one of those persons who actually enjoys water and opts for it over most other beverages. Plus I've read that drinking an ample amount of water can produce benefits, such as, for example, reducing the chance of kidney stones.

- I eat fresh fruit almost every day. My home usually has at least three or four kinds in stock at any given time. What I have depends on availability and quality. Typical fruits that can be found in my house include: bananas, apples, pears, peaches, grapes, strawberries, blueberries, raspberries, blackberries, cherries, oranges, tangerines, grapefruit, and melon.

- Supper almost always includes a tossed, or garden, salad and at least one vegetable or vegetable-based ingredient. It also usually includes a starch item, either potato, rice, or pasta. The potato is almost always a baked or roasted version, as opposed to fried. I realize some people frown on eating starchy items, but I eat them for supper. They are, however, prepared with healthy-style cooking methods, which typically means without deep-frying or sautéing.

- I eat reduced-fat or low-fat peanut butter instead of regular or "full-fat" peanut butter. Yup, I do enjoy a peanut butter and jelly sandwich. For that I typically use a reduced-sugar grape or strawberry jelly. Presently, my favorite reduced-fat peanut butter brands are Natural Jif, Reduced-fat Jif, and Smart Balance. All three have great peanut flavor. They, by the way, have nearly identical ingredients. Also, I find that Welch's brand reduced-sugar jellies and spreads suit my taste.

- I use Miracle Whip Light, or reduced fat, in place of regular Miracle Whip for many of my meat, cheese, and tuna fish sandwiches. I also often use mustard as my spread in sandwiches.

- I use low-fat, nitrate/nitrite-free deli sliced turkey for most of my meat sandwiches.

- For making hamburgers, chili, tacos, and the like I go with low-fat ground beef — that is, ground beef made to contain no more than about 4–6 percent fat. And, in most of my home cooking I tend to avoid "regular" ground beef or hamburger, which typically has a fat content of 20 percent or more.

- I often include a can of "light" or "heart healthy" soup for lunch. I typically go with something like vegetable beef or chicken noodle or chicken rice or Manhattan-style seafood chowder, for examples. Light-style soups typically contain two servings per can and have a per-serving calorie load in the 80–110 range, or 160–220 calories per can.

Sometimes when I'm extra hungry I'll "fortify" the soup with some canned vegetables or leftover vegetables from the prior night's dinner. Or, in the case of seafood chowder I might add a small (3 oz) can of tuna fish, or in the case of chicken soup a small (3 oz) can of chicken.

- When I get a hankering for a cookie I typically eat a low-fat graham cracker or perhaps a few animal crackers. Believe it or not, animal crackers are one of my favorite cookies. Plus they're relatively low in fat and sugar, as cookies go. I like the Stauffer's brand best, but find the Nabisco version to be good, too.

- For home-stocked ice cream I gravitate toward the fat-free and reduced-fat versions. To me, Breyers fat-free ice cream—chocolate, vanilla, or strawberry—and also Edy's "1/2 the fat" ice cream have decent flavor and texture. I usually eat my ice cream in a cake cone rather than in a dish, thereby prolonging eating pleasure.

- Sometimes I have popcorn. I go with the low-fat varieties, which have about 100–120 calories per serving. This is a great way to satisfy a salty-snack hankering with relatively few calories and very little "harmful" ingredient. I eat it one kernel at a time, thereby prolonging eating pleasure.

- Occasionally I have a fried egg sandwich. Actually, it's not a true fried egg as I use no fat but, instead, I "fry" it with a non-stick skillet, with little or no fat added. I put the fried egg on top of a piece of unbuttered low-cal whole wheat toast and add a slice of fat-free or low-fat cheese on top of the egg. When the slice of cheese is applied while the egg is still hot the cheese slightly melts over the egg. The result is a tasty open-faced egg sandwich. Sometimes for variety I'll grill up a couple slices of low-fat soy-protein "bacon," which my family lovingly calls "fakin' bacon," and add that on top of the cheese. And, when I feel like going all-out I include a couple slices of tomato between the bread and egg. This results in a nutritious, tasty, low fat egg-bacon-tomato-cheese sandwich.

- While I can't say I eat soy-protein foods extensively, I do enjoy them now and then. Two items stocked in my freezer are soy-protein Bacon Strips (mentioned above) and soy-protein Black Bean Burger, both made by Morning Star Farms. According to the manufacturer, the Bacon Strips have 44 percent less fat than regular pork bacon and the Black Bean Burger has 73 percent less fat than regular ground beef.

When heated in a skillet, as opposed to a microwave, both products are tasty and satisfying. The bean burger is especially good when topped with a dab of thousand island dressing plus the usual burger condiments of dill pickle, cheese, and sliced tomato. Lastly, please know that I mention the Morning Star Farms name as a point of reference and not to imply that it's the only maker of good soy-protein-based foods.

- To obtain the right amount of daily fiber I go with whole psyllium husk as a supplement. I prefer it over other fiber sources because it provides both types of fiber: soluble and insoluble — in a ratio of about 75% soluble, 25% insoluble. I purchase it in bulk form — large can, bottle, or bag — from a health food store or a well-stocked supermarket. Psyllium husk, by the way, happens to be the main fiber-providing ingredient in Metamucil.

I include the psyllium husk with my breakfast and supper meals. At breakfast I add a *rounded* tablespoon to my bowl of oatmeal. This provides about four grams of added fiber. But, if I deem it to be desirable I'll increase the portion slightly. For supper I combine the same amount into a small portion of cold cereal, usually Grape-nuts Flakes, and eat it as a "dessert" after supper. Or, in place of that, I might sprinkle it over a tossed salad, after the dressing has been added. Or, I might stir the psyllium into a large glass of water and drink it right before starting eating. Note: Psyllium husk is nearly taste-free, so it leaves the flavor of whatever it's added to — like a salad or bowl of cereal — virtually unchanged.

At supper I might adjust the psyllium portion amount based on what I figure my fiber intake has been for that day. If it seems like I've consumed an above-average amount of fiber, via the foods I've eaten, I reduce the psyllium portion slightly at suppertime. Conversely, if I figure I consumed a below-average amount of fiber in that day I increase the psyllium portion slightly.

Clarifying Comments

In the above description I use the word "I" extensively, as in "I prepare" this and "I stock" that. This conveys an impression that I'm a one-man dietary dynamo doing everything myself. In actuality, my wife and life partner Janet does most of our food shopping, which happens to be her preference, and also prepares most of our at-home supper meals, which is her preference.

This conveys the impression that I do nothing regarding dietary decision-making, food shopping, and kitchen duties. But that's not the case, either. I make trips to the market for certain foods, and will convey to Janet, via our weekly shopping list, requests for specific foods. Fortunately for me, she's accommodating of my food-related requests and suggestions, and even sometimes takes the initiative to buy or prepare something new that she thinks I might like to "test out."

Also, by the way, as regards suppertime kitchen duties Janet and I take a team approach. She does meal preparation; I do after-meal clean-up. It typically requires 30 to 60 minutes on her part to prepare a supper, and 20 to 30 minutes on my part for clean-up. So I figure I'm getting a good deal.

I now reiterate a point made at the opening of this chapter. Which is: By relating my personal approach to eating I am *not* suggesting that it's necessarily the most productive approach for you. And, just because I happen to apply a self-designed dietary program, as opposed to one of the established programs, I am *not* saying that a self-designed eating program is the best way to go for you. In fact, I happen to believe that for many persons an established dietary program is the easiest, most effective, most rewarding way to do dieting, or dietary management.

But regardless of what dietary program or strategy you apply — and regardless of whether you go the design-it-yourself route or the established program route — there's an additional thing you should do. Along with doing your preferred dietary program *also* do the five daily actions of the Weight Success Method at the same time. Doing this likely will make the dietary program of your choice easier and more effective.

CONCLUDING QUESTION: What Should Be the Rule?

When it comes to good health and weight control, what you do only now and then seldom makes a difference. Rather, what usually makes the big difference is what you do most of the time. So, unless it's something you can absolutely attain, it might be best to forego absolute-type rules like "never engage in overeating" or "always and forever do non-overeating."

Instead, a more productive approach might be to have non-overeating be your main type of eating, as opposed to being your only type of eating. So when now and then you accidentally or deliberately happen to engage in a small amount of overeating, there's no need to feel angry, guilty, discouraged, sinful, weak, or any other counterproductive negative emotion. In short, the question is this.

What's the Most PRODUCTIVE Approach to Eating and Weight Control?

Perfection **OR** Enough Right Eating to Achieve Good Health and Healthy-weight Living

What's Your #1 Eating Goal?

For most persons their #1 eating goal is maximize pleasure. But this leads to overeating and weight gain. So, I suggest you make your #1 eating goal to be: maintain body weight in your healthy-weight range. Then, within that context, make goal #2 to be: promote good health, and goal #3 to be: gain maximal eating pleasure from right eating — in that order of priority. When you do this you'll find that creating healthy-weight living becomes much *EASIER.*

The Choice is Yours: Which Approach Should You Opt For?

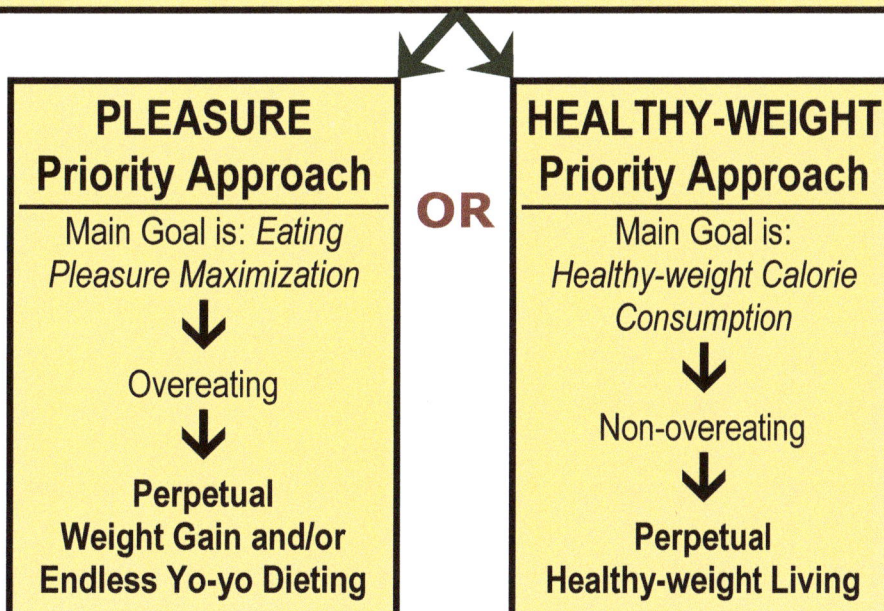

PLEASURE Priority Approach		HEALTHY-WEIGHT Priority Approach
Main Goal is: *Eating Pleasure Maximization*	**OR**	Main Goal is: *Healthy-weight Calorie Consumption*
⬇		⬇
Overeating		Non-overeating
⬇		⬇
Perpetual Weight Gain and/or Endless Yo-yo Dieting		**Perpetual Healthy-weight Living**

CHAPTER 12: Eight Actions for Easier Calorie Control

Calorie control can be easier and more enjoyable than you likely imagine, if you go about it the right way.

IF YOU DESIRE to maximize eating pleasure while also controlling calorie intake, apply the eight simple actions in this chapter. These actions pertain to my second eating principle: maximize pleasure while minimizing calories (p. 75).

When it comes to calorie control most people hold an erroneous belief. They believe controlling calorie intake is hard to do. So, they hate pursuing any dietary program that involves calorie control, which many programs do. Truth is, controlling daily calorie intake is easier and more enjoyable with a certain approach. This chapter describes that approach. But before disclosing it I must lay some groundwork.

The Dilemma in Eating

Most of us eat to satisfy two objectives: (1) to acquire nourishment and energy and (2) to derive eating pleasure. But while deriving eating pleasure a nasty side-effect usually crops up: *weight gain.* Weight gain comes from consuming more calories than our body is metabolizing, or "burning up." We call this overeating. Initially this weight gain is merely a nuisance. Eventually, however, it grows into a problem. When this happens some persons adopt a third objective: *weight control.*

Most weight-control programs involve one or both of two strategies. The first strategy is to enact a higher level of physical activity, called exercise. This results in burning up the "extra calories" we're consuming.

The second strategy is to consume an amount of daily calories that's equal to the amount of calories our body has been burning up. This involves daily calorie control.

Many persons find using both strategies in combination produces the quickest results. But you need to know that the first strategy — exercise — is optional, while the second strategy — calorie control — is must-do. Why? Because it's possible for most folks to achieve and maintain their desired healthy weight without exercise. But, except for those engaged in very high levels of physical activity, most of us cannot achieve and maintain our desired weight without controlling calorie intake. So, contrary to what many people assume, calorie control is a vital requirement for weight management success, and exercise is not. Which, of course, is not to say you should forget about exercise.

Unfortunately, when most of us attempt to enact calorie control a problem arises. In our effort to reduce calories we end up consuming less food. In consuming less food we derive less eating pleasure. This reduction in eating pleasure creates a feeling of pleasure deprivation, or withdrawal. Finally, this feeling of pleasure deprivation drives us back to eating the types and the amount of food we previously derived pleasure from. The result: We fail at calorie control and, thereby, fail at weight control.

What makes calorie control so tricky is it involves a dilemma. It happens to be a universal dilemma of dieters. That dilemma is this. When we consume an amount of calories that results in putting or keeping our body weight in our desired weight range we end up with a reduced amount of eating pleasure and also nagging hunger pangs much of the time. On the other hand, when we consume the amount of food that gives us maximum eating pleasure and a feeling of fullness we end up overeating and acquiring fat.

So, the dilemma comes down to this. Should I live with a reduced calorie intake, which results in eating pleasure deprivation *or* should I live with a non-reduced calorie intake, which results in endless overeating and fat gain? Each is a bad option.

Most people assume there's no way out of this dilemma. But there is a way. It involves a third option: Adopt a two-prong eating strategy of maximizing eating pleasure while controlling calorie intake. Applying this strategy involves a certain perspective. So I'm now going to describe that perspective. After that comes the "secret to easier calorie control."

Best Perspective for Controlling Calories

For maximal effectiveness, approach calorie control like this. Pretend that when you arise each morning you're given a bag of calories to use for that day. This bag of calories is your *healthy-weight calorie allotment.* It's the maximum number of calories you can consume each day and still achieve or maintain your desired healthy weight. Each day you may use all the allotted calories or only part of them. But you absolutely are not allowed to consume more calories than are in your "healthy-weight calorie allotment bag." Lastly, it's up to you and your qualified health advisor to determine how many calories your healthy-weight calorie allotment should consist of.

What's more, pretend that you have an eating mission. Assume that this mission is to derive maximum eating pleasure from the bag of calories you've been allotted for each day. To succeed at this mission you must treat your allotment of daily calories like precious currency. That is, you must spend it wisely. You must spend it in a way that maximizes your eating pleasure.

When you do this you avoid, or at least greatly reduce, eating pleasure deprivation. This, in turn, makes it easier for you to control your calorie intake and stick with your preferred dietary program; thus, making it easier for you to create healthy-weight living.

So, how do you accomplish your eating mission? You apply seven eating actions. I call them *pleasure-maximizing eating actions.* By applying these seven actions you maximize the eating pleasure from your healthy-weight calorie allotment and, thereby, make calorie control non-painful and easier.

So, in a nutshell the secret to easier calorie control is: *Each day maximize the eating pleasure of your healthy-weight calorie allotment.*

Now, here in summary form are seven actions for doing that.

1. Dispense with low-pleasure, high-calorie add-ons.
2. Reduce the portion amount of high-pleasure, high-calorie add-ons.
3. Replace high-calorie foods with lower-calorie foods that still yield eating pleasure.
4. Choose foods that deliver a longer duration of eating pleasure per calorie consumed.
5. Eat in a way that lengthens the duration of eating pleasure per calorie consumed.
6. Season foods in a way that increases the amount of pleasurable palate sensation.
7. Replace high-cal snacks with low-cal and no-cal snacks.

Apply these seven actions on a daily basis. It enables you to each day maximize the eating pleasure of your healthy-weight calorie allotment. Which, in turn, makes for easier calorie control. Also, along with these seven actions include one more action: Action 8. I'll now describe these eight actions, which lead to easier calorie-control success.

> ### ACTION 1: Dispense with low-pleasure, high-calorie add-ons.

Virtually every item you eat provides pleasure. But items differ in the amount of pleasure per calorie that they provide. Some deliver a large amount of pleasure for a small amount of calories. Others deliver a small amount of pleasure for a large amount of calories. Since you have only a certain number of calories to work with — that being your healthy-weight calorie allotment — you should do these two things. Firstly, focus on foods that deliver a greater amount of pleasure per calorie. Secondly, shun foods that deliver a lesser amount of pleasure per calorie, while maintaining a healthy balanced diet, of course. View the situation like this.

Greater pleasure per calorie = *Good Food*

Lesser pleasure per calorie = *Bad Food*

Good Foods create **maximal** pleasure for your healthy-weight calorie allotment

Bad Foods create **minimal** pleasure for your healthy-weight calorie allotment

So, focus on "good foods" — those that deliver greater eating pleasure per calorie. And, shun "bad foods" — those that deliver lesser eating pleasure per calorie.

One of the easiest ways to reduce your consumption of "bad foods" is eliminate add-ons. Indeed, omitting an add-on often turns a "bad food" into a "good food." An *add-on* is something that's added to another food to change its taste or texture. Many of the calories most persons consume come from add-ons. These items tend to be high in fat or, in some cases, consist totally of fat. Examples of high-calorie add-ons include fat-based spreads, such as butter and margarine, and high-fat dressings, sauces, and condiments. For certain food items, add-ons can constitute 20, 30, or even 50 percent or more of the total calorie load of the food. Ditto for an entire meal.

Examples

I'll illustrate. To begin, consider how most persons make a sandwich. First they get a slice of bread. It contains between 50 to 100 calories. Then they apply one to two tablespoons of butter or margarine to the slice. This constitutes 100 to 200 calories. So let's see — original slice of bread equals 100 calories, add-on equals 100 calories, total calories for the modified slice: 200 calories. Wow, is this add-on really needed? Why not just make the sandwich without the 100 to 200 calories of low-pleasure butter spread? The sandwich's taste will be nearly identical to what it is with the add-on. Within a week or two, especially after delivering a mini-directive to your mind, you'll not miss the butter or margarine you once had in your sandwiches.

Here's another example. Consider how most people eat a pancake or waffle or French toast. The first thing they do is slather it with butter or marga-

rine. So, what they end up with is this. Original pancake equals 200 calories, butter equals 200 calories, total calories for the modified pancake: 400 calories. This is crazy. Why not just eat the pancake without the 200 calories of add-on butter spread? Just add a little of your usual sweetener — like some reduced-sugar syrup, or reduced-sugar jam, or sliced fruit, or government-approved artificial sweetener — and enjoy the pancake without the added calories and, by the way, without the added saturated fat. The pancake's taste will be nearly identical to what it is with the butter or margarine. After eating it this way a few times you'll not miss the butter.

A similar thing often happens with eating a roll or a muffin. Many persons apply a thick dollop of butter or margarine to it. Instead, try eating these foods plain, or with nothing on them. You might be surprised. You might discover, as I did, that the bread, roll, or muffin tastes as good without the add-on as with it.

Ditto for potatoes and vegetables. A quality potato or vegetable, properly prepared and with a touch of seasoning, tastes great — every bit as good as one floating in a sea of butter or smothered with sauce, gravy, sour cream, or any of the many other taste-altering, calorie-adding add-ons.

There's a reason why this is so. It's because add-ons don't always enhance the flavor of a food. We just erroneously assume they do. Instead, an add-on often masks a food's original flavor rather than improves it. When you dispense with the add-on you can enjoy the pure taste of the original food. Sometimes the pure taste is even more enjoyable than the masked or altered taste of the modified food. We just never learned to enjoy the original flavor because we've been eating food smothered with add-ons from about age two.

Question

Now here's the key question. In any of these examples, are the 100 to 200 calories of add-on really worth it? If the answer's "no," *dispense with it.*

Another way of framing the question is: Can I get a bigger pleasure bang from my healthy-weight calorie allotment by dispensing with this low-pleasure add-on? Or, in other words: Can I make better use of the 100 or 200 calories consumed by this add-on? By "better use" I mean, using the add-on's calories in a way that produces greater eating pleasure.

If the answer's "yes," dispense with the add-on. Put those saved calories to better use. You have two options. First, use the saved calories for consuming some other food that provides greater pleasure than the low-pleasure add-on. Second, don't use the calories at all. That is, reduce your calorie intake for the day by the amount of calories you saved. Either option enables you to more easily achieve your calorie intake goal.

ACTION 2: Reduce the portion amount of high-pleasure, high-calorie add-ons.

So, what about add-ons that are high calorie but also deliver high pleasure for you? For these items reduce the portion amount. As explained in Action 1, many persons use huge portions of add-ons. They use way more than what's needed to impart the desired flavor. So, for these cut the portion of high-pleasure add-ons by half or more.

You'll discover that a 50 percent reduction in portion amount often results in only about a 10 percent reduction in flavor. In other words, with many add-ons the first 50 percent of the portion amount creates 90 percent of the flavor enhancement. And, the second 50 percent adds little or nothing. As a result, the second 50 percent of the portion amount can be viewed as wasted calories that can be put to better use. So, cut the portion amount of high-pleasure, high-calorie add-ons by half or more. Amazingly, you won't miss this portion of the add-on.

Also, try substituting a portion of the high-calorie add-on with a low-calorie or no-calorie add-on. For example, with salads you can cut the portion amount of dressing in half and then add a squeeze of lemon juice or sprinkle of vinegar to the salad to replace the flavor that's lost from the missing half-portion of dressing. It works great. And, you're consuming only half as many calories in

salad dressing. This can greatly reduce the overall calorie load of a salad.

Then, put those saved calories to better use. Either (a) use them to up your eating pleasure by enjoying some other food that delivers greater pleasure or (b) don't use them at all and, thereby, reduce your calorie intake for that day.

ACTION 3: Replace high-calorie foods with lower-calorie foods that still yield eating pleasure.

Much of what I've said about add-ons also applies to an entire food type. Many foods, including beverages, come in high, medium, and low calorie levels. The high level is usually labeled "regular" or "traditional" or "original" or "classic." Medium is often labeled "reduced calorie." And, low is labeled "low-calorie" or "no-calorie" or "calorie-free".

Milk is a good example. You can get it in 3-percent fat (whole milk), 2-percent fat (reduced fat milk), ½-percent fat (low fat milk), and no-fat (skim milk). Many persons turn up their nose at reduced-fat and no-fat milk. But you can use it to reduce calorie intake. Whole milk (3-percent fat) is 145 calories per cup or eight ounces. Skim milk is just 85 calories per cup — nearly 40 percent fewer calories. If you're a milk drinker, as I am, switching from whole milk to skim milk frees up a lot of calories per day that could be put to some other possibly more productive use. It also greatly reduces your saturated fat intake. Check the Nutrition Facts box on the label. The saturated fat difference is eye-opening.

A similar situation applies to many other food products. They come in high-calorie versions, reduced-calorie versions, and low-calorie versions. Examples include beer, ice cream, cheese, bread, salad dressings, spreads, soups, and dessert items or sweet treats. It goes on and on. In many cases the reduced-calorie version — and sometimes even the low-calorie version — carries nearly as much pleasing taste as the high-calorie version.

ACTION **4**: Choose foods that deliver a longer duration of eating pleasure per calorie consumed.

Foods vary in duration of eating pleasure they provide. Some provide no more than a few seconds of eating pleasure. Others provide several minutes or more. Plus here's the catch. Oftentimes both foods contain the same amount of calories. So, which food do you want to be eating? The one that delivers 10 seconds of eating pleasure for **X** amount of calories? *Or*, the one that delivers, say, five minutes of eating pleasure for the same **X** amount of calories? Obviously, you gain more eating pleasure per calorie with the second one. So, choose that one and avoid the first one.

So evaluate your food choices in terms of calories consumed per minute of eating pleasure. The fewer calories consumed per minute of eating pleasure, the better. Here's the formula for it:

Calorie Load of the Food ÷ Minutes of Eating Time = Calories Per Minute of Eating Pleasure

I call it *Calories Per Minute of Pleasure* formula. I'll illustrate how it works.

EXAMPLE 1: Ice Cream. You can eat ice cream one of two ways: in a bowl or in a cone. In a bowl you consume the ice cream in about one minute. The same amount in a cone takes you three to five minutes. So, you gain two to four extra minutes of eating pleasure with the cone. Here's how it works with the calories per minute of pleasure formula. Let's assume the ice cream portion contains 200 calories and the cone is 10 calories.

Calories Per Minute of Pleasure with the bowl = **200** calories per minute (200 calories ÷ 1 minute)

Calories Per Minute of Pleasure with the cone = **52** calories per minute (210 calories ÷ 4 minutes)

I'll take the cone every time.

EXAMPLE 2: Popsicles. To get three or four minutes of low-calorie eating pleasure have a popsicle. You loved 'em when you were a kid and, guess what, they still taste great. To achieve maximum pleasure bang per calorie, check out the no-sugar-added versions, which are about 15

calories. It's like three minutes of eating pleasure for free!

EXAMPLE 3: Reduced-fat popcorn. A bowl of individual-portion popcorn can take 10 to 15 minutes to eat when eaten one kernel at a time. A typical individual portion of reduced-fat popcorn has about 100 calories. If it takes you 10 minutes to eat, that amounts to just 10 calories per minute of eating pleasure (100 calories divided by 10 minutes). By comparison, if you eat a typical cookie in, say, one minute, that could amount to 100 or more calories per minute of eating pleasure. This is ten times more calories per minute than in eating reduced-fat popcorn.

So, when making food choices use the calories per minute of pleasure formula. It's a nifty way of gaining maximum eating pleasure from your healthy-weight calorie allotment.

ACTION **5**: Eat in a way that lengthens the duration of eating pleasure per calorie consumed.

This action goes hand-in-hand with Action 4. In Action 4 you select foods that take longer to eat. In this action you eat foods in a way that results in lengthened eating time. In both cases the goal is the same: to derive more pleasure bang for your daily calorie allotment by lengthening the duration of pleasure-producing eating time.

You can lengthen the duration of eating three ways. First, take smaller bites and smaller swallows. Second, chew slower or longer. Third, pause between bites. For this you might have a sip of water or a little conversation. In short, try to avoid gobbling food and gulping beverage and, instead, savor it.

ACTION **6**: Season foods in a way that increases the amount of pleasurable palate sensation.

Seasoning often determines the amount of pleasure you derive from a food. The most common seasoning is salt. After that, black pepper. But other seasoning options abound. Consider the many herbs, spices, hot sauces, condiments, and vinegars. Nearly all are low in calories. Many are calorie-free.

Use these seasonings to increase the pleasure you derive from food. For an example, here's a snack tactic I sometimes use to satisfy a "craving for flavor" without consuming a lot of calories. I get some tomato juice and pour about six ounces into a glass. Then, I stir in some ground black pepper, oregano, hot sauce, a squeeze of lemon, and perhaps a dash of Worcestershire sauce. I use enough of the hot items to create a fiery flavor. Then I enjoy this along with a dill pickle or some other high-flavor, low-calorie snack item. If when I'm done my mouth isn't screaming "Great, great ... enough, enough ... I'm happy now," it means I probably didn't put enough seasoning and hot sauce into the tomato juice. Next time I experiment with upping the seasoning or hot sauce.

ACTION 7: Replace high-cal snacks with low-cal and no-cal snacks.

Some diet programs tell you to eliminate snacking between meals. For many people this is good advice. But if ending all between-meal snacking results in eating pleasure deprivation, which in turn results in leaving the diet program, then this might be not-so-good advice.

When the latter condition applies, do this Action 7: Switch from high-calorie between-meal snacks to low-calorie or no-calorie snacks. Use these snacks to neutralize a craving or a nagging desire to experience eating pleasure.

Also, combine this Action 7 with Action 5. That is, eat your low-cal snacks in small bites or small sips to maximize the duration of eating pleasure you derive.

So to sum up this far, the secret to easier calorie control is: *Each day maximize the eating pleasure of your healthy-weight calorie allotment.* Do it by applying the above Actions 1–7. Plus, also apply this Action 8.

ACTION 8: Know the calorie load of what you're eating (or about to eat).

To achieve easier calorie control, bear in mind the calorie load of the food you're consuming or are thinking of consuming. By doing this it causes your mind to steer you toward correct calorie consumption. It also makes it easier for you to maximize the pleasure of your healthy-weight calorie allotment with Actions 1, 3, 4, and 7. Here are two ways you can know the calorie load of what you eat.

1 – Look at the Nutrition Facts Box
The easiest way to get calorie info is check the **Nutrition Facts** box. It appears on the package of nearly every food item. It will tell you the *calories per portion* and also total calories for the entire container. Make it a habit to check this information and to know the calorie load of what you eat or are thinking of eating.

Also, restaurants are starting to tell us the calorie amount of their menu items. Sometimes it can be found on the menu or on the back of a placemat or in a pamphlet. Many post it on their website.

For the rare food item that comes without printed nutrition info you can usually find this information on the Internet, such as, for example at:

calorieking.com

Also, when making a decision about whether to eat something it can help to know the amount of exercise that would be required to burn up the number of calories consumed by eating it. So, when you see the *calories per serving* number on a menu or in the Nutrition Facts box on a package it sometimes can help to refer to this chart.

Calories Burned Per Hour				
	BODY WEIGHT			
ACTIVITY (1 hr.)	130 lb	155 lb	180 lb	205 lb
Brisk Walking (3.5 mph)	224	267	311	354
Slow Running (5 mph)	472	563	654	745
Mod. Cycling (12–13.9 mph)	472	563	654	745
Weight-lifting, light workout	177	211	245	279

This chart lists four exercise activities. For each of the activities it tells you the number of calories you burn in one hour. So, for example, if you weigh around 155 pounds and do brisk walking for one hour you burn about 267 calories. To extend the example, if you eat something that contains 267 calories and you weigh in the neighborhood of 155 pounds you would have to do one hour of brisk walking to burn the calories in that portion of food. Suggestion: Make a copy of this chart and carry it in your wallet or purse for quick reference. For info on calories burned by other types of activities, go to: **nutristrategy.com**
The numbers in this chart come from there.

2 – Use Food-measuring Tools at Home

As with most every pursuit, to excel at it it helps to have the right tools. To excel at calorie control, especially if you do a lot of home cooking, these three food measuring tools can be helpful:

1. Set of measuring spoons and perhaps a set of dry-measure measuring cups;
2. Liquid-measure measuring cup; and
3. Portion scale with at least a sixteen ounce maximum capacity divided into quarter-ounce increments or smaller — or, in metric, at least a 500 gram maximum capacity divided into five-gram increments or smaller.

TIP: If you're serious about calorie control, a portion scale and measuring cups can be very helpful.

Concluding Summary

The secret to easier calorie control is: *Each day maximize the eating pleasure of your healthy-weight calorie allotment* (Actions 1–7), plus bear in mind the calorie load of what you eat (Action 8). As an infographic it works like this.

Eight Key Calorie-control Activities

1. Dispense with low-pleasure, high-cal add-ons.
2. Reduce the portion amount of high-pleasure, high-calorie add-ons.
3. Replace high-calorie foods with lower-calorie foods that still yield eating pleasure.
4. Choose foods that deliver a longer duration of eating pleasure per calorie consumed.
5. Eat in a way that lengthens the duration of eating pleasure per calorie consumed.
6. Season foods in a way that increases the amount of pleasurable palate sensation.
7. Replace high-cal snacks with low-cal snacks.
8. Know the calorie load of what you're eating.

↓

Creates maximum eating pleasure from your healthy-weight calorie allotment.

↓

Results in you more easily controlling calorie intake and achieving right eating and, ultimately, healthy-weight living — especially when done in conjunction with the Weight Success Method.

Either you control calories or calories control you. The easiest way to gain control over calories is (a) wring maximum pleasure from those you should be eating, then (b) spurn the rest.

What's Your #1 Priority in Eating?

Having *pleasure maximization* as a #1 priority in eating promotes overeating and weight gain. To avoid this, make ***healthy-weight calorie consumption*** your #1 priority. Then make your #2 and #3 priorities the deriving of optimal health and maximal pleasure from those calories. When you do this you'll find that creating healthy-weight living becomes easier. For more, see the Right Eating section in Startup Action 6 (p. 18).

So often it seems to come back to this ...

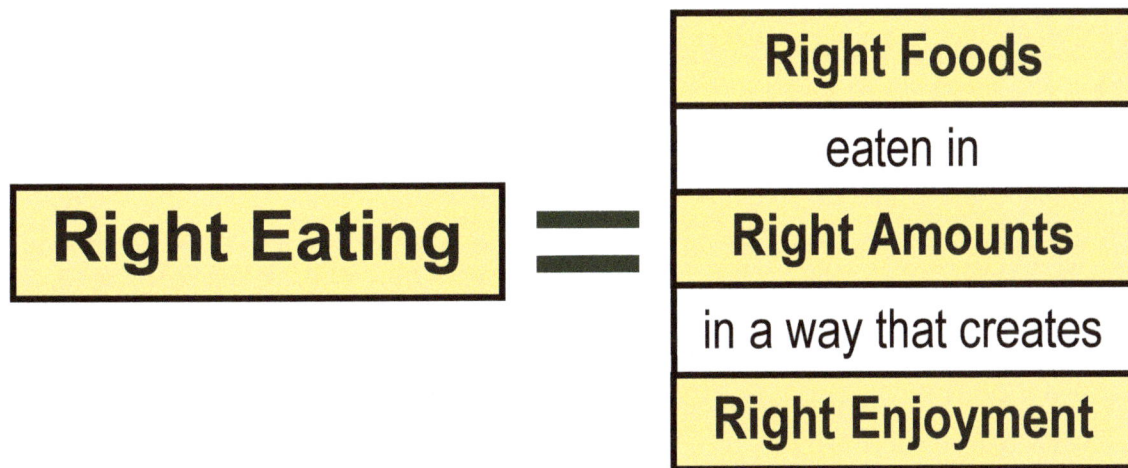

Right Eating **=**

> **Right Foods**
> eaten in
> **Right Amounts**
> in a way that creates
> **Right Enjoyment**

Do the **Five Daily Actions** <u>every</u> day . . .
and **Lifelong Weight Success** will be <u>Yours</u>.

Typically takes <u>less than</u> **8** minutes of dedicated time per day.

CHAPTER 13: Six More Mind Motivators

To some people more is better. So here's MORE — six additional, optional, powerful ways to motivate your mind to assist you with creating healthy-weight success.

MOST PEOPLE will find that doing the five daily actions of the Weight Success Method is sufficient to motivate their mind to steer them toward living in their healthy-weight range. But in every pursuit there are those who desire to progress a little faster or gain extra expertise. If you happen to be one of these persons, this chapter is for you. All you need do is apply one or more of these six optional mind motivators. In doing this you might use the test-it-out approach. That is, pick one of the six and try it for a week. If it increases your healthy-weight focus and effectiveness, make that motivator an add-on to the five daily actions of the Weight Success Method. If it doesn't do much for you, drop it and test another one. Here now are six optional mind motivators.

MOTIVATOR 1:
High-frequency Goal Statement

Say your Healthy-weight Goal Statement *more than* 25 times a day.

Daily Action 4 of the Weight Success Method instructs you to say your Healthy-weight Goal Statement at least 25 times each day. Note: "at least 25 times each day" defines a minimum, not a maximum. So if you'd like to increase your mind's focus on realizing healthy-weight living say the Goal Statement more than 25 times a day. Like, say it 40 or 50 or even 100 times a day. As explained in Daily Action 4, you can easily do this by fitting Goal Statement iterations into the "free time" periods of your day, or into those times when you can do Statement iterations while also doing something else at the same time. Regarding that, here's a couple powerful suggestions to try.

Nighttime Iterations

Some persons sleep through an entire night without waking. But many arise at least once to go to the bathroom. If you do that, take advantage of it. Silently deliver either your Healthy-weight Goal Statement or a backup depiction statement after you come back to bed. (Upcoming Motivator 2 lists backup depiction statements.) Do this by repeating the statement in your mind as you're falling asleep. Delivering healthy-weight messages at this time can produce powerful results.

Waking-up Iterations

When you awaken in the morning, and while still lying in bed with your eyes closed and mind relaxed, say your Healthy-weight Goal Statement three times in your mind. Or, for extra effect, say it ten times, which takes only about 40 to 50 seconds.

Saying your Healthy-weight Goal Statement at these two times — when you awaken at night and first thing in the morning while waking up — can produce a powerful effect.

Plus, in addition to increasing the number of times you say your Healthy-weight Goal Statement also increase your emotional intensity when saying it. You need not do this for all iterations but it could be worthwhile to do it for at least a few.

MOTIVATOR 2:
Backup Depiction Statements

Say a backup depiction statement at least 10 times a day.

Your Healthy-weight Goal Statement (in Daily Action 4) is a form of verbal depiction. A verbal depiction is a word description of a situation. Typically the situation being depicted is either (a) an imagined desired situation you want to actualize, or make real or (b) a desirable present situation you want to perpetuate, such as continuing to live in your healthy-weight range.

Your Healthy-weight Goal Statement is the primary verbal depiction used — or daily iterated —

in the Weight Success Method. It produces great results. But by including iterations of a backup depiction statement each day you can *increase* results. Coming up is a list of backup statements.

How Backup Statements Work. Backup depiction statements work with your Healthy-weight Goal Statement to expedite healthy-weight living. Your Goal Statement portrays your ultimate goal. Which is, to live your life as a person of your healthy weight. Each of the backup depiction statements describes a means or situation for helping bring about this ultimate goal. When a backup depiction statement is said on the same day as your Healthy-weight Goal Statement it causes your mind to focus on both your ultimate goal and a means for getting it. This can be powerful.

What to Do. Pick a backup depiction statement that looks interesting, or that appears like it might help fix a certain problem or achieve a certain goal. For example, if you're having trouble with over-snacking you might find backup depiction statement #5 (in the list below) to be effective, or if you're eating too much at meals you might use statement #6.

Then use the chosen statement for a week. *Say it at least 10 times each day.* Do this along with saying your Healthy-weight Goal Statement, not in place of it. If it produces desired results, keep using it. If it doesn't, drop it and test another one. Note: It's okay to use two or more depiction statements the same day. Also, the power of depiction statements derives from repetition. The more repetition, the greater the power. Here are eleven sample statements to choose from.

11 Optional Backup Depiction Statements

1. *I am right now in a guided-eating week. I do guided eating every time I eat.*
   (Note: Guided eating is described in Daily Action 5.)

2. *I am right now in a right-eating day — a right-eating day in every single way.*

3. *I am right now in a right-eating day — less than _____ calories is what I eat today.*
   (In the blank space, insert a number of calories.)

4. *I am right now forever <u>free</u> of every wrong-eating habit that's ever been with me.*

5. *I am right now forever <u>free</u> of the over-snacking habit that used to be with me.*

6. *I am right now forever <u>free</u> of the mealtime gluttony-eating that once appealed to me.*

7. *Healthy weight, BENEFITS — Overweight, PAIN. <u>Steer</u> me to the benefits — <u>Save</u> me from the pain.*

8. *I control eating — eating doesn't control me.*

9. *I'm living each day in my healthy-weight range.*

10. *I focus each day on healthy-weight living.*

11. *I weigh _____, _____, _____.*
    (In each of the three blank spaces, insert your ideal weight number.)

Optional Wording. Feel free to modify any statement to best fit your situation. For example, in statements 2 and 3 you can replace the word "right-eating" with "healthy-eating," if you wish. Also, in statement 4 you can replace "wrong-eating" with "overeating." And, in statements #4 and #5 you can replace "habit" with "urge."

Make Your Own. Also, reading the above statements might give you ideas for backup depiction statements of your own creation. If so, write them up and test them. Tip: The "listening audience" for depiction statements is your mind — in particular your subconscious mind. Remember this when crafting the wording for your statements.

Definition of Key Terms Used in the Depiction Statements

Right-eating day (a.k.a. healthy-eating day): A day in which your overall eating for the day amounts to right eating (a.k.a. healthy-weight eating).

Wrong eating (a.k.a. non-healthy eating): Eating that hinders good health or hinders living in your healthy-weight range.

Over-snacking: Eating too much or too many times between meals, resulting in overeating for the day.

Mealtime gluttony-eating: Eating until stuffed, or until your stomach can hold no more; or overeating during meals.

Healthy-weight living (a.k.a. right-weight living): Living in your healthy-weight range.

MOTIVATOR 3:
Upcoming-day Description

In the morning right after waking, tell your mind how you want the upcoming day to happen.

Many people often lie in bed for a few minutes in the morning after waking up. If you happen to be one who does this you can use that time for powerful results.

While lying in bed, with your eyes closed and mind relaxed, sometimes called resting-mind mode, silently — in your mind — say your Healthy-weight Goal Statement three times.

Then, with your eyes still closed, communicate to your mind — or, more specifically, to your subconscious mind — how you want the upcoming day to turn out, especially as pertains to eating. Tell it *exactly* what you want it to help make happen.

So, what do you describe? To answer this question consider the following.

Would you like to go through the day without being harassed by the over-snacking habit or by the mealtime gluttony-eating habit or by unwanted cravings and hunger pangs? Sure you would. So, tell your subconscious mind that.

What else would you like? How about finding it easy to follow your preferred dietary program?

Or ... how about feeling totally filled up and satisfied every time after eating a right amount of food, or the amount prescribed by your preferred dietary program?

Or ... how about finding right foods, or the foods prescribed by your dietary program, to be tasty and satisfying?

Or ... how about finding wrong foods, or the foods prohibited by your dietary program, to be unappealing and tasteless?

Or ... how about each meal turning out to be a "healthy-meal victory" and you having a great feeling of satisfaction after each one?

Or ... how about finding your daily exercise activity to be enjoyable and invigorating?

Or ... how about your subconscious mind reminding you to do all five daily actions of the Weight Success Method, plus automatically performing every action described in the Weight Success Benefits Directive?

Would you like one or more of these things to happen? Sure you would. So, tell your subconscious mind exactly what you want it to help make happen in the upcoming day. Doing this takes less than 60 seconds. But the results can astound.

Try Resting-mind Mode

Now here's an optional tip for possibly enhancing the impact of your upcoming-day descriptions. Your conscious mind mainly functions in two modes: awake and sleeping. In the awake mode it's active. As such, it's busy receiving and processing stimuli and responding to events going on around you. During this time it directs most or all of your words and actions. We call this *awake-mind mode.*

In the sleeping mode your conscious mind is inactive. As such, it pays little or no attention to stimuli around you, except that which it interprets as being an emergency.

However, you have periods where you aren't completely sleeping but also not fully functioning in awake-mind mode. These periods often occur when you're in the process of either waking up or falling asleep, or between awake-mind and sleeping modes. For reference purpose we'll call such periods *resting-mind mode.*

Resting-mind mode usually lasts for a short period, like a few minutes. But sometimes it can go longer. It mainly occurs when you're (a) drifting off to sleep, (b) waking up in the night, such as before going to the bathroom or otherwise arising for something, (c) going back to sleep in the night (such as after going to the bathroom), and (d) waking up in the morning, or when you're awake but haven't yet opened your eyes and arisen from bed.

During resting-mind mode your conscious mind is functioning but it's not focusing on and dealing with stimuli and events of the world around you. So, what's the difference between awake-mind mode and resting-mind mode? In awake-mind mode your conscious mind is mainly focusing on the events of the outer world. In resting-mind mode it's mainly focusing on the events of the inner world, or the activity of your subconscious mind.

A unique feature of resting-mind mode is the opportunity for enhanced communication between you and your subconscious mind. For some reason, messages sent to your subconscious mind during resting-mind mode often have a stronger impact on your subconscious mind. It's as if your subconscious mind focuses on these messages more intently, or views them as being of higher importance.

If you find communicating to your subconscious mind during resting-mind mode to be effective *and* you'd like to do this type of communication at times other than at night or in the morning, or during sleep time, you can easily do so. Just do this. Close your eyes, relax your conscious mind, and begin silently talking to your subconscious mind. The more relaxed you are and the more your conscious mind is detached from focusing on external stimuli, the easier and more effective the communication will be. Becoming proficient at this is easy to do. All you do is practice it a few times, and deliver positive reinforcement to yourself after your conscious mind follows instructions and goes into resting-mind mode.

How to Get Input from Your Subconscious

Here's an additional thing you can do in resting-mind mode. It's not directly related to weight control, but it's something you might be able to apply for personal benefit. (Note: I've been using it for years in creative pursuits, such as, for example, in creating inventions and patents and also in book writing.) Basically, it's an easy way to get timely input — mainly, ideas and suggestions — from your subconscious mind. Messages from your subconscious mind seem to come through more distinctly in resting-mind mode than in awake-mind mode. Here's how to do it.

First, put your conscious mind into resting-mind mode. Then, to get an answer or idea on a specific topic, pose a simple clearly-worded question to your subconscious mind. Make the question as clear and specific as possible. Why? Because your subconscious typically can't or won't respond to a vague ambiguous question.

Often your subconscious will send back an answer almost instantly. If it doesn't, set a deadline for it to deliver a response — like, for example, "by 9:00 a.m. tomorrow morning."

The message that comes back from your subconscious mind will likely be in the form of a fleeting thought, or idea or realization, or phrase, or image, or feeling, or hunch, or musical lyric, or memory of a past event. At this point it's up to you to interpret what it means. Much of the time the meaning is crystal clear; it's a "do this" type of message. Other times it's symbolic, so it requires some interpretation. And, now and then it seems inexplicable. When this happens ask your subconscious mind to send a clarifying message, which it usually will do. Or, rephrase the question. Oftentimes when you get an incomprehensible response it's because you posed a confusing question. To get a simple, specific, unambiguous answer, pose a simple, specific, unambiguous question. Lastly, *thank* your subconscious mind for sending the answer.

To get maximum benefit from this process, keep a pad and pencil by your bedside or chairside, and also a small table light or flashlight for night use. When your subconscious mind sends some insightful or useful info, open your eyes, turn on the light, and write down the message on the pad. When finished writing, lay down, close your eyes, and go back to resting-mind mode. If you like, you can continue the communication where you left off.

I've found that the best pencil for this is an automatic pencil with erasure. The best pad is a 6-by-9 inch steno pad with a wire coil at the top. You can handily store the automatic pencil by sliding it into the end of the wire coil, with the pencil's clip engaging the wire. If you use this process often you might find it helpful to put the date at the top of the first page of each session. This makes it easier to refer back to a message at a later date.

MOTIVATOR 4:
Day-end Thanks

At the end of the day, right before going to sleep, thank your subconscious mind for at least one desired action it performed that day.

A "desired action" would be any action that assisted you with achieving right eating or healthy-weight living. Another name for this is "weight success action."

Thanking your subconscious mind after it performs a desired action, along with telling it to repeat that action in the future, motivates it to repeat the action in the future. This dynamic is a key factor in Daily Actions 2A and 5.

Unfortunately, most people are oblivious to the desired actions their subconscious mind performs throughout each day. As such, they never thank it for these actions. The result: They miss out on a big opportunity to motivate their subconscious mind to *more frequently* perform desired actions. But, you can go a long way toward rectifying this situation by applying this Motivator 4. Here's how. After going to bed for the night, close your eyes and relax your mind. Then do these two things.

FIRST, mentally review the past day. In doing this, identify one or more specific weight success actions performed by your subconscious mind. Note: When your subconscious mind does any of the actions described in your Weight Success Benefits Directive, that's a *weight success action.*

SECOND, deliver thanks to your subconscious mind for having performed this desired action. For this, deliver a short Thank You, Keep It Up message. You can deliver your thanks either by speaking silently in your mind or by speaking aloud. Note: whispering counts as speaking aloud. Do it whatever way feels most natural and meaningful at the time. Doing this Motivator 4 takes less than 30 seconds. But the results can be powerful.

MOTIVATOR 5:
Benefits Visualization

For at least 60 seconds, visualize one of your exciting weight success benefits as an accomplished fact, at least once a day.

In delivering your Weight Success Benefits Directive (for Daily Action 3) you briefly visualize the attainment of a weight success benefit. With this Motivator 5 you do it more in depth. Here's how. Sit in a relaxing chair or lay in bed, close your eyes, and visualize one of your exciting weight success benefits as an accomplished fact. That is, visualize the benefit being fully achieved and you enjoying it that very moment. Mentally fill the scene with pleasant details. Create a good feeling in yourself — this is important. Visualize for at least a minute.

Also, do at least one visualization a day. You can visualize the same weight success benefit each time *or* you can visualize a different benefit each time — your choice.

Visualization exists in two forms: still image and moving image. A still-image visualization is a mental picture of a single situation or thing, like a mental photograph. A moving-image visualization is a mental picture of a moving action or event, like a mental video or movie. This mental movie can be in either third person or first person. In **third** person you're *viewing* yourself performing the action, like watching a movie. In **first** person you're imagining yourself being in the process of *doing* the action, like making the movie. Some persons believe the first-person approach is more effective than the third-person. Do it whichever way creates the most enjoyable feeling.

MOTIVATOR 6:
Goal Reminders

View goal-reminding images each day.

Each day view images and messages pertaining to your healthy-weight goal and ongoing realization of that goal. Whenever you see such an image it causes three events to occur.

First, it momentarily focuses your mind, including subconscious mind, on the continuing realization of that goal.

Second, it reminds you to do all five Daily Actions of the Weight Success Method that day.

Third, it reminds you of your substantial accomplishment in sustaining ongoing daily realization of your healthy-weight goal. This can — and should — give you a surging feeling of joy and pride.

These three events motivate you and your subconscious mind to make that day be a Weight Success Day — that is, a day that contributes to creating weight success.

So, what might you use for visual reminders of your healthy-weight goal and of your ongoing realization of that goal? For illustration, here are three examples of visual goal reminders:

1 – A prominently displayed note or sign depicting the number of years (months or weeks) you've been living in your healthy-weight range. In the Part 1–A section of Chapter 1 is an example of such a note (p. 8). It's my "Years Living in My Healthy-weight Range" note. An updated new note goes up each December 31. It's pinned to my bulletin board and is viewed by me every day. It's a *very* powerful reminder.

2 – A prominently displayed Win-Day Calendar, which is contained in Ch. **27** (p. 154) and also in the Toolkit at:

correllconcepts.com/toolkit.pdf

3 – A prominently displayed Weight Success Actions Scorecard, which is in Ch. **27** and also in the Toolkit.

Those are three examples. It's likely you can create visual goal and progress reminders of your own design. Finally, "post" your visual reminders not only on paper but also on your digital devices. In short, put them "all over," so that you see them *throughout each day.*

Most people underestimate the faculties of their subconscious mind. And, their subconscious mind — always eager to fulfill expectations — responds in accordance with the underestimation.

~

When you apply the full faculties of your whole mind to a pursuit, such as the pursuit of Weight Success Creation, the accomplishment of that pursuit becomes easy, or at least way easier than you've likely been imagining it to be.

CHAPTER 14: How to Adapt the Weight Success Method to Fix Problems

Be dogged in fixing weight management problems, and you'll *succeed* at surmounting every one.

THE WEIGHT SUCCESS Method provides exact procedures for the five daily actions. But in spots it tells you to feel free to improvise. This is for two reasons: (1) so you might make the Method more closely fit your situation, and (2) so that if you confront a special problem — such as a troublesome eating urge, craving, or habit — you might create a special solution that enables you to more readily surmount that problem.

To help you apply reason #2, this chapter gives eleven special problem resolution tactics, any of which you might apply for helping resolve an occasional special problem that could arise.

TACTIC 1: In Daily Action 2A–Reinforcement, when delivering the Thank You, Keep It Up message, include a special instruction to your subconscious mind that tells it what you want done regarding resolution of the special problem.

TACTIC 2: In Daily Action 3–Benefits Directive, when delivering the Weight Success Benefits Directive include some ad lib instruction to your subconscious mind that tells it what you want done regarding resolution of the special problem.

TACTIC 3: For the Weight Success Benefits Directive, write up an additional healthy-weight action. Word it so it tells your subconscious mind what to do regarding resolving the special problem on an ongoing basis. Make it action #6 and incorporate it into the Directive after action #5. You can write it in or type it up and tape it in.

TACTIC 4: In Daily Action 5–Guided Eating, apply a custom guided-eating self-talk statement. In Step 1 of the Action (the Communication step), two sample statements are provided. But for resolving a special eating-related problem you could create your own customized self-talk statement for neutralizing that problem.

Upcoming Tactics #5–9 are adaptations of the six optional mind motivators described in the Six More Mind Motivators chapter (p. 90).

TACTIC 5: Apply Motivator 1: High-frequency Goal Statement (p. 90). For this, say your Healthy-weight Goal Statement a hundred times a day. Sometimes an intense focus on the ultimate goal of your weight success journey can have the effect of neutralizing, or "drowning," a special problem.

TACTIC 6: Apply Motivator 2: Backup Depiction Statements (p. 90). For this, create a custom backup depiction statement aimed at neutralizing the special problem. Make it describe an action or outcome you want your subconscious to do, or describe some affirmation you want your whole mind to take heed of and actualize. Say the statement many times per day.

TACTIC 7: Apply Motivator 3: Upcoming-day Description (p. 92). For this, do an upcoming-day depiction that describes the special problem being resolved, and what it will be like after it's resolved.

TACTIC 8: Apply Motivator 4: Day-end Thanks (p. 94). For this, at the end of the day reflect back on the special problem. Did you, or your subconscious mind, perform any action that amounted to progress in resolving the problem? If so, deliver appreciation and thanks to your subconscious mind (use a type of Thank You, Keep It Up message).

TACTIC 9: Apply Motivator 5: Benefits Visualization (p. 94). For this, use the visualization technique described for Motivator 5 and visualize the problem resolved and you enjoying it.

TACTIC 10: Ask your subconscious mind to tell you the best way to solve the problem. To do this, use the technique described in the section titled "How to Get Input from Your Subconscious" (p. 93).

TACTIC 11: Ask God to disclose to you an insight, tactic, or opportunity you might use for resolving the special problem and, thereby, creating easier lifelong healthy-weight living. This method consists of three parts: Communicate, Believe, Appreciate. (Sound familiar?) It can be done anytime, but a particularly good time is before going to sleep for the night.

Three Steps to Getting and Using Input from God

Here's what to do.

Step 1 – COMMUNICATE. *Communicate to God the full situation regarding the problem you want to resolve, and then request God to disclose a solution to you.* ❧ As you convey the message, imagine, or assume, that God, or God's spirit, is invisibly present in the room with you at that very moment. Then, include the following information in your communication:

(1) an *exact description* of the problem you want to resolve,

(2) an expression of *strong desire* for God to disclose to you an insight, tactic, or opportunity that, if employed by you, would resolve the problem,

(3) the *reason why* you want the problem resolved, or how having the problem resolved will greatly benefit you and your life,

(4) an expression of your firm *belief* that God will be acting on your request,

and then after doing parts 1–4,

(5) *ask God* to please disclose the input you're seeking by a certain time (like, for example, "by 9 a.m. tomorrow morning").

Step 2 – BELIEVE. *Fully believe that God will be following through on your request and that the input will be forthcoming within the requested time.* ❧ Hold this belief both while making the request and afterward as well. Also, keep these three points in mind:

(1) God's response or input can come at any time, including (a) immediately, like within a min-ute after making the request, or (b) just before the specified deadline, or (c) in a dream, or (d) while you're waking up or right after waking up.

(2) When the response comes, immediately write it down on a piece of paper (or perhaps on a digital device), so keep paper and pencil or digital device handy — that is, by your bedside (if you don't write it down you'll likely find it hard to remember later, or the next morning).

(3) The message that comes back from God can be in the form of a fleeting thought, or idea or realization, or phrase, or image, or feeling, or hunch, or musical lyric, or memory of a past event. At this point it's up to you to interpret what it means. Much of the time the meaning is crystal clear; it's a "do this" type of message. Other times it's symbolic, so it requires some interpretation. And, now and then it seems inexplicable. When this happens ask God to send a clarifying message.

Step 3 – APPRECIATE. *When the requested input comes, thank God for it; then* <u>*proceed to apply it.*</u> ❧ If this insight involves ongoing action of some sort, incorporate the action into your daily application of the Weight Success Method.

> NOTE: To the best of my conjecture, God doesn't get involved in directing a person to impose harm or negative consequences on their self or on another person. So, when I say "apply God's input" I'm not suggesting you pursue something that's rude or illegal or immoral or potentially harmful to you or to someone else, or that would constitute an imposition or trespass on someone or their property. If such a thought should come to mind, convert it into a version that's courteous, legal, moral, and non-harmful to you and others; then pursue this legal, harmless version. In other words, pursue only harm-free activities.

As you now know, the key to succeeding at lifelong healthy-weight living is:

Do Weight Success Actions <u>every day</u>.

For maximal effectiveness in doing this, be creative in applying the Weight Success Method for surmounting any problem that arises, and don't hesitate to use every available resource and Tactic (#1–11 described in this chapter) for realizing your healthy-weight goal. <u>This</u> is how problems are resolved and weight success is most easily and enjoyably accomplished.

WEIGHT SUCCESS
is the GOAL

WEIGHT SUCCESS METHOD™
is the MEANS

Goal+Means+<u>Action</u>=WEIGHT SUCCESS™

WEIGHT SUCCESS = Living most or all of one's days
in one's desired healthy-weight range AND
deriving benefits, enjoyment, and
fulfillment from it.

CHAPTER 15: Achieving Exercise Success

**An exercise program could expedite healthy-weight living, but it's not a requirement.
By applying the Weight Success Method you can live at your desired weight without exercising,
although you might need to eat a little less food to do it.**

MOST PERSONS view exercise as a "non-essential" to achieving good health and a good life. So they don't do it on a regular basis. Truth is, for most of us exercise enhances virtually every aspect of our being, for the entire duration of our life. Few activities benefit us as much as daily exercise does. Plus it does one other interesting thing: It can make weight reduction and weight management *easier*.

Also, before beginning a new exercise program or making a major change to a present program you should consult with your physician to ensure you're physically capable of performing the program without personal harm or medical issues.

Seven Keys to Exercise Success

Use these seven keys for starting, sticking with, and enjoying the daily exercise activity of your choice. These pointers apply to virtually every type of exercise.

KEY 1: *Pursue exercise activities you enjoy doing.* ~ When you don't enjoy doing a particular exercise you likely won't stick with it. When you *do* enjoy doing a particular exercise you have a greater chance of succeeding with it. Also, you don't need to limit yourself to doing the same type of exercise every day. To avoid boredom, have a "stable" of exercises you can choose from. My exercise stable, for example, includes walking, weight-resistance workout, bicycling, and a recumbent training bike.

KEY 2: *Start small and build up gradually.* ~ The biggest mistake most people make when undertaking an exercise program is they start wrong. They (a) attempt too much in the first day or week or (b) build up too quickly or (c) do both. In doing this they either sustain an injury or become so exhausted they mentally burn out. So start small, build up gradually. That's how you succeed at exercise.

KEY 3: *Use the right technique and gear.* ~ For virtually every type of exercise there's a right way and a wrong way to do it. The wrong way almost always creates problems, sometimes big ones. So, learn the correct way to perform your chosen exercise. You might get a book or DVD on it. Also, using the right gear and apparel can help. In short, don't take chances with wrong technique or gear. Avoid problems by doing it the right way from the start.

KEY 4: *Record your exercise sessions.* ~ On a calendar or a chart, record what you did and when you did it. This gives you added opportunity to feel good about what you're doing. It's called positive reinforcement. It motivates you to continue doing the thing that made you feel good.

KEY 5: *Keep it fun.* ~ If a particular exercise session is turning out to be not-fun you might end it early. Don't force yourself to have a bad experience. This only de-motivates you in the future. Also, if your chosen exercise activity begins to grow stale or become not-fun, modify it to be fun again. Or, adopt a different type of exercise. Do whatever it takes to keep your exercising fun ... or, at least, to keep it from becoming an unpleasant experience.

KEY 6: *Make doing your chosen exercise a top priority.* ~ When doing your exercise isn't a top priority it always ends up being bumped out of line by some other "more important thing." So, you end up not sticking with it — or, at best, doing it hit-and-miss. To succeed at exercising you must view getting your regular exercise as being mandatory, not optional. Scheduling it for a certain timeslot in the day can help. For many persons, doing it at the start of the day works best.

KEY 7: *Try to do at least some exercise every day, or most days, of the week.* ~ To succeed at exercise, exercise must be a habit with you. To maintain exercise as a habit it helps to engage in some form of exercise at least several days a week.

How to Make Yourself Start and Stay with It

Every activity has both an upside and a downside. The upside is that aspect of the activity that you like or enjoy. The downside is that aspect that you dislike or don't enjoy. When the downside looms large in your mind you find it hard to make yourself do the activity.

Often, the hardest part to doing an exercise program is making yourself take the first step. This results from the perceived downside — or hassle, aggravation, annoyance, discomfort — attached to doing the exercise. Which means, if the downside were to be reduced to insignificance, *you would start doing the exercise!* So, the key to beginning an exercise program is reduce the downside to insignificance.

You can use an easy 2-step technique for reducing the downside to insignificance — and, thereby, making yourself start and stick with a particular exercise:

1. Reduce the exercise to a miniscule amount, and start at that amount;
2. Increase the exercise amount in miniscule increments and very gradually over time.

How to Enhance the Upside

The above technique reduces the downside of exercising. Now what you also should do is enhance the upside. You can do this one or both of two ways.

One, before each exercise session deliver a short directive to your mind. In this directive tell your mind to make the exercise feel enjoyable. That is, tell it to minimize any emotional discomfort you might feel from exercising. Also, tell it to cause you to derive a feeling of pleasure and satisfaction from the act of exercising — both while exercising and afterward. To help make this happen, while exercising visualize yourself being in possession of one or more of your weight success benefits, which are the items listed in the benefits section of your Weight Success Benefits Directive.

Two, after the exercising deliver to your self — or your mind — a Thank You, Keep It Up message. Thank it for reminding you to do the exercise. Also thank it for assisting you with making the exercise enjoyable. In short, after each exercise session deliver to yourself a generous dose of positive self-reinforcement. The main idea is to generate a good feeling after each session.

Summing up: Regular exercise is one of the most beneficial activities you can engage in. One of those benefits is easier weight loss and weight control. You can enhance your chance of exercise success by doing certain things. It works like this.

Seven Keys to Exercise Success
1. Pursue exercise activities you enjoy doing.
2. Start small and build up gradually.
3. Use the right technique and gear.
4. Record your exercise sessions.
5. Keep it fun, or at least keep it from being unpleasant.
6. Make doing your chosen exercise a top priority.
7. Try to do at least some exercise every day (or most days).

Results in exercise success which, in turn, creates numerous benefits including easier weight loss and weight control.

CHAPTER 16: Escaping Schadenfreude

(and also escaping reverse-schadenfreude)

SCHADENFREUDE is a German word. Literally, it means "damage-joy" (schaden = damage; freude = joy). But a dictionary-type definition would be: *delight, joy, or pleasure derived from seeing or hearing about someone else's troubles, failures, or misfortunes.*

So, what does this have to do with healthy-weight living? More than you might imagine. You might assume that your family and friends would want to see you succeed in your weight success journey. You might assume that once you've made the decision to change your life from overweight living to healthy-weight living that they'd be cheering you on. You might assume that after you've switched from wrong eating to right eating they'd take joy in you doing this, and delight in hearing about your progress, and want to encourage and assist you. You might assume that as your body slowly morphs from overweight to right weight that they'd be happy to see you that way, and offer sincere compliments and encouraging words.

Some family members and friends will respond that way. But also it's likely some will not. Their typical response will be no response. What's more, the more progress you make the more "no response" there will be.

Now, you might assume that the reason for this "no response" is that these people have no interest in what you're doing, no interest in learning about what's happening in your life.

But probably that's not the case. They likely have considerable interest in hearing about what's happening with you. But it's not an interest in hearing about what you're succeeding with; it's an interest in hearing about what you're struggling and failing with. Which means, as regards your weight success journey, these people will show little interest in hearing about your progress and successes but will have keen interest in learning of your troubles and setbacks and, perhaps most of all, your ultimate failure.

Why do some people respond this way? Schadenfreude! Every time they hear about how you might be struggling with losing weight or with maintaining your desired weight it creates a pleasurable feeling in them. Further, every time they hear about how you might be succeeding in your weight-loss program it creates a not-so-pleasurable feeling in them. I call this *reverse-schadenfreude.* (I don't know what the German word for "success-misery" would be.) In short, for some people your weight management failure = their joy; your weight management success = their misery. So they love hearing about your weight struggles and setbacks, and hate hearing about your weight progress and accomplishments.

What's the most productive way to deal with this perverse situation? Do these four things.

1 – As regards the "no-positive-response folks," realize that schadenfreude and reverse-schadenfreude are what is driving their response. Meaning, recognize that their negative response to your weight management pursuit is not because of you but because of some deviant schadenfreude (or reverse-schadenfreude) dynamic they carry in their head.

2 – Ignore the no-response/negative response of the "schadenfreuders." Meaning, don't let this response deter or discourage you. Realize that this is just the way some people are. Bear in mind that (a) you're on the right track with your pursuit of healthy-weight living and (b) they're on some other track with their seeming inability to view the pursuit of healthy-weight living in a positive light.

3 – Embrace those family members and friends who view your weight success journey in a positive light. Maintain, or perhaps build, your relationship with them.

4 – If you feel overwhelmed or discouraged by some peoples' negative response to your weight success journey, consider joining a dietary program that involves interaction with others — that is, with instructors and co-dieters who provide encourage-ment and support. This will offset the potentially-discouraging negative response of those who secretly desire to see you struggle with creating healthy-weight living.

Always, always bear in mind:

Despite what anyone might say or believe, you <u>have</u> the capability to live your life in your healthy-weight range *and* you have the capability to do it <u>easily</u>, or at least way more easily than you, or they, might be imagining.

Do the **Five Daily Actions**
<u>every</u> day . . .
and **Lifelong Weight Success**
will be <u>Yours</u>.

Typically takes <u>less than</u> **8** minutes
of dedicated time per day.

CHAPTER 17: Why the Weight Success Method is Enjoyable

Most people assume weight management is painful. But, actually, doing the Weight Success Method (described in Chapter 1) can be enjoyable and uplifting.

SHORTLY after starting the Weight Success Method in 2007 I made an eye-opening discovery. I realized that the *process* of doing the Method can be enjoyable and gratifying in itself. Here's how it happens.

Enjoyment from the PROCESS

All five daily actions of the Weight Success Method produce enjoyment.

Daily Action 1 – Weighing (p. 22)

You might find this hard to believe, but it's true. Each day I look forward to my daily weighing. Now, some people might deride this. They could say "you're weight obsessed" or "you're vain and self-absorbed over how you look."

But such conclusions miss the point. I don't spend time obsessing over body weight. And, I'm not one to be vain and self-absorbed over personal appearance, or at least no more than anyone else.

Rather, what I *am* absorbed with is giving myself opportunity to become the finest person I can be and to create the most beneficial life I can create. This includes realizing the many benefits that come with living in my healthy-weight range. In short, becoming the finest person I can be and creating the most beneficial life I can create is a top priority of mine.

So, it's obvious why I enjoy weighing myself each day. It's because my daily weighing gives me timely feedback on the daily progress I'm making toward realization of one of my top priorities. I find this to be enjoyable. Indeed, not only do I find it enjoyable I find it motivating and uplifting, as well — a great way to start a day.

Now, you might be thinking: What about when you get a scale reading that shows your weight being above your healthy-weight range? How do you feel then?

Well, naturally, I feel disappointment. But in no way am I sad or discouraged. I view it as an opportunity — an opportunity to gain extra enjoyment at the next day's weighing. Whenever I get a desired weight reading the day after getting an undesired one, or return to my healthy-weight range after straying from it, it doesn't just make me feel good, it makes me feel *very* good. So, on the infrequent occasion when my weight slips outside my healthy-weight range I take immediate, vigorous corrective action in the next 24 or 48 hours (Daily Action 2B). This immediately brings my body weight back into line, which brings me extra enjoyment at a subsequent day's weighing.

To add to this discussion I note that most persons hate stepping onto a scale. That's because it too often results in a painful experience. But this painful experience occurs because they're doing weighing and weight control the wrong way.

By applying the approach described in Daily Action 1, I actually derive enjoyment from daily weighing. And, in turn, this enjoyment makes it easier for me to motivate my mind to stick with my healthy-weight living activities and program. In short, doing Daily Action 1 is an enjoyable, motivating, uplifting experience for me. It can be this way for you, too.

Daily Action 2A – Reinforcement (p. 23)

Each time I deliver the Thank You, Keep It Up message after the daily weighing, I deliver it with happiness and exuberance. I make it a joyous moment. This, in turn, builds on the great feeling I derived from getting the positive feedback, or desired weight reading, that came with the daily weighing. In short, doing Daily Action 2A is an enjoyable, motivating, uplifting experience.

Daily Action 2B – Correction (p. 26)

Perhaps it's hard to see how doing Daily Action 2B could be enjoyable. But, believe it or not, I actually derive pleasure and gratification from it. It's all in the perspective.

If I view doing this action as "proof that I'm a weight-control failure" then, as you might expect, I feel badly. But, on the other hand, when I view it as "proof that I'm a weight-control winner" I feel good. A winner, after all, isn't someone who never experiences setbacks or makes mistakes or misses the mark now and then. Rather, a winner is one who learns from mistakes, bounces back after setbacks, and persists in spite of missteps. More precisely, a winner is one who, after a setback, ratchets up their focus and intensity to the point where they surmount the setback and, once having done so, emerges as a stronger, smarter person than they were before the setback. That's the viewpoint and approach I take when doing Daily Action 2B. It works every time — meaning, every time it puts me instantly back on track *and* generates a good feeling, too.

So, I pursue Daily Action 2B with intensity and resoluteness. I view it as a positive experience. And, I view it as proof that I'm a winner in general and a healthy-weight winner in particular. Approaching it this way makes doing Daily Action 2B enjoyable and motivating.

What this comes down to is positive approach to a setback versus negative approach. With a positive approach — described above — the correction process is pleasurable and successful. With a negative approach — opposite of the above — the correction process usually turns out to be painful and often unsuccessful. Plus, applying the positive approach requires no more time and effort than applying a negative one. So, I opt for the positive perspective — and derive enjoyment and benefit from it.

Daily Action 3 – Benefits Directive (p. 28)

In terms of time, Daily Action 3 requires the most commitment. It involves setting aside two to three minutes a day of dedicated time for delivering the Weight Success Benefits Directive. So one could view it as being a time-consuming inconvenience. And when something's viewed as an inconvenience it tends to be non-enjoyable.

But it needn't be this way. I've found that delivering the Directive can be an enjoyable experience if I do one or more of these three things.

First, I act as-if my mind — in particular my subconscious mind — is right then, as I'm reading the Directive, in the process of acting on every instruction I'm giving it. Which means the present day is going to be a right-eating day — also known as healthy-eating day. This is a pleasure-producing thought.

Second, I bear in mind the many weight success benefits I gain from living in my healthy-weight range. This is another pleasure-producing thought. These benefits are cited in the Directive.

Third, I apply a creative delivery technique now and then, as described in action #7 of the Seven Actions for Delivering the Directive for Maximum Effect (p. **67**). Indeed, the cliché is correct: Variety is the spice of life.

Doing any of these three things increases the enjoyment I derive from Daily Action 3. It makes the action less like a chore and more like a pleasure.

Daily Action 4 – Goal Statement (p. 34)

Saying the Healthy-weight Goal Statement 25 — or 40 or 50 or 100 — times a day might seem like repetitive drudgery. And drudgery isn't fun. But it doesn't have to be this way. There are three things I do to change this potential drudgery into enjoyment.

First, each time I say my Healthy-weight Goal Statement I *act as-if* I am at that very moment the person depicted in the statement. That is, I act as-if I'm "the person of my healthy weight" and one who's "healthy, happy, and doing great." Or, put another way, whenever I say my Healthy-weight Goal Statement I realize that I am, indeed, the actual person depicted in the Statement. This imparts a good feeling within me.

Second, as I'm saying the Statement I call to mind one or two exciting weight success benefits. And then I act as-if my mind is right then in the process of actualizing these benefits with every iteration of my Healthy-weight Goal Statement. This also gives me a good feeling.

Third, I change up my delivery style from time to time. For example, the Statement can be said rapidly or slowly. And different words can be emphasized at different times.

Doing these three things, especially the first two, make Daily Action 4 enjoyable, motivating, and uplifting.

Daily Action 5 – Guided Eating (p. 35)

Daily Action 5 involves applying the Guided Eating Process to each eating session. The Guided Eating Process consists of Communicate, Believe, Appreciate. In acronym form, I call it the C-B-A process (which is A-B-C in reverse). To review, doing this process involves these three steps.

Communicate Step. As the eating begins — and perhaps during the meal too — I deliver guided-eating self-talk to my self, or my mind.

Believe Step. As I'm eating I hold the belief, and also act as-if, my mind is right then, at that very moment, in the process of performing the actions described in my guided-eating self-talk; so I'm on the lookout for a stop-eating signal, which usually includes the full-stomach feeling.

Appreciate Step. If a stop-eating signal comes I thank my mind — or, more specifically, my subconscious mind — for sending the signal; then I follow the signal — that is, I stop eating. When I do this the urge to continue eating immediately begins to fade away.

Now we come to the main point. Doing this 3-step process — especially the third step — gives me a feeling of accomplishment. It makes me realize that I control my eating and my eating isn't controlling me. And, this makes me feel good. It makes me feel like a healthy-weight winner. I like that feeling. It's enjoyable, gratifying, and uplifting.

Summary of Process Enjoyment

So to sum up, here are the six kinds of enjoyment I derive from the process of doing the Weight Success Method.

1 – *Enjoyment from Daily Progress.* ❧ Each time I get a desired weight reading when doing my daily weighing (Daily Action 1) it tells me I've achieved yet another day of progress toward the further realization of lifelong healthy-weight living. I find this to be enjoyable, motivating, and uplifting.

2 – *Enjoyment from Daily Reinforcement.* ❧ Each time that I deliver and receive positive self-reinforcement I find it to be enjoyable, motivating, and uplifting. This comes from delivering an exuberant Thank You, Keep It Up message to my self — or my mind — after each desired weight reading (Daily Action 2A).

3 – *Enjoyment from Triumphing over Adversity or Setback.* ❧ Each time that I do Daily Action 2B I triumph over a setback and also derive a benefit from the process. Doing this I find to be enjoyable, motivating, and uplifting.

4 – *Enjoyment from Being Director of My Eating.* ❧ In any given eating situation, either I'm the director of my eating *or* my eating is the director of me. I accomplish being director of my eating by applying the Weight Success Method, and especially by doing Daily Actions 3 and 5. I find that being director of my eating is enjoyable, motivating, and uplifting.

5 – *Enjoyment from Focusing on an Exciting Ultimate Goal.* ❧ My days seem to go better and obstacles and annoyances seem to be smaller when I'm focusing on an exciting ultimate goal. Doing the five daily actions of the Weight Success Method focuses me each day on one of my ultimate goals — specifically, being the person of my healthy weight and living my life in my healthy-weight range. Doing Daily Action 4 keeps me focused on this goal. I find this to be enjoyable, motivating, and uplifting.

6 – *Enjoyment from Viewing Myself as a Winner.* ❧ I like viewing myself as a winner. Or, more directly, I like being a winner. And what's a winner? A winner is someone who performs winning actions. The Weight Success Method is full of opportunities for winning actions. Each time I do one of the five daily actions I'm performing a winning action. Also, each time I do one of the actions described in any of the optional chapters of this book (Ch. 2–27) I'm doing a winning action. I find doing winning actions and feeling like a winner to be enjoyable, motivating, and uplifting.

To sum up, doing the five daily actions of the Weight Success Method involves interacting with my self in a way that motivates my mind — including subconscious mind — to steer me toward living in my healthy-weight range. For the reasons just described, I find this interaction process enjoyable, motivating, and uplifting.

Enjoyment from the OUTCOME

Along with deriving enjoyment from the process of doing the five daily actions, I also get it from the outcome. This outcome manifests in two forms: general and specific.

The general outcome is: living my life in my healthy-weight range. Presently, the act of putting one's weight into a healthy-weight range and then *maintaining* it there for the rest of one's life is a rare accomplishment. Which means any person who's accomplishing it is a healthy-weight high-achiever. Living my life as such a person I find to be enjoyable, motivating, and uplifting.

From this general outcome arises a specific outcome: the realization of my weight success benefits. The benefit I find to be most motivating and uplifting is benefit #1: a greater chance of living healthier longer, or greater chance of living free of debilitating accidents, illnesses, diseases, and bodily malfunction.

Now here's a big point. Enjoyment from bene-fits comes two ways: (1) from *actualization* of the benefit and (2) from being *aware* of the benefit on a daily basis. Doing the Weight Success Method, especially Daily Actions 3 and 4, maintains my awareness of my weight success benefits on a daily basis. As a result, I derive substantial enjoyment and motivation from my weight success benefits.

To sum up, I enjoy the outcome of the Weight Success Method *and* I enjoy the process of creating the outcome. So, in terms of enjoyment, gratifica-tion, and fulfillment, the Weight Success Method is

a double-win. This double-win — plus the fact that creating it typically requires less than eight minutes of dedicated time per day — is why I continue doing the Method day after day, year after year. It's also why I decided to publish it in this book.

Bad Pleasure | Good Pleasure

For the first six decades of my life I held a certain limiting assumption. The assumption was that the main purpose of my life was to do things that resulted in personal enjoyment, happiness, success, and fulfillment. This assumption seemed inherently obvious to me.

But there was a slippery little question lurking in the bushes of my mind. That being: What, exactly, are the activities that (will) result in creat-ing personal enjoyment, happiness, success, and fulfillment? In a sense, I spent the first 60 years of my life trying to find the answer to that question. And the answer eluded me.

Then, one day while writing my first weight management book — which, believe it or not, spanned a period of over six years (yes, there were numerous versions and re-writes) — the answer came.

And, what came is this. The purpose of my life is to (a) strive to become the finest person I'm capable of being, (b) strive to create the most beneficial life I'm capable of creating, and (c) help as many others as I can to do the same. I then realized that performing these three actions is the reason my life exists — and perhaps the reason why all human lives exist. Then I further realized that it's through performance of these three actions that I — and perhaps humankind — experience maximal peace, love, joy, and fulfillment in life.

After that, I realized that all pleasures and pursuits can be divided into two groups: (1) those that assist me in performing those three actions and (2) those that hinder me in performing those actions.

For identification purposes I dubbed the first group *good pleasures and pursuits* and the second group *bad pleasures and pursuits*. Alternatively, these two groups could be called *productive* pleasures and pursuits and *counterproductive* pleasures and pursuits.

And then I realized that a pivotal factor in determining the course of my life were the decisions I had made regarding what pleasures to pursue. And, further, I realized it was not only a deciding factor in *my* life but was also a factor in determining the prior history, and perhaps the "future history," of humankind.

All this raised a question. When we humans confront an either/or decision regarding pursuing an activity that yields a bad pleasure versus an activity that yields a good pleasure, why do we sometimes, or perhaps much of the time, opt to pursue the bad activity? It's because of this. The pleasures derived from performing an activity in the bad activity group tend to be large at the start; while the pleasures derived from performing an activity in the good activity group tend to be smaller at the start. So, we're often motivated to pursue a bad activity over an opposing good activity because the bad activity affords the most pleasure *right now.*

There is, however, an additional distinction between these two types of pleasure-producing activities. Although the bad activity often yields the largest immediate pleasure this pleasure tends to diminish over time — and often eventually diminishes to the point of being a "negative pleasure," or pain and handicap.

On the other hand, although the good activity might yield a smaller immediate pleasure this pleasure tends to expand over time — and often continues expanding to the end of a person's life — and ultimately provides large lasting benefits.

So, why have I included this discussion in a book on eating and weight management? It's because, like so many aspects of human life, eating and weight management come down to "choosing our pleasures," or deciding whether to (a) pursue a counterproductive activity that produces a large immediate pleasure but eventually creates a large future penalty or (b) pursue a productive activity that produces a smaller immediate pleasure but eventually yields large future benefits.

As pertains to this book, what I'm talking about is the choice between overeating and non-overeating. Overeating affords, or appears to afford, the opportunity for greater eating pleasure in the present but brings on long-term penalty and suffering that *hinders* me in my pursuit to become the finest person I can be and create the most beneficial life I can create.

Non-overeating, on the other hand, might afford lesser eating pleasure in the present but it brings major long-term benefits, those benefits being my weight success benefits. In doing so, non-overeating *assists* me in becoming the finest person I can be and in creating the most beneficial life I can create.

Plus, it enables me to "help others do the same." And how does it enable me to help others? Many people hold the belief that how they live their life affects only them. But that's self-deceiving rationalization, and grossly incorrect. *Their life impacts every life around them,* whether they want it to or not. What they do that's not-so-good inflicts not-so-good impact on those around them. And what they do that's good bestows good on those around them. This is especially the case when one is a parent, grandparent, spouse, sibling, or close friend.

One of the most powerful ways we impact the lives of those around us, for better or for worse, is by *how* we live our life. Like it or not, *how* we live our life — including what we do and the type of person we choose to be — is a powerful *role model* that impacts the lives of others, especially children, grandchildren, siblings, and close friends.

So, for all the reasons cited above, several years ago I made the decision that for the rest of my life I would pursue non-overeating and weight control over overeating and weight non-control. I figured it would help me become the finest person I can be, create the most beneficial life I can create, and possibly help others do the same.

An Interesting Discovery

In the six-year span of creating, testing, and refining the Weight Success Method an interesting thing happened. I discovered that the amount of immediate pleasure and enjoyment derived from a particular good activity — in this case, right eating and weight control — isn't necessarily a fixed amount. I realized that the immediate enjoyment to be derived from right eating and weight control can be *expanded.* For some ways of doing that, go to the Eight Actions for Easier Calorie Control chapter (p. **82**).

Summing Up

Here in a nutshell is how healthy-weight enjoyment happens. I derive daily enjoyment and motivation from doing the five daily actions of the Weight Success Method because by doing these actions I experience enjoyment from (a) achieving and seeing daily personal progress, (b) delivering and receiving positive self-reinforcement, (c) triumphing over occasional adversity or setback, (d) being director of my eating, (e) daily focusing on an exciting ultimate goal, and (f) feeling like a winner by performing daily winning actions.

I also derive enjoyment and motivation from (g) succeeding at living in my healthy-weight range, which makes me feel like a high-achiever, (h) realizing exciting weight success benefits from living at my healthy weight, and (i) maintaining awareness of these benefits on a daily basis.

And, finally, I derive enjoyment and gratification from (j) the act of improving my self and my life by pursuing a productive activity in place of a counterproductive one, or by living in my healthy-weight range rather than outside it, and from (k) being a living example that achieving *easier* healthy-weight living is *doable*, thereby inspiring others to "give it a go."

So, the Weight Success Method is not only the easiest and most effective way to healthy-weight living, it's also probably the most enjoyable and gratifying.

Easiest **+** Most Effective **+** Most Enjoyable & Gratifying **=**
Super Weight-management Tool

One of the secrets to lifelong happiness is: Savor and mentally expand good pleasures, and ignore and avoid bad pleasures. *Good pleasures* are those pleasures that contribute to you becoming a finer person, creating a more beneficial life, and helping others do the same. *Bad pleasures* are those that detract from those three things. This applies to virtually every aspect of living, including relationships, work, recreation, exercise, and eating.

CHAPTER 18: Why the Weight Success Method Gets Your Whole Mind Involved

This chapter explains the interaction between the Weight Success Method and your mind. It could be eye-opening ... or, perhaps more correctly, mind-opening.

FOR THE PAST 50 years we've been seeking "the easy way to weight control." We've been expecting it to be some new-tech, new-pill, new-surgery, new-food, new-diet, new-exercise, new-gimmick thing. But no one has found it. One reason is, a main key to easier weight control isn't in the physical world; it's in the <u>mind</u> world. It's this: Have your *whole* mind — that is, both conscious <u>and</u> subconscious mind — involved each day in the pursuit of living in your healthy-weight range. This is a main driver of successful weight management. (For more on this, see the Whole Mind Involvement section in the Success Drivers section in Ch. **19**, page 121.)

Those who are succeeding at creating easier healthy-weight living are applying this dynamic — either knowingly or unknowingly, intentionally or non-intentionally. Those who are not yet succeeding at creating healthy-weight living are not yet applying this dynamic.

As previously stated, the easiest way to get both your conscious *and* subconscious mind involved in the daily pursuit of living in your healthy-weight range is apply the five daily actions of the Weight Success Method each day. I'm now going to explain why this is. It involves knowing how the mind — in particular, the subconscious mind — works.

How Your Mind Works: An Overview

Here's a "weird little thing" you may have not yet realized: The conception you hold of your own mind determines to a large extent the way your mind performs. Yes, it's true. So here's a conception that can lead to getting optimal performance and benefits from your mind.

View your mind as a two-part entity with each part possessing certain faculties and performing certain functions.

Further, view these two parts of your mind as working together as a team, with one part being the upfront member of the team, which we'll call *conscious mind,* and the other part being the behind-the-scenes member of the team, which we'll call *subconscious mind.* Further assume that you are a unique human being that possesses a certain unique spiritual identity, which we'll call *I* or *self.* Assume that this *I* or *self* identity resides mainly in the conscious part of your mind.

Further, assume that this conscious–subconscious mind team performs a certain set of team functions — that is, functions that the team members perform jointly.

Still further, assume that one of these team functions is a function that lies at the core of everything the team does. We'll call it *creation function.*

Further, assume that this creation function involves two processes: the first process being to identify creation opportunities and the second process being to actualize those creation opportunities that have been identified. Your conscious mind mainly works on the first process; your subconscious mind mainly works on the second one. We'll call the first process *conceptualizing* and the second process *actualizing.* Each results in a certain type of outcome. The outcome of conceptualizing is conceptualizations, or *imagined situations.* The outcome of actualizing is actualizations, or *actual situations.*

So, a main role of your conscious mind is to identify imagined situations for actualizing and a main role of your subconscious mind is to actualize these imagined situations. Or, put more concisely, a main role of your subconscious mind is to *actualize the content of your conscious mind.*

Now here's a key point. Your subconscious mind strives to perform this actualizing role automatically and diligently. It goes at it 24/7, and you can't stop it, and it continues up to the moment you die.

Most people are unaware of the actualizing function and power of their subconscious mind. This is because this activity goes on "behind the scenes," or in a realm apart from the conscious mind. But, even though it may go largely unnoticed by most people, the actualizing action of your subconscious mind has been playing a major role in determining what you do each day of your life, including what and how much you eat.

Conscious Mind Content

So, a main function of your subconscious mind is to actualize the content of your conscious mind. This leads to a question: What is the "content" of your conscious mind? Simply put, the main content of your conscious mind is desires and perspectives.

I define *desire* as an imagined situation that you'd like to see become an actual situation. We apply various labels to our desires. Some of the most common are: goal, dream, plan, aspiration, hope, wish, and, of course, desire.

I define *perspective* as a mental view or depiction you hold about some aspect of your self, your mind, your life, or the world about you. We apply various labels to our perspectives. Some of the most common are: belief, assumption, conviction, conjecture, conception, attitude, outlook, viewpoint, and, of course, perspective. Also, an interpretation of something we believe happened in the past is a form of perspective, and an expectation of something we believe will happen in the future is a form of perspective.

How Your Subconscious Mind Actualizes

So, your subconscious mind strives 24/7 to actualize the dominant desires and perspectives, or dominant imagined situations, held in your conscious

mind. This now leads to the next key question: How, exactly, does your subconscious mind actualize a particular desire or perspective (a.k.a. imagined situation) held in your conscious mind?

Answer: It does it through performing one or both of these two processes:

1 – It acts to *validate* the particular desire or perspective; and/or,

2 – It acts to *materialize* the particular desire or perspective.

To **validate** a particular desire or perspective your subconscious mind creates *thoughts* and *feelings* that align with, or corroborate, the desire or perspective.

To **materialize** a particular desire or perspective your subconscious mind creates *thoughts* and *feelings* that guide you to perform actions that lead to the creation of an actual situation that corresponds to the imagined situation (desire or perspective).

By one or both of these two processes your subconscious mind works to actualize, or "make real," any particular dominant desire or perspective (a.k.a. imagined situation) held in your conscious mind.

So, the way your subconscious mind brings about easier healthy-weight living is: When motivated to do so, it creates *thoughts* and *feelings* that steer you toward performing actions that lead to the actualization of healthy-weight living. Here are examples of how this can happen.

If, for example, you were to motivate your subconscious mind to assist you with doing more right eating and less wrong eating it would create thoughts and feelings that steer you toward right eating and away from wrong eating.

If you were to motivate it (your subconscious mind) to assist with surmounting a certain impediment to creating healthy-weight living, it would create thoughts and feelings that steer you toward sidestepping or surmounting that impediment. By the way, any fat-promoting factor, such as one of those cited in the Fat-promoting Factors list at the beginning of Chapter 20, is a surmountable "impediment."

If you were to motivate it (your subconscious mind) to assist with finding a more effective dietary program it would create thoughts and feelings that steer you toward finding or contacting such a program.

If you were to motivate it to assist with acquiring some additional know-how or information it would create thoughts and feelings that steer you toward discovering a source that contains that know-how or information.

If you were to motivate it to assist with getting a certain type of input or assistance it would create thoughts and feelings that steer you toward finding or making contact with a person or program that specializes in providing such assistance.

If you were to motivate it to assist with helping you adopt a certain perspective necessary for expediting easier healthy-weight living, it would create thoughts and feelings that steer you toward a situation that results in you gaining that perspective.

And, finally, if you were to motivate your subconscious mind to assist with squelching a certain overeating habit and replacing it with a right-eating habit, it would create thoughts and feelings that assist with subduing the overeating habit and with installing the right-eating habit. (For more on habits, go to the Key to Beating the Bad Habit of Unguided Eating chapter, page **132**.)

To sum up, to create healthy-weight living more easily you must involve your WHOLE mind, including subconscious mind, in your pursuit of healthy-weight living. Once you do this your mind applies its *full* faculties to the process. And, when your mind's full faculties are at work, healthy-weight living happens and happens *easily,* or at least more easily than you've likely ever thought possible. Coming up is an infographic that sums up this discussion on how easier healthy-weight living happens.

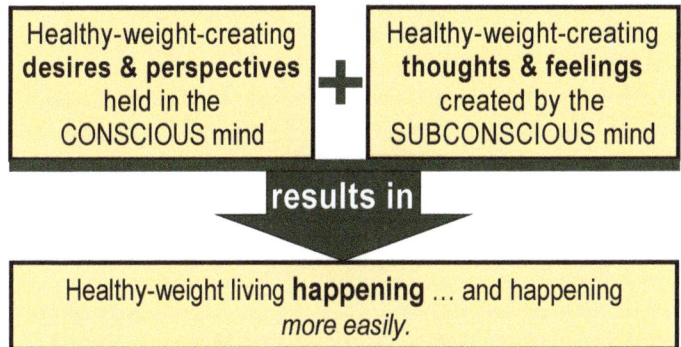

In short, the more involved your subconscious mind is in your pursuit of healthy-weight living, the easier the creation of healthy-weight living becomes.

How Easier Healthy-weight Living Happens

Healthy-weight-creating **desires & perspectives** held in the CONSCIOUS mind	**+**	Healthy-weight-creating **thoughts & feelings** created by the SUBCONSCIOUS mind

results in

Healthy-weight living **happening** ... and happening *more easily.*

So, in this section I've provided a general overview of how your mind works. Now I need to describe how your subconscious mind affects eating and weight management. For this I must add some specifics, which includes further insights into the subconscious mind and how it works.

A Perspective on the Subconscious Mind

A hundred years or so ago psychologists tended to depict the subconscious mind as a capricious, wild, inscrutable, infantile, non-directable "force." Since then other perspectives of it have emerged. Which raises the question: Of all the various perspectives of the subconscious mind, which one is the correct one? My answer: Perhaps each of them, *depending on the situation.*

How can that be? It's for this reason. My experience tells me that my subconscious mind will essentially perform in a manner consistent with the way I envision it performing. Meaning, whatever perspective I might hold of my subconscious mind, my subconscious mind pursues actualizing that perspective. This concept — if universally true, and I believe it is — carries significant ramification.

So, realizing that my subconscious mind strives to actualize, or make happen, the perspective I hold of it, I should be holding the following perspective. I view my subconscious mind as a responsive, reliable, helpful, directable, logical, creative, insightful, wise, dedicated partner perpetually committed to assisting me in becoming the finest person I can be and creating the most beneficial life I can create, and possessing vast powers and connections for answering the questions I pose to it and for actualizing the goals, directives, and expectations I submit to it. In short, I view it in the most positive, productive perspective possible. I urge you to view your subconscious mind in a similar way. I predict you'll be pleased — even amazed — by what happens.

How Your Subconscious Mind Determines What It Will Actualize

I just explained in general concept how you influence what your subconscious mind does. Now I explain it more specifically.

To decide on what it will actualize your subconscious mind takes cues from your conscious mind. These cues exist as two types: (1) deliberate communication sent from your conscious mind to your subconscious mind, and (2) observation by your subconscious mind of what your conscious mind is focusing on. I'll describe each.

Cue Type #1: DELIBERATE COMMUNICATION

Few people provide this type of cue to their subconscious mind. This is because few know about it. But sending deliberate communication to your subconscious mind is a powerful way to motivate it to do what you want it to be doing.

It's especially useful and effective when your subconscious mind has been spending years actualizing a particular undesirable situation, such as, for example, wrong eating, or overeating.

You can send deliberate communication to your subconscious mind three ways: by words, by images, by actions — otherwise called verbalization, visualization, and demonstration. Here's how each works.

Communication Way #1: Verbalization

Verbalization involves expressing a communication with words. It can be done either by speaking aloud, including in a whisper, or by "speaking silently in your mind." The five main types of verbalization messages are feedback, self-

reinforcement, directive, depiction, and feeling expression. I'll describe each.

Feedback. *Feedback* is information about past performance that enables us to achieve or maintain desired performance in the future. Along with being communicated verbally, feedback can also be expressed numerically and graphically. In the Weight Success Method timely feedback mainly derives from the daily weighing done in Daily Action 1. It also can derive from any of the tools presented in Ch. **27** (p. 154).

Self-reinforcement. When you convey appreciation and thanks to your self — or your mind — for having performed a certain desired action, or for having actualized a certain imagined desired situation, we call it *verbal self-reinforcement.* To add strength to the reinforcement we often include instructions to keep on doing the desired action. Our special label for this type of reinforcement communication is Thank You, Keep It Up message. A main example is the Thank You, Keep It Up message used in Daily Action 2A. It's also used in the Guided Eating Process of Daily Action 5–Guided Eating.

Directive. When the communication takes the form of an instruction, order, or request conveyed to your subconscious mind we call it a *directive.* The Weight Success Method makes powerful use of directive-type communication. A main example is the Weight Success Benefits Directive used in Daily Action 3–Benefits Directive. Also, directive-type communication is used in the Guided Eating Process of Daily Action 5–Guided Eating.

Depiction. A *depiction* is a word description of a particular imagined situation. Typically it's of an imagined situation you want your subconscious mind to actualize (which it does by creating an actual situation that corresponds to the imagined situation). The Weight Success Method makes extensive powerful use of depiction statements. A main example is the Healthy-weight Goal Statement described in Daily Action 4–Goal. It's also sometimes used in the Guided Eating Process of Daily Action 5.

Feeling Expression. When a verbalization conveys how you feel about a certain situation we call it a *feeling expression.* This type of communication tells your subconscious mind how you feel, or want to be feeling, about a situation. Feeling expressions that promote right eating and living in one's healthy-weight range occur within the five daily actions of the Weight Success Method.

Communication Way #2: Visualization

Visualization involves expressing a communication with images, or mental pictures. It comes in two forms: still image and moving image. A still image is a mental picture of a single situation or thing; basically a mental photograph. A moving image is a mental picture of a moving action or series of events; basically a mental movie or video. The mental movie can be in either third person or first person. In third person you're viewing yourself acting in the movie. In first person you're an actor in the process of making the movie. Some persons believe the first-person approach is more effective than the third-person.

Typically a visualization is of an imagined situation you want your subconscious mind to actualize, which it does by creating an actual situation that corresponds to the imagined situation. In the Weight Success Method you're sending a visualization communication to your subconscious mind every time you visualize the realization of one of your weight success benefits or visualize yourself being at your healthy weight.

Communication Way #3: Demonstration (or Acting As-if)

Demonstration — also called **acting as-if** — involves communicating with actions. The actions include both physical actions <u>and</u> mental actions. Precisely defined, acting as-if is the act of holding in mind an assumption that a particular situation presently exists or is in the process of coming about, *and then conducting your thinking, feelings, and actions in accordance with that assumption.* Put another way, it's doing a "real-life role-play" of a situation you want to exist or have happen.

Expressing a particular imagined situation via demonstration or acting as-if is a little known but very powerful means of communicating to your subconscious mind what you want it to be doing. It's used throughout the Weight Success Method. For more on acting as-if, go to the Acting As-if section in Startup Action 5 (p. 17).

Three Communication-enhancing Factors

Three factors determine the degree of impact your deliberate communications of cue type #1 have on motivating your subconscious mind to actualize a particular imagined situation. These three factors are: variety, frequency, and intensity.

Variety. The more ways you communicate a particular imagined situation to your subconscious mind, the more diligently your subconscious mind works at actualizing the particular imagined situation. In doing the five daily actions of the Weight Success Method you use *all three* of the ways I just described — that is, verbalization, visualization, and demonstration or acting as-if.

Frequency. The more frequently you express a particular imagined situation to your subconscious mind, the more diligently your subconscious mind works at actualizing the particular imagined situation. In doing the five daily actions of the Weight Success Method you express certain imagined situations — mainly, right eating and healthy-weight living — *numerous* times throughout each day.

Lesser FREQUENCY of right-eating communication by the **conscious** mind — results in — lesser ASSISTANCE with creating right eating & healthy-weight living by the **subconscious** mind.	**&**	Greater FREQUENCY of right-eating communication by the **conscious** mind — results in — greater ASSISTANCE with creating right eating & healthy-weight living by the **subconscious** mind.

Intensity. The more intensely, or emotionally, you express a particular imagined situation to your subconscious mind, the more diligently your subconscious mind works at actualizing the particular imagined situation. When you do the five daily actions of the Weight Success Method you express certain healthy-weight-creating communications with emotional intensity at various times every day.

So to sum up, to maximize the impact of deliberate communication on motivating your subconscious mind to actualize a particular imagined situation — such as right eating and healthy-weight living — you do three things:

1. Communicate in *multiple* ways the imagined situation you want actualized;

2. Communicate *frequently* the imagined situation you want actualized;

3. Communicate with *emotional intensity* (at times) the imagined situation you want actualized.

What this means is: When you'd like your mind to diligently pursue actualizing a particular imagined situation or goal — such as the goal of living in your healthy-weight range the rest of your life — make this goal a highly important priority in the "eyes" of your subconscious mind. To do this, (a) communicate this priority to your subconscious mind in multiple ways, and (b) communicate it numerous times every day, and (c) at least some times every day communicate it with emotional intensity. Doing the five daily actions of the Weight Success Method each day results in you doing these three things as regards achieving the goal of healthy-weight living.

But, as powerful as deliberate communication is for directing one's subconscious mind, most persons never use it. So for these people how does their subconscious mind determine what it will actualize? It's by cue type #2.

Cue Type #2: *CONSCIOUS MIND FOCUS*

Although only a few people use cue type #1, cue type #2 operates with everyone. This cue consists of what the conscious mind regularly focuses on. It works like this.

There are hundreds of possible imagined situations your subconscious mind could pursue

actualizing. But it will actualize only a few at a time. That's because if it tried to pursue actualizing hundreds of imagined situations at the same time it would result in you being an ineffectual person living a confused, chaotic life.

So, how does your subconscious mind determine which imagined situations it will pursue actualizing? Answer: It strives to actualize those imagined situations that appear to it to be *most important* to you. And, how does it determine which imagined situations are most important to you? It observes what your conscious mind spends the *most time* focusing on — that is, thinking about, talking about, pursuing, and enjoyably doing. In short, as regards any particular imagined situation, *your subconscious mind assumes that greater amount of focus time means greater importance, and lesser amount means lesser importance.*

As a result, those imagined situations that receive the most amount of conscious mind focus time get the most "actualization effort" by your subconscious mind, and those situations that receive the least amount of conscious mind focus time get the least "actualization effort" by your subconscious mind. So how does this apply to the pursuit of healthy-weight living? It works like this.

Lesser FOCUS on right eating & healthy-weight living by the **conscious** mind — results in — lesser ASSISTANCE with creating right eating & healthy-weight living by the **subconscious** mind.	**&**	Greater FOCUS on right eating & healthy-weight living by the **conscious** mind — results in — greater ASSISTANCE with creating right eating & healthy-weight living by the **subconscious** mind.

What's more, if two imagined situations happen to be mutually exclusive — that is, only one can be actualized and not both — your subconscious mind will pursue actualizing the one that appears to it to be the most important of the two, and will ignore actualizing the other one. For example, right eating and wrong eating, or non-overeating and overeating, are mutually exclusive. So which one will your subconscious mind choose to actualize? *It will pursue actualizing the one that's receiving the greatest amount of conscious mind focus time,* or is being thought about, talked about, pursued, and enjoyed the greatest amount of time — and will ignore pursuing the opposing imagined situation.

All of which means, if you've been spending more time focusing on wrong eating than on right eating, your subconscious mind has been concluding that wrong eating is more important to you than right eating and, so, it has been focusing on actualizing wrong eating and ignoring actualizing right eating. Such a situation makes doing daily right eating nearly impossible, at least on a sustained basis, and makes doing daily wrong eating inevitable. This, by the way, explains why most folks are engaging in daily overeating.

It also explains why some are successful at losing weight but fail at keeping it off. While pursuing weight loss they have their conscious mind focusing intently each day on actualizing their weight-loss goal. But, once they achieve that goal they conclude that it's "job done" and, in doing so, they let their conscious mind cease its daily focus on weight management. This results in their subconscious mind ceasing to perform weight management activities. Which results in them failing to keep off the weight they lost. In short, they succeeded at weight loss because they focused daily on weight loss; they fail at weight maintenance because they *don't* focus daily on weight maintenance. (For more, go to the Part 1–A section of Chapter 1, page 7.)

So, to summarize, if your conscious mind has been spending years focusing on wrong eating, your subconscious mind has been spending years concluding that wrong eating is what you want it to be actualizing, or bringing about. In such a situation, the easiest, quickest, most effective way to change your eating habits from wrong eating to right eating, or from overeating to non-overeating, is do two things:

1 – *Increase FOCUS.* Spend more conscious mind time focusing on right eating than on wrong eating — that is, spend more time thinking about, talking about, pursuing, and enjoyably doing right eating than wrong eating (this is cue type #2); and

2 – *Increase COMMUNICATION.* Send deliberate daily communications to your subconscious mind — specifically, communications that motivate it to (a) pursue right eating and avoid wrong eating and (b) pursue living in your healthy-weight range (cue type #1).

Or, in other words, use *both* cue types to motivate your subconscious mind to actualize your goal of easily engaging in right eating and living in your healthy-weight range.

Why the Five Daily Actions Work

One of the reasons the five daily actions of the Weight Success Method work and work easily is because these actions do two things: (1) they send *multiple kinds* of powerful healthy-weight-promoting communications *numerous times* each day to your subconscious mind, with some of these communications being delivered with *emotional* intensity and (2) they cause you to spend *more time* focusing on right eating than on wrong eating, and *more time* focusing on living in your healthy-weight range.

In the "eyes" of your subconscious mind, all this makes right eating to be more important than wrong eating, and makes living in your healthy-weight range to be very, *very* important. This, in turn, motivates your subconscious mind to actualize right eating and healthy-weight living for the rest of your life. And, by your subconscious mind doing this, healthy-weight living happens easily — or way more easily than you've ever imagined.

In short, by doing the Weight Success Method each day you each day involve your *whole* mind — that is, both conscious <u>and</u> subconscious mind — in the pursuit of living in your healthy-weight range. This results in your mind steering you away from overeating and toward non-overeating which, in turn, results in creating healthy-weight living for life. The following infographic depicts how this works.

A Reason Why the Weight Success Method Works

Doing the Weight Success Method each day

creates → **Increased right-eating FOCUS by the conscious mind**

&

creates → **Increased right-eating COMMUNICATION delivered to subconscious mind**

creates ↓   *creates* ↓

Increased right-eating ACTION by the whole mind — including the subconscious mind — which results in achieving right eating and healthy-weight living for life

Right-eating FOCUS = Time spent thinking about, talking about, pursuing, and enjoyably doing right eating and healthy-weight living.

Right-eating COMMUNICATION = Communication that tells your subconscious mind to steer you toward right eating and healthy-weight living.

Three Concepts to Keep in Mind

1 – The more daily **focus** you put on right eating and healthy-weight living <u>and</u> the more right-eating **communication** you express, the more vigorously your mind — including subconscious mind — works at bringing about right eating and healthy-weight living.

2 – The more vigorously your subconscious mind works at bringing about right eating and healthy-weight living, the *easier* it becomes for you to achieve right eating and healthy-weight living.

3 – It doesn't matter how strong your overeating habits might be, there is a point at which a certain amount of right-eating **focus** and right-eating **communication** will result in your subconscious mind installing right-eating habits and urges that overwhelm and surmount the overeating habits and urges, and also surmount any fat-promoting factor that might apply to you or your life.

> Do the **Five Daily Actions** <u>every</u> day . . .
> and **Lifelong Weight Success** will be <u>Yours</u>.

Typically takes <u>less than</u> **8** minutes of dedicated time per day.

CHAPTER 19: Success Drivers and Success Killers in Depth

Doing the Weight Success Method installs and maintains success *drivers* in your weight success pursuit — and also diminishes success *killers*.

CHAPTER 1 lists 19 vital elements for succeeding at weight control and healthy-weight living (p. 10). We dubbed them *success drivers*. This chapter 19 describes them in depth.

Success Driver 1:
ACHIEVEMENT GOAL

This driver involves identifying a desired ultimate outcome pertaining to a particular pursuit.

We call this desired ultimate outcome *achievement goal*. The vital function of an achievement goal is it provides an imagined desired situation that's held in the mind. When one holds an imagined desired situation (a.k.a. achievement goal) in mind it triggers one's mind, including one's subconscious mind, to create thoughts and feelings that guide one to perform actions that lead to achievement of the goal — or, in short, that lead to creation of an <u>actual</u> situation that corresponds to the <u>imagined desired</u> situation.

As pertains to your weight success pursuit, the Achievement Goal is: *To be the person of your healthy weight and be healthy, happy, and doing great.* (Note: Your *healthy weight* is every weight in your desired healthy-weight range.) We call this the Healthy-weight Goal. More on healthy-weight goal is described in Daily Action 4 (p. **34**).

Success Driver 2:
FAILURE CAUSE AWARENESS

This driver involves recognizing the root activity or factor that causes setback — and perhaps failure — in a particular pursuit.

As pertains to the pursuit of weight control and healthy-weight living, the root activity causing failure is: *Overperformance* of a certain three-action process, the process of:

1 – Opening one's mouth;

2 – Inserting a piece of metabolizable calorie-containing food into one's mouth; and

3 – Swallowing the piece of food.

Overperformance of this process is the <u>real</u> cause and <u>only</u> cause of (a) weight gain and (b) weight control failure. And, it's *totally controllable* by each person. Recognizing this is the first step to succeeding at weight control and healthy-weight living. (More on failure cause awareness is described in Startup Action 1, page **14**.)

> **Note:** In this book the word *eating* encompasses drinking. And the word *food* encompasses beverages. So wherever you read the terms *eating* and *food* know that it includes drinking and beverages.

Success Driver 3:
GOAL-ACHIEVING MINDSET

This driver involves holding a mindset of goal-promoting views and beliefs, and acting as-if these views and beliefs are a true depiction of reality.

Along with working to actualize important goals, your mind — including subconscious mind — also works to actualize your dominant views and beliefs, especially those beliefs you *act on* each day, or act as-if are a true depiction of reality.

As pertains to your healthy-weight living Achievement Goal — there are two types of beliefs: goal-promoting and goal-hindering. Beliefs that steer you toward accomplishment of the goal we call *goal-promoting beliefs*. Beliefs that steer you away from goal accomplishment we call *goal-hindering beliefs*.

The more goal-promoting beliefs you hold in mind and act as-if are true the more your subconscious mind works at creating thoughts and feelings that steer you toward goal achievement.

> More on weight success mindset is described in Startup Action 5 (p. **15**).

Mindset → Actions → Outcome

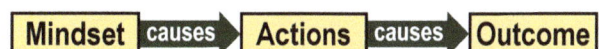

Mindset causes **Actions** causes **Outcome**

Success Driver 4:
ENJOYMENT OF PROCESS

This driver involves identifying or creating a process, or set of actions, by which daily enjoyment is derived from daily pursuit and realization of the Achievement Goal.

When you find the activity involved in achieving a goal to be fun, enjoyable, or otherwise gratifying to do, it makes it easier for you to accomplish the goal because you automatically put more time, focus, and energy into the process. So, as much as feasible you should strive to make the goal-achieving process of healthy-weight living to be fun, enjoyable, and/or gratifying. Yes, it *is* possible to do. To learn how, go to the Why the Weight Success Method is Enjoyable chapter (p. **103**.)

Success Driver 5:
MOTIVATING REASON

This driver involves identifying the main reason or reasons for pursuing the Achievement Goal.

As pertains to your weight success pursuit, the "main reasons" you have for doing it are the benefits you gain from living in your healthy-weight range. We call these benefits *weight success benefits.* The more clearly and frequently you envision them, the more good reason you have for striving to achieve lifelong weight success. Which, in turn, translates into greater daily motivation for living in your healthy-weight range.

More on weight success benefits is described in Startup Action 3 (p. 15) and in Ch. **7** (p. 60).

Success Driver 6:
MANDATE DECISION

This driver involves deciding that accomplishment of the Achievement Goal is a *mandatory* feature of one's life.

As pertains to your weight success pursuit, you must make the firm decision that living at your healthy weight is a <u>non</u>-optional, <u>will</u>-do, <u>must</u>-have aspect of your existence. You must make this decision and commit to realizing it. Why? Because, if you don't you'll almost certainly fail at creating healthy-weight living.

Success Driver 7:
FEEDBACK SYSTEM

This driver involves identifying or creating a way of measuring daily performance pertaining to realization of the Achievement Goal.

As pertains to your weight success pursuit, the most powerful daily feedback system you can employ is: *daily weighing with an accurate bathroom scale.*

What do you do with this daily feedback? When the daily weight reading is a *desired* reading you deliver positive reinforcement to your self — that is, to your mind. When the reading is an *undesired* reading you respond by taking immediate corrective action.

An accurate daily weighing system that's *properly* used <u>each</u> day is the <u>most</u> powerful healthy-weight creation tool there is.

More on feedback, reinforcement, and correction is described in Daily Action 1 (p. **22**), in Daily Action 2A (p. **23**), and in Daily Action 2B (p. **26**).

Success Driver 8:
REMINDER SYSTEM

This driver involves installing a failproof reminder system.

As pertains to your weight success pursuit, this is a system that never fails to remind you each day to apply your preferred dietary program and daily action plan. This is critical for healthy-weight living success. Why? Because, failure to *remember* to do what one should be doing is a major cause of project failure.

More on failproof reminder system is in Startup Action 8 (p. **20**).

Success Driver 9:
GOAL-ACHIEVING KNOWLEDGE

This driver involves acquiring knowledge vital to achievement of the Achievement Goal.

As pertains to creating weight success, the main goal-achieving knowledge you'll need for doing that is contained in Chapter 1. So, the way you acquire vital goal-achieving knowledge for healthy-weight living is: Read Chapter 1. Also, depending on the Preferred Dietary Program that you select, you might find it helpful to familiarize yourself with any special information pertaining to that program.

Success Driver 10: ESSENTIAL SUCCESS ACTIONS

This driver involves making sure the essential success actions for realizing the Achievement Goal are done each day.

Some success actions are "helpful to do." Others are "critical to do every day" — meaning, if they're not done, the likelihood of achieving the Achievement Goal is greatly diminished. We call them *essential success actions.* It's imperative that you do the essential success actions every day.

What are the essential success actions in your weight success journey? They're Daily Actions 1–5 of the Weight Success Method.

Doing essential success actions performs two vital functions. First, it maintains your *daily focus and motivation.* Second, it creates ongoing *daily progress* toward goal achievement. It's worth noting that doing essential success actions each day is at the core of virtually every successful significant personal pursuit.

So, *every day* for the rest of your life do the essential success actions aimed at achieving the goal of lifelong healthy-weight living. This is one of the ultimate keys to succeeding at creating lifelong weight success. Doing the Weight Success Method *makes this happen.*

Success Driver 11: DESIRE

This driver involves holding strong daily desire for realizing the Achievement Goal.

It also involves each day fueling this desire by calling to mind the reason for (or benefits to be derived from) goal achievement. Typically, the bigger the goal, the more desire is needed for accomplishing it.

> Other terms for "desire" are passion, eagerness, determination.

As pertains to your weight success pursuit, this means if you want to succeed at realizing your Healthy-weight Goal, you need to hold *strong daily desire* for its accomplishment. If you don't you'll likely drift away from pursuing the goal and end up quitting. So, how do you hold strong daily desire for achieving your healthy-weight goal? You do these three things.

Firstly, you decide that achieving your healthy-weight goal is a *mandatory* feature of your existence.

Secondly, you hold the assumption — and also act as-if — achieving the goal is doable (and perhaps even *easily* doable).

Thirdly, each day you call to mind the *benefits* of goal achievement, and you visualize how good your life will be with these benefits. And, you hold the belief that these benefits are in the process of coming about each day.

The more times you think about, or visualize, the benefits of accomplishing your healthy-weight goal, the more you fuel your daily desire to achieve the goal. And, the stronger your daily desire is, the more your mind — including subconscious mind — assists with goal realization by creating thoughts and feelings that steer you toward that realization. In your weight success journey, we call these benefits *weight success benefits.*

> More on weight success benefits is described in the Weight Success Benefits in Detail chapter (p. **60**).

Success Driver 12: FOCUS

This driver involves each day focusing on the Achievement Goal.

Or, put another way, it involves each day thinking about, talking about, pursuing, and/or deriving enjoyment from the accomplishment or progressive realization of the goal.

The more time you spend focusing on, or paying attention to, a particular goal, the more importance your subconscious mind attaches to that goal. And, the more importance your subconscious mind attaches to the goal, the more it acts to create thoughts and feelings that steer you toward accomplishment of the goal.

So, as pertains to your weight success journey, you must spend time each day *focusing* on the ongoing realization of your healthy-weight goal. A main purpose of doing the Weight Success Method is to cause this daily focusing to happen.

> For more on focus, go to the "Cue Type #2: Conscious Mind Focus" section, p. **114**.

Success Driver 13: SELF-COMMUNICATION

This driver involves sending goal-promoting communications to one's self each day.

Communications you send to your self we call *self-communications.* They are communications you send to your mind — including your subconscious mind. Self-communications are delivered three ways: verbalization, visualization, and demonstration or acting as-if. These communications tell your mind what you want it to be doing.

A main type of self-communication is goal-promoting communication. A *goal-promoting communication* is a communication that tells your mind what it should be doing in way of assisting with achieving a certain goal. The purpose of this communication is to trigger your subconscious mind to create thoughts and feelings that make goal realization happen, or happen more easily. The more goal-promoting communication you send, the more you motivate your mind — including subconscious mind — to assist with goal achievement.

As pertains to your weight success pursuit, goal-promoting communications trigger your subconscious mind to create thoughts and feelings that guide you to performing right eating actions and to achieving your goal of lifelong healthy-weight living. A main purpose of doing the Weight Success Method is to cause goal-promoting communications to occur. (Note: In the Weight Success Method, another term for goal-promoting communication is "right-eating communication.")

> For more on self-communication, go to "Cue Type #1: Deliberate Communication" section, p. **112**.

Success Driver 14: PROGRESS TRACKING AND RESPONSE

This driver involves tracking one's daily performance and providing immediate positive response.

For tracking progress one needs feedback. *Feedback* is information that depicts past performance. When the feedback depicts *desired* past performance — a.k.a. progress — you deliver immediate self-reinforcement. When the feedback depicts *undesired* past performance you initiate immediate corrective action. Each is a positive response that expedites goal achievement. Also, for progress tracking to be optimally useful it must be timely. Meaning, for example, daily progress tracking (a.k.a. daily feedback) is usually more useful than, say, weekly progress tracking. In your weight success pursuit, the weight number you get from Daily Action 1 (daily weighing) is the most useful tracking feedback in your weight success journey.

> For other examples of progress measuring tools, go to the Handy Extra Tools chapter (p. **154**).

Success Driver 15: SELF-REINFORCEMENT

This driver involves delivering reinforcement — such as appreciation and praise — to one's self after daily progress happens, and telling oneself to keep up the good work.

What is reinforcement? The act of giving someone something they like as a response or consequence for performing a certain action or creating a certain result is known as *reinforcement* — a.k.a. positive reinforcement. When that "someone" is our self, or our mind, we call it *self-reinforcement.*

When you deliver self-reinforcement, or appreciation and praise, to your mind — in particular, to your subconscious mind — after it provides assistance with creating a certain desired performance or result, it motivates your mind to continue providing that assistance in the future. In short, desired performance plus reinforcement creates more desired performance. (More on reinforcement is described in Daily Action 2A, page **23**.)

Success Driver 16:
SETBACK SURMOUNTING

This driver involves holding a productive perspective whenever there's a setback, and also enacting immediate corrective action and converting the setback into a progress action.

In every major endeavor — including the pursuit of weight success — setbacks occur. Success depends on the response to these setbacks. When one responds in a counterproductive way it results in turmoil, frustration, and defeat. But when one responds in a productive way it results in (a) learning from the setback and (b) converting it into a progress action.

> More on setback surmounting is described in Daily Action 2B (p. **26**) and also in the Setback Reversal Made Easier chapter (p. **68**).

Success Driver 17:
PERSISTENCE

This driver involves persistently pursuing the Achievement Goal, and pressing on in spite of challenges, setbacks, or discouragement.

The realization that unceasing persistence is a key to achieving any major goal isn't new; it has been around for decades. Many names have been used for it. Examples include: persistence, perseverance, determination, tenacity, doggedness, pressing on, stick-to-it-ness, gutting-it-out, and grit.

So, as pertains to your weight success journey, *don't give up.* Instead, each day press on toward accomplishment of your worthy healthy-weight goal. If you do this, along with doing the Weight Success Method, you *will* achieve your goal.

Success Driver 18:
GOAL-ACHIEVING RELATIONSHIPS

This driver involves discovering and building relationships that encourage and assist one in accomplishing the Achievement Goal.

This success driver does not apply to every type of pursuit. But it can be made to apply to most. And, when it is applied it can be powerful.

As pertains to your weight success pursuit, productive relationships can expedite realization of your healthy-weight goal at least two ways. First, they can be a means for sustaining motivation and productive mindset during the pursuit of the goal. Second, they can be a means for obtaining valuable assistance — such as, advice, know-how, key resources — that can be helpful in expediting goal achievement. This assistance can be obtained from productive interaction with people and also God.

Lastly, it's important to note that one might find it helpful to downplay relationships or interactions that run counter to achievement of one's life-enhancing goals.

> For more on relationships, see the Escaping Schadenfreude chapter (p. **101**) and the relationships section (p. **140**) of the How the Weight Success Method Enhances Your Life Journey chapter, and the Three Steps to Getting Input from God section (p. **97**).

Success Driver 19:
WHOLE-MIND INVOLVEMENT

This driver involves having one's whole mind — that is, both conscious <u>and</u> subconscious mind — involved each day in the pursuit of the Achievement Goal.

As pertains to your weight success pursuit, when your whole mind is involved each day in the pursuit of your healthy-weight goal something powerful happens. It results in your subconscious mind stepping up and assisting with the achievement of that goal. Your subconscious mind does this by creating thoughts and feelings that make you more effective at (a) surmounting obstacles and (b) obtaining what you need for goal achievement. Which means, the more involved your subconscious mind is in the achievement of your healthy-weight goal, the easier the achievement of that goal becomes.

When your subconscious mind is working to steer you toward living in your healthy-weight range it creates healthy-weight-promoting thoughts and feelings that guide you toward healthy-weight living. This results in you doing right eating and weight control. Conversely, when your subconscious mind *isn't* involved in steering you toward living in your healthy-weight range it *doesn't* create healthy-weight-promoting thoughts and feelings. This results in overeating and weight gain. And, when you cycle between the two — that is, your subconscious mind is involved for a period, stops being involved for a period, starts again, stops again — you lose weight, gain weight, lose weight, gain weight — a condition called yo-yo dieting.

I call all that *The Whole-mind Dynamic of Healthy-weight Living.* Most people are unaware of this dynamic. So, they don't realize that a main success driver of healthy-weight living is:

Have your WHOLE mind — that is, both conscious and subconscious mind — involved *each day* in the pursuit of living in your healthy-weight range.

As an infographic the Whole-mind Dynamic looks like this.

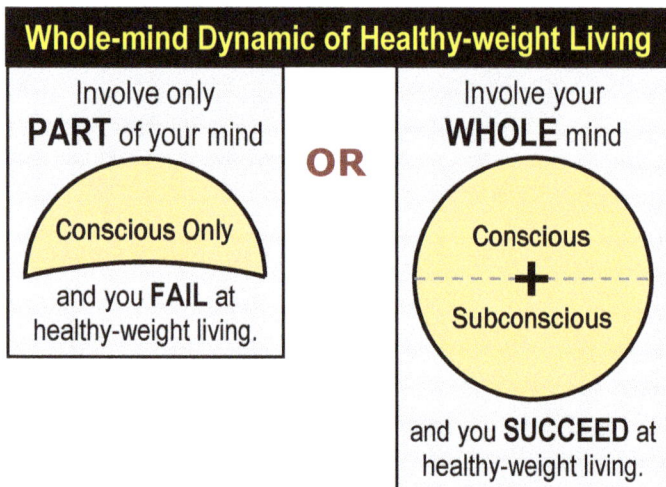

Whole-mind Dynamic of Healthy-weight Living

Involve only **PART** of your mind — Conscious Only — and you **FAIL** at healthy-weight living.

OR

Involve your **WHOLE** mind — Conscious **+** Subconscious — and you **SUCCEED** at healthy-weight living.

So, be sure to include this Success Driver 19 in your weight success journey.

Does the thought of "having your whole mind involved each day in the pursuit of living in your healthy-weight range" seem complex or hard to do? Well, good news, it's not. It's actually simple and easy **if** you do this: Apply the Weight Success Method. Doing the five daily actions of the Weight Success Method typically takes less than eight minutes a day. Yet it causes you to have your WHOLE mind involved *each day* in the pursuit of

healthy-weight living. And this, in turn, *greatly* increases the likelihood of you succeeding at creating healthy-weight living for life.

> For more on whole mind involvement, go to the Why the Weight Success Method Gets Your Whole Mind Involved chapter (p. **109**).

Societal Impact of the Whole Mind Dynamic

Here's how the Whole-mind Dynamic applies society-wide. Those few people who are living in their healthy-weight range likely have their *whole* mind — or both conscious and subconscious mind — involved each day in the pursuit of healthy-weight living. This involvement of their whole mind comes about either intentionally or non-intentionally or both.

Conversely, most of those people who are continuing to live above their healthy-weight range do *not* have their whole mind involved each day in the pursuit of healthy-weight living.

What's more, those who lost weight *while* dieting and then gained the weight back *after* the dieting had their whole mind involved *during* the dieting but stopped having their whole mind involved *after* the dieting!

Trying to achieve your biggest goals using only the "conscious half" of your mind is like trying to take a canoe trip using "half a canoe." Applying the Weight Success Method is the easiest way to ensure you're taking your whole canoe on your weight success journey.

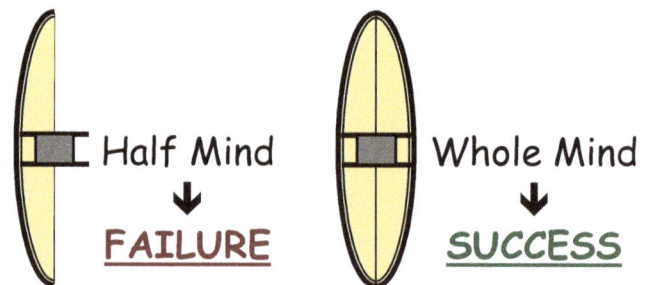

Half Mind → FAILURE

Whole Mind → SUCCESS

21 Success Killers

This section examines the flip-side of the weight success coin. It describes 21 activities that can promote failure at weight control and healthy-weight living or, at least, cause a person to experience needless hassle and difficulty in achieving weight control. We dub these 21 activities *success killers.*

Put simply, the easiest, most effective way to succeed at healthy-weight living is this: (a) *include* as many success drivers as you can and (b) *exclude* or avoid as many success killers as you can. Doing this expands to the max the likelihood of creating lifelong healthy-weight living.

You'll note that many of these success killers are an "opposite action" to a success driver. So, doing the particular success driver automatically eliminates the opposing success killer.

Here are the 21 success killers you should strive to avoid:

1 – Believing that there's "no problem" in being "a little bit" overweight. ✏ This success killer causes one to do nothing when only slightly overweight. This is a problem, because being slightly overweight usually is the first step to becoming *a lot* overweight. So avoid this success killer by eliminating overweightness in any amount.

2 – Believing that there are factors beyond one's control that are making one overeat and gain weight. Or, put another way, it's holding the belief that weight control is impossible. ✏ This success killer causes one to avoid pursuing weight control because it promotes the rationalization that no matter what one does there are uncontrollable factors that will make one fail at weight control. So avoid this success killer by realizing that you have full control of your healthy-weight living destiny. (For the real cause of weight gain, see Success Driver 2, page 117.)

3 – Believing that weight control is hard to do. ✏ This factor isn't as harmful as #2, but it's still a weight control saboteur. It causes one to procrastinate on weight control because humans shun hardship, at least as involves eating. Plus it's self-fulfilling. When we believe something will be hard to do our mind often ensures that it is. How so? It's because our subconscious mind automatically creates thoughts, feelings, and actions that align with or actualize our dominant views and beliefs. So avoid this success killer by realizing that most likely weight control is easier than you ever imagined it could be.

4 – Believing that doing weight control is unpleasant and enjoyment-robbing. ✏ Weight control requires making changes, and change is often unpleasant, especially when it involves giving up a daily pleasure. This causes one to procrastinate on weight control because most of us don't like losing a daily pleasure. So avoid this success killer by realizing that weight control can actually be pleasurable and enjoyable.

> Truth is, when done the right way, weight control and healthy-weight living creates *more* enjoyment than is lost — meaning, it can be an enjoyment *builder.* For more on this, see Ch. **17** (p. 103) and also the Right Eating section in Startup Action 6 (p. 18).

5 – Believing that lack of exercise causes overweightness and that more exercise is a requirement for creating weight control and weight success. ✏ This success killer causes one to fail at weight control because it blinds one to the real cause of weight gain (for that, see Success Driver 2, page **117**). So avoid this success killer by realizing that even though exercise is a beneficial activity a lack of exercise is not the cause of overweightness and more exercise is not the guaranteed cure.

> One of the biggest false assumptions of our society is that weight gain and overweightness is a result of too little exercise. This is a myth. Weight gain can occur even with a lot of exercise. Conversely, weight control and healthy-weight living can happen even with no exercise.

6 – Not realizing that the first step to weight-control success is *mindset* change. ✏ Overweightness is a physical condition. But the first step to conquering overweightness doesn't involve taking a physical action. Rather, it involves taking a *mental* action, or making a change in one's mindset — that is, a change in one's views and beliefs regarding eating and weight control. Without this first step, lifelong weight control and healthy-weight living usually don't happen. So avoid this success killer by making one of your first steps be the adoption of a healthy-weight-promoting mindset. (For more on this, see Startup Action 5, page 15.)

7 – Not identifying one's desired healthy-weight range. Or, put another way, it's using a single weight number as one's target, or goal. ✎ Here's how this success killer undermines weight control. By having a single weight number as one's target, or goal, it makes one be a weight management loser on many days. This, in turn, tends to make one quit the pursuit of weight control. To enable yourself to be a weight management winner on most days, define a reasonable weight *range* as your goal. (For more on this, see Startup Action 2, page 14.)

8 – Not deciding that healthy-weight living is *mandatory*. ✎ If you don't make the firm decision that healthy-weight living is a <u>non</u>-optional, <u>will</u>-do, <u>must</u>-have aspect of your existence, you will give up and quit as soon as the first inevitable little setback or discouragement arises. So avoid this success killer by deciding that healthy-weight living is a *mandatory* feature of your existence. (For more on this, see Startup Action 4, page 15.)

9 – Not identifying one's weight success benefits. ✎ If you don't have strong, ample reason for pursuing weight control and healthy-weight living, you will lack full motivation for pursuing it. And, lacking full motivation will result in less than full results. So avoid this success killer by identifying all your weight success benefits. (For more on this, see Startup Action 3, page 15, and also the Weight Success Benefits in Detail chapter, page 60.)

10 – Not identifying healthy-weight calorie consumption as the top priority of eating. ✎ There are two mutually exclusive top priorities in eating: (1) eating pleasure maximization and

(2) healthy-weight calorie consumption. The first priority leads to overeating and weight gain. The second leads to non-overeating and healthy-weight living. To succeed at creating lifelong healthy-weight living one must embrace healthy-weight calorie consumption as the top priority. So avoid this success killer by adopting healthy-weight calorie consumption as your foremost eating priority. (For more on this, see Startup Action 6, page 17.)

11 – Not adopting a dietary program that fits *you*. ✎ To achieve optimal success at weight control and healthy-weight living, most persons must apply a preferred dietary program. Further, this program must be applied fully. Finally, the easiest dietary program to apply fully is one that fits *you*, or that best fits your personal needs, desires, and lifestyle. So avoid this success killer by adopting a dietary program that best fits *you.* (For more on this, see Startup Action 7, page 19.)

12 – Not remembering to do what one needs to be doing every day. ✎ You can have the best daily action plan in the world. But if you often fail to remember to apply it, all is lost. So, as pertains to your healthy-weight living daily action plan (which is the Weight Success Method), you need to have a failproof reminder mechanism that guarantees that you remember to do the Method each day. So avoid this success killer by installing a failproof reminder mechanism. (For more on this, see Startup Action 8, page 20.)

13 – Not getting daily feedback derived from daily weighing. ✎ Without having *daily* feedback on one's body weight one lacks information for dispensing daily self-reinforcement and for taking daily corrective action when needed. And, without daily self-reinforcement and corrective action, one's weight control and healthy-weight living effectiveness suffers. So avoid this success killer by correctly weighing yourself *every* day. (For more on daily weighing, see Daily Action 1, page 22.)

14 – Not keeping healthy-weight living a *top* priority. ✎ To succeed at any significant pursuit — including healthy-weight living — achieving success at the pursuit must be a top priority. If it's not, your mind — including subconscious mind — won't vigorously contribute the thoughts and feelings needed for creating that success. So avoid this success killer by holding healthy-weight living as a top priority in your life.

15 — Not responding to setbacks in a productive way. ❧ In every major pursuit, including the pursuit of healthy-weight living, setbacks happen. When one fails to respond productively to setbacks something bad happens. Discouragement and continued bad performance set in, and eventually one quits. So avoid this success killer by responding productively to every setback. (For more on this, see Daily Action 2B, page 26.)

16 — Not ignoring negative comments by others. ❧ Receiving negative, discouraging comment from others — especially those close to you — can be a demotivator and major drag on one's weight control efforts. So, if you happen to be the target of such comment, do your best to ignore it. (For more on this, see the Escaping Schadenfreude chapter, page 101.)

17 — Not doing guided eating most of the time. Or, put another way, doing <u>unguided</u> eating most of the time. ❧ In terms of control, there are two types of eating: unguided and guided. Unguided eating leads to overeating and weight gain. Guided eating leads to weight control and healthy-weight living. To avoid unguided eating apply the Guided Eating Process described in Daily Action 5 (p. 35).

18 — Not viewing healthy-weight maintenance as a noteworthy achievement. ❧ As a people, we applaud persons for the amount of weight they lose; then say nothing when they succeed at keeping the lost weight off. This reaction is cockeyed. Even though losing weight is commendable, *maintaining* one's desired healthy weight is the truly exceptional accomplishment. When you fail to view it that way, you rob yourself of deserved joy and motivation. So avoid this success killer by deriving a good feeling each day from your noteworthy accomplishment of contin-

uing to live in your healthy-weight range. (For more on this, see The No-change Secret of Maintenance Achievement chapter, page 146.)

19 — Not involving one's whole mind each day. ❧ When your whole mind — or both conscious <u>and</u> subconscious mind — is involved each day in the pursuit of healthy-weight living it results in your subconscious mind creating thoughts and feelings that guide you toward achievement of that goal. Conversely, when your subconscious mind *isn't* involved it results in you being less-than-fully effective at creating healthy-weight living. So avoid this success killer by having your whole mind involved in your weight success pursuit. (For more on this, see Success Driver 19, page 121.)

20 — Not applying a *daily* success methodology for pursuing healthy-weight living. ❧ Applying a properly-constructed success methodology — a.k.a. daily success action plan — is one of the key tools for succeeding in any major personal pursuit. So avoid this success killer by applying a daily success methodology in your weight success pursuit. Tip: The easiest, most effective success methodology I know for pursuing healthy-weight living is the Weight Success Method, described in Chapter 1.

21 — Not doing Weight Success Actions *every* day, or not making each day be a Weight Success Day. ❧ When you don't pursue weight control and healthy-weight living as an ongoing daily success process — that is, as an ongoing process of doing vital Weight Success Actions each day — you eventually fail at healthy-weight living. So avoid this success killer by doing the five Daily Actions of the Weight Success Method each day for the rest of your life. It typically takes *less than* **8** minutes of dedicated time per day.

WEIGHT SUCCESS
——— is the GOAL ———

WEIGHT SUCCESS METHOD™
——— is the MEANS ———

Goal+Means+<u>Action</u>=WEIGHT SUCCESS™

CHAPTER 20: 16 False Assumptions that Are Sabotaging Us

When it comes to weight management, it's US versus a World of False Assumptions, Delusions, and Wrong-headed Thinking.

THE WORLD abounds in false assumptions and misguided thinking pertaining to eating, weight gain, and weight management. This is one of the biggest obstacles we have to conquering over-weightness. Eradicating and circumventing these false assumptions is an essential step to creating nationwide healthy-weight living.

Within our society there exists 16 such assumptions that have been sabotaging our individual and national efforts at creating healthy-weight living and weight success. But we can break free of these beasts. Taking the approach of the Weight Success Method helps us identify these assumptions for what they are: harmful *false* beliefs.

So here are 16 false assumptions within our society that have been sabotaging our healthy-weight living and weight success efforts.

False Assumption 1: *Certain factors beyond individual control are causing us to overeat and be overweight.* ❧ There's an insidious trend afoot. This trend is spawning a crazy delusion that's sabotaging our efforts to conquer overweightness and create healthy-weight living. The trend I'm referring to is the "movement to discover factors that cause overeating and fat gain." I call these factors **fat-promoting factors.** Here are some that, so far, have been cited as things that are "causing" overeating and fat gain: genes, hormones, heredity, body chemistry, brain function, gender, age, menopause, lifestyle, too slow rate of metabolism, expanded appetite or food cravings, decreased smoking, anxiety, stress, depression, lack of sleep, lack of fiber, lack of fatty acids, eating at the wrong time, skipping breakfast, eating foods in the wrong sequence, eating too fast, eating foods derived from grains, eating foods containing "hidden carbs," low-fat foods, salt, sugar, artificial sweeteners, potato chips, food advertising, fast-food restaurants, availability of packaged foods made with too much sugar, artificial additives in

food, low cost of food due to agricultural innovation, taste buds insensitivity, too little exercise, working night shifts, unhealthy friends and family, glamorization of overweightness, criticism of over-weightness, hearing people talk about body weight, thinking you're overweight, too many plus-sized models, yo-yo dieting, age and weight of your mother when you were born, level of carbon monoxide in the atmosphere, indoor temperature too high, lack of air conditioning during hot months, living near a noisy highway or railway or airline flight path, doing repeated decision-making at work, certain environmental factors that promote eating, endocrine disrupting chemicals such as bisphenol A and phthalates, certain environmental chemicals such as flame retardants, types of bacteria in your intestine, increasing abundance of food in modern society, certain viruses such as adenoviruses, and certain drugs such as medications that treat depression, heartburn, diabetes, inflammation, allergies, hypothyroidism, hypertension, contraception, and mental illness. Yes, every one has been cited as a factor causing overeating or over-weightness.

And, amazingly, the list keeps growing! The above array of fat-promoting factors is current as of *December 2015.* It's much larger as of the date you're reading this, because since 2015 the obsessive quest to "discover" new scapegoat fat-promoting factors has been surging onward.

Not surprisingly, this "science of fat-promoting factors" is super-seductive. When I first encountered it it seemed like some of these factors pertained to me. It seemed like they might be the cause of my overeating and weight gain. Finally, I realized that this "discovering fat-promoting factors craze" is creating one of the craziest, most harmful national delusions in history. It's the *"I can't control my weight"* delusion. This is a *very* dangerous thing. It's dangerous because it leads to the copout conclusion "There's no point in me even trying."

Don't be sucked into the growing fat-promoting factors movement. Don't let the media hype that publicizes it make you believe you don't control your destiny when it comes to healthy-weight living. Because, you *do* control it.

Sure, some of these fat-promoting factors might promote overeating and make it easier to gain weight. But not a one *causes* a person to overeat or be overweight. Overeating and over-weightness are caused by one thing only: overper-formance of a certain 3-action process, the process of opening our mouth, inserting food into our mouth, and swallowing the food — a process that happens to be *totally controllable* by each of us. Our failure to recognize and act on this truth is a main factor preventing our creating healthy-weight living. And, this false assumption #1 is a main factor that's causing us to not act on that truth.

False Assumption 2: *If you're only slightly overweight it's okay because there are no bad consequences to it.* ✍ This is a self-comforting myth. Yes, it's true that being only slightly over-weight is not as harmful as being greatly over-weight. But, any degree of overweightness is still a problem, if for no other reason than this: Being slightly overweight seldom stays that way. It almost always leads to *greater* overweightness, or, at the least, to a lifetime of endless yo-yo dieting.

False Assumption 3: *Most humans lack the capability to control how much they eat.* ✍ This insidious assumption drives much of what's hap-pening in today's world of weight control. Much of what's being proposed and pushed by government, corporations, and health organizations is based on this assumption. But, because it's inherently offensive it's seldom articulated; it's implicit, not explicit.

And, why is it offensive? Because if it were true, we'd no longer be human beings; we'd be something other than human. Worms, fish, pigs, dogs, and every other animal lacks the capability to deliberately determine how much it should eat. They eat by instinct or inborn behavior. But humans possess the capability to determine and control how much they eat. It comes with "being

human." So, we should squelch the unarticulated implicit assumption that we lack this capability, otherwise folks might eventually start believing it ... and then start *acting as-if it's true.*

False Assumption 4: *Healthy-weight eating, or right eating, is hard to do.* ✍ This assumption is one of the great deterrents to people striving for healthy-weight living. They believe eating right foods in the right amount has just got to be painful and difficult. So they procrastinate on pursuing healthy-weight living. Fact is, healthy-weight eating is <u>not</u> hard to do. Or, if you prefer, it doesn't have to be hard to do. It all depends on what one believes and desires. When a person believes it will be easy to do, and strongly desires for it to be that way, they can and will find a way to make it that way.

False Assumption 5: *Healthy-weight eating is a pleasure-lacking, enjoyment-robbing experience.* ✍ As with Assumption 4, this assumption is also a deterrent to striving for healthy-weight living. But, healthy-weight eating, or right eating, doesn't have to be pleasure-lacking and enjoyment-robbing. It depends on what one believes and desires. When a person believes that healthy-weight eating can and will be enjoyable, and strongly desires for it to be that way, they can and will find a way to make it that way. Perhaps what we need is a new style of cuisine, a cuisine dedicated to creating foods that promote right eating — in other words, a *right-eating cuisine.*

False Assumption 6: *The main priority of eating is — or should be — pleasure maximization.* ✍ This assumption is one of the most pernicious. Why? Because, when a person's <u>main</u> eating priority, goal, or focus is pleasure maximization, their eating always extends into *overeating* — if not all the time at least enough of the time to create ongoing weight gain. This assumption is a stealthy manipulator that makes overeating *inevitable.*

It's also one of the hardest to debunk. This is because it's widespread and deeply entrenched in our society. So most people unquestionably accept it as fact. And, when you suggest that it's not the best way to approach eating, for the reason cited above, they tend to launch a host of defense mechanisms. Not least of which is trying to turn the suggestion into a joke. So, what's the best way to approach eating? It's to make your main eating priority to be healthy-weight calorie consumption. This involves the three priorities of *right eating.* (For more this, go to Startup Action 6, page 17.)

False Assumption 7: *The main key to weight-control success is to find the right diet program.* ✎ Many people hold the belief that the key to their creating healthy-weight living lies in finding that one perfect diet program that works best. And, they further hold the belief that without finding such a program they're doomed to failure. So they spend years searching for the perfect program. But, ultimately, they never find a program that works for them. Why is that?

It's because, what makes any bona fide diet program work *isn't* the program, per se. Rather, it's whether or not the program is *fully* applied.

When a person applies a bona fide diet program fully, or the way it's intended to be applied, it usually works. When a person doesn't apply a program fully, it usually doesn't work, or works only partially. In short, partial application creates partial or no results; full application creates full results. So, we would be better served to spend less time focusing on the "which diet program is best" question and more time on the "how do we motivate our self to fully apply the dietary program of our choice" question.

Now, to ensure I'm not being misinterpreted, I point out that some diet programs are a better fit for you and your situation than are other programs. And, these "better fitting" programs are easier for you to fully apply. So they're the programs you might want to focus on. But, again, any bona fide diet program that's applied fully typically works fully and any that's not applied fully typically doesn't work fully. And, now, a reminder question: What's the easiest way to motivate yourself to do a diet program fully? Do the Weight Success Method.

False Assumption 8: *Lack of exercise is the cause of overweightness and more exercise is the solution.* ✎ Certainly, regular exercise is helpful

and good. And every person would be well advised to do it. But, the belief that lack of exercise is the cause of overweightness and more exercise is the solution is erroneous and sometimes self-defeating. It can be self-defeating because *overweightness is caused by overeating, not by under-exercising!* What makes this Assumption 8 so harmful is it diverts people's attention from the real cause of overweightness: eating too much. This dooms many persons to years of frenetic exercising while still gaining weight — a discouraging situation, indeed. In short, exercise can work well as a *complement* to right eating, but in the long run it doesn't replace it.

False Assumption 9: *Weighing yourself each day is counterproductive, so avoid it.* ✎ This is one of the most misguided myths of the weight management world. Yes, daily weighing can be counterproductive when it's done the wrong way. But, virtually every activity in life is counterproductive when done the wrong way. Daily Action 1 (p. 22) describes the right way. Do it the right way and daily weighing becomes one of the most powerful tools there is for conquering weight gain and creating healthy-weight living.

False Assumption 10: *Food advertising causes people to eat more, so if we reduce food advertising we'll reduce people's overeating.* ✎ Decades ago we outlawed certain types of cigarette and liquor advertising. Did that put an end to smoking, drinking, and over-drinking? Obviously not. So why are some folks suggesting that the way to curb overeating and weight gain is to limit food and restaurant advertising?

Truth is, blaming business advertising is a red herring that obfuscates what really needs to be done to achieve nationwide healthy-weight living. Instead of blaming businesses for our weight failure situation the blame — if any is to be ascribed — should rest on the government leaders who have thus far failed to create a national program designed to motivate and equip people to voluntarily engage in right eating. Having such a program would actually result in reducing nationwide overweightness. The "outlaw food advertising" circus is politicians' feckless ruse.

False Assumption 11: *Enacting food taxation and consumption laws will make people "eat right."* ❧ For decades now we've imposed heavy taxes on cigarettes and liquor. Has it stopped cigarette smoking and liquor drinking? Obviously not. So, why are the proponents of this assumption thinking that taxing "bad" foods will end consumption of "bad" foods when taxing hasn't ended smoking and drinking?

Getting the people of our nation to minimize wrong eating and increase right eating won't happen by outlawing food advertising and piling heavy taxes on "bad" foods. Rather, it will happen when our government leaders enact a national program that equips people with the resources, know-how, and motivation to voluntarily engage in right eating. For more, see the Going Nationwide chapter (p. **162**).

And, speaking of motivating people to eat right, one of the most powerful motivators would be a leadership *role model* — that is, it would be *every* key person who's working in our federal congressional and executive branches setting an *example* by doing daily right eating and achieving personal healthy-weight living. Such a model would be a big step toward motivating the people of our nation to engage in right eating and healthy-weight living. It would be far more motivating than the "tax bad foods" circus that some politicians are trying to foist on us.

False Assumption 12: *Overweightness is a physical problem, so the solution must be a physical solution.* ❧ For years we've been spending thousands of hours and millions of dollars trying to discover a physical fix to the burgeoning overweightness condition. But we haven't discovered it. Why? Because it doesn't exist. Yes, overweightness is, indeed, a physical issue. But the fix to this physical issue happens to involve a *mind* solution. Enacting this solution is the key to ending overweight living. This book was written to describe the easiest, most enjoyable, most effective form of this solution.

False Assumption 13: *Succeeding at losing weight is the main achievement and most important thing.* ❧ In the world of weight control we have our priorities askew. Losing weight is important and applaud-worthy but it's not the end of each individual weight story, as most people assume it to be. Rather, it's the *beginning* of the story; it's Chapter 1. What happens next in the years *after* the weight loss is the main thing. This is the big story, the story that needs to be told, and read about, and applauded, because this is when creation of healthy-weight living actually happens. I suggest that if we viewed weight control from this perspective we would be more effective at conquering overweightness and creating both individual and nationwide healthy-weight living.

False Assumption 14: *You don't understand what it takes to create healthy-weight living until you've gained a lot of weight and lost it.* ❧ One of the most entrenched assumptions in the world of weight control is that one doesn't, or perhaps can't, understand what it takes to create healthy-weight living until one has first become hugely overweight and then lost the excess weight. We tend to assume that having this experience somehow endows a person with special insight into the process of healthy weight achievement.

That assumption is false. This is proven by the fact that, at the present time, over ninety percent of people who go through the experience of gaining and then losing a lot of weight eventually become overweight again. So, clearly, if the process of losing a large amount of weight automatically endowed a person with special insight into the process of creating healthy-weight living, everyone who succeeds at losing a large amount of weight would be living out the rest of their life in their healthy-weight range.

So who should we be looking to for a role model? There are two groups of people who have undergone a certain experience that's even more enlightening and noteworthy than that of gaining and then losing a huge amount of weight.

The first group consists of people who decided early in their life that they would live out their life in their healthy-weight range, and then committed their self to doing that, and created a personal life plan or healthy-weight strategy for accomplishing it, and then implemented that strategy throughout their life and achieved lifelong healthy-weight living as a result.

The second group consists of people who began gaining weight at some point in their life and then, after putting on 10 or 20 excess pounds, decided to change the situation and to live out the rest of their life in their healthy-weight range, and then created a personal life plan or healthy-weight living strategy for accomplishing it, and then implemented that strategy for the rest of their life and, as a result, lived out the remainder of their life in their healthy-weight range.

Both these groups fly under the radar, so to speak. We pay little attention to them because, for the most part, the people in these two groups just quietly go about "doing their thing." So no one's noticing their unique accomplishment, and certainly no one's applauding it. And, on the rare occasion when one of these weight winners becomes known, or decides to share their healthy-weight strategy or story, very few people take note of it.

This is too bad, because the people in these two small groups have acquired even more valuable insight into the process of creating healthy-weight living than have those who became highly overweight and lost the weight. These people have discovered — either knowingly or unknowingly, intentionally or non-intentionally — what it takes to achieve lifelong healthy-weight living, and then are *doing it.* They're the ones we should be "studying," listening to, and learning from.

False Assumption 15: *Since 70 percent of us are overweight, 30 percent of us aren't affected by overweightness.* ❧ Federal government survey as of 2017 indicates that about 70 percent of adults (those over age 18) are overweight and 30 percent are non-overweight. These numbers are alarming, yet they likely greatly <u>under</u>represent the magnitude of the overweightness situation. Here's why.

The "30% non-overweight" number depicts a slice in time, a moment when a survey occurred. But when we view the overweight situation over a span of years we can see the truth. Which is, many

of the people in the "30% non-overweight" category will, in the future, *be overweight.*

The 30% non-overweight category mainly comprises four groups of persons: **(1)** yo-yo dieters who are at the low-weight end of the yo-yo cycle but who will be overweight again in about twelve months, **(2)** young people who are *presently* non-overweight but will become overweight in just a few years as they live more of "the good life," **(3)** hyper-exercisers who are beating back fat gain with vigorous calorie-burning activity but who will eventually find it doesn't work as they grow older, and **(4)** people who have adopted a lifelong eating management strategy that results in consuming an amount of calories that's equal to the amount their body is metabolizing.

I estimate that groups one through three constitute at least half of the "30% non-overweight" category (which would equal 15% of total population), and group four constitutes the other half (15% of population).

So, to sum up, the magnitude of the overweightness situation isn't accurately portrayed by the tidy "70% overweight, 30% non-overweight" ratio. The reality is, it's likely that about *85 percent* of the population ends up living their life stricken with overweightness (70% + 15% = 85%). So, for about 85 percent of us, becoming overweight isn't a matter of IF — rather, it's a matter of *when* and *how much.*

This is a sobering scenario. So how do we break it? Simply put, we equip, teach, and motivate the people of our nation — and perhaps the world — to do what group 4 is doing. That is, we teach, equip, and motivate them to apply an eating management strategy that enables them to *easily, enjoyably* manage their eating in a way that results in consuming an amount of calories that's equal to the amount their body is metabolizing. A main aim of this book is to explain this process.

False Assumption 16: *Our overweightness is caused by a complex multifactor condition.* ❧ For decades now, governmental bodies, academia, the scientific–medical community, and society-at-large have been seeking the cause of and solution to our growing overweightness. We've sunk thousands of hours and millions of dollars into it. And yet — by the evidence and by the opinion of some experts — we're no closer today to understanding and discovering the elusive "cause and solution" to our growing weight failure than we were when we started looking for it decades ago.

The only thing that has resulted from it all is a delusion-creating mire of fat-promoting factors (p. **126**), which has led us to the copout conclusion "There's no point in us even trying to personally control our weight."

So, why is it that after all the time and money spent on trying to identify the cause of our overweightness we haven't found it until now — until the creation of this book? It's because of this. As a nation we've been holding a powerful false assumption: the assumption that weight failure is caused by a *complex multifactor condition.* Holding this assumption has created a bizarre, counterproductive situation. It has made us unable to recognize the real cause of our overweightness. In short, we're not "seeing" this real cause because it's a *simple single-factor* condition instead of being the complex multifactor condition that most researchers assume exists and are looking for.

This simple single-factor condition — explained in False Assumption 1 (p. 126) — happens to be *overperformance of the three-action process of opening one's mouth, inserting food into one's mouth, and swallowing the food.* This is the REAL cause — and also the most productive explanation — of why overweightness exists.

So, why are researchers perpetually not recognizing the real cause of overweightness? The reason is simple. It's because this single-factor explanation contradicts the complex multi-factors assumption held by most weight researchers. Or, put another way, they're not recognizing the obvious simple answer because they're assuming this answer doesn't exist. Or, put still another way, they're not seeing reality because this reality is not what they expect, or want, to see.

All this would be amusing except for one thing. It's sad that we're wasting such vast amounts of time and money in pursuit of trying to discover something that doesn't exist. So, what should we be doing instead? Two things. First, we should cease our feckless pursuit of the imaginary multi-factor fat-causing condition. Second, we should take a portion of the time and money we save by ceasing our pointless pursuit of the non-existent condition and allocate it to doing the only thing that will enable us to achieve both personal and nationwide healthy-weight living. We should equip people with the wherewithal — motivation, resources, and method — for easily guiding themselves each day to right eating and healthy-weight living. For more, see the Going Nationwide chapter (p. **162**).

Once we escape our false beliefs regarding eating and weight we'll be in position to more quickly achieve nationwide healthy-weight living. The approach of the Weight Success Method ignores and/or circumvents these false beliefs rather than accepting and embracing them. This is one reason why the Method is so effective at creating lifelong healthy-weight living.

CHAPTER 21: Key to Beating the Bad Habit of Unguided Eating

Most people find it hard to end unguided eating. But doing the Weight Success Method makes it easier.

WOULD YOU like to know what's causing most people to engage in unguided eating ... and why they find it so hard to free themselves from it? Would you like to know why the Weight Success Method enables one to more easily escape unguided eating and, thereby, more easily create healthy-weight living for life? If so, read on.

The Eating Triggers

Most eating occurs as a habitual response to one of six conditions. I call these conditions *eating triggers*. They are: food, hunger feeling, desire for eating-derived pleasure, time period, situation, and mood. I'll explain.

1 – Food. The presence of food or pictures of food can trigger eating. Also, an aroma of food can do it, too.

2 – Hunger Feeling. The presence of hunger, also known as hunger pang, can trigger eating. It works like this. Hunger is an unpleasant feeling; the desire to remove this unpleasant feeling prompts us to eat.

3 – Desire for Eating-derived Pleasure. A desire to experience pleasure by way of consuming food can trigger eating. When this desire is strong and pertains to a certain type of food we call it a craving. This trigger happens to be a big promoter of unguided eating for many people. The pleasure-priority approach to eating, which is described in Startup Action 6 (p. 17), derives from the desire to experience eating pleasure.

4 – Time Period. The arrival of a certain time period — such as, for example, lunchtime, dinnertime, snack time — can trigger eating.

5 – Situation. The presence of a certain situation can trigger eating. For examples, a holiday, social event, or tense situation might be an eating trigger for some persons.

6 – Mood: The presence of a certain mood or feeling can trigger eating. For examples, happiness, anxiety, or sadness might be an eating promoter for some persons.

All six triggers don't necessarily apply to every person. Plus, each trigger affects various persons in different ways. For one person a certain trigger might have minimal impact and for another person a huge impact. So, whether a trigger is strong or weak depends on the person.

Three Responses to Eating Triggers

Now we come to the vital point. How a person *responds* to the eating triggers in their life determines whether they live *in* their healthy-weight range or *outside* their healthy-weight range. Most people assume there's only one response to these triggers: automatic, or unguided, eating. But that's not correct. There are *three* possible responses: (1) unguided eating, (2) guided eating, (3) no eating. Here's what's involved with each.

Unguided Eating. In unguided eating we don't guide our eating actions. Instead, the eating triggers do it, especially trigger #1: *the presence of food*. Food items are visual cues. The cues trigger a certain behavior. This certain behavior consists of performing a series of unguided-eating actions that result in consuming the cues. We mostly perform this unguided-eating behavior automatically, or with very little deliberation or conscious direction. (Note: Other names for unguided eating are automatic eating, undirected eating, and non-controlled eating.)

So, unguided eating is a 3-action process. First, we confront food items, which are cues. Second, the food cues trigger an automatic-eating response. Third, we engage in undirected or automatic eating until the cues disappear from being eaten. During this time we aren't thinking about what we're doing. As a result, we're not guiding our eating activity. And, whenever we're not guiding our eating activity, our eating activity is <u>uncon-</u>

trolled. Which is why unguided eating leads to overeating and eventual failure at creating lifelong healthy-weight living. So, we should replace unguided eating with guided eating.

Guided Eating. In guided eating *we* guide the eating process. Meaning, instead of the food items determining what and how much we eat, *we* do it. This might sound hard to do, but it's not. You can easily create guided eating any time you want. All you need do is apply a certain 3-action process, which we call *Guided Eating Process.* (Other names for guided eating are directed eating and controlled eating.) This Process is described in Daily Action 5 (p. 35). Guided eating is a major key to replacing overweight living with healthy-weight living for life.

> **Note:** In this book the word "eating" encompasses drinking. And the word "food" encompasses beverages. So wherever you read the terms "eating" and "food" know that it includes drinking and beverages.

No Eating. In addition to unguided eating and guided eating there's a third possible response to the eating triggers: no eating.

Each response produces a certain outcome. *Unguided eating,* done daily or frequently, leads to living <u>above</u> your healthy-weight range. *Guided eating,* done daily or frequently, leads to living <u>in</u> your healthy-weight range. And, *no eating,* done in moderation, might also lead to living *in* your healthy-weight range, <u>or</u> when done to excess lead to living *below* your healthy-weight range.

The Habit of Unguided Eating

A person's response to any particular eating trigger is determined one of two ways: either by deliberate choice or by habit. A *habit* is an automatic frequently repeated behavior or activity. So, the *habit of unguided eating* is unguided eating done automatically and repeatedly.

Most persons respond to the eating triggers of their life not by deliberate choice but by habit. Further, the particular habit that's most in play is the habit of unguided eating. Which means, for most people, every time an eating trigger appears they automatically engage in habit-driven unguided eating. Unfortunately, this ultimately results in

overweight living. So, a main Cause–Effect Dynamic of Overweight Living is this:

Eating Triggers prompt **Habit-driven Unguided Eating** which causes Overweight Living

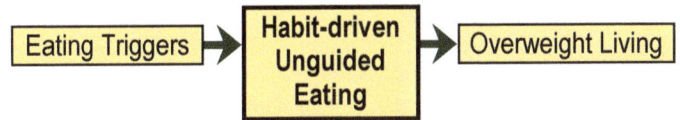

This means, to more easily live the rest of your life in your healthy-weight range you need to override or nullify the habit of unguided eating. And, then, replace that habit with deliberate guided eating and, eventually, a guided-eating habit. By doing this the unguided-eating problem would be instantly solved.

But this is easier said than done. Why so? Because most likely your habit of unguided eating is a *strong* habit. And why is it strong? Because the more a habit is repeated the stronger it becomes. So, if you're like most folks, by the time you decide to switch from unguided eating to guided eating your habit of unguided eating has been repeated for *numerous* years, which comprises *thousands* of days and <u>*tens of thousands*</u> of unguided eating sessions. The result of all this repetition is: Your habit of unguided eating has become a strong, *deeply engrained* habit. Which means, for many people the strength of their unguided-eating habit is a main impediment to easily conquering overweightness and creating healthy-weight living.

A Habit Is a Beast of Two Components

In addition to the habit of unguided eating being strong, most people don't know how to defeat an unwanted habit. This is because they don't know the anatomy of a habit. They don't realize that every habit consists of two parts: a physical component and a mental component. The physical component, which I call *action-habit,* is a certain automatic repeating physical activity. The mental component, which I call *mind-habit,* is a certain automatic repeating mental process. Now here's the big point: The mind-habit underlies and drives the action-habit. It works like this.

Two-part Anatomy of a Habit

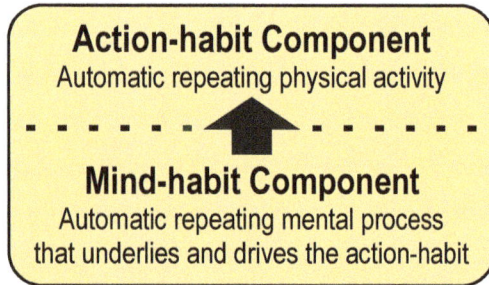

Action-habit Component
Automatic repeating physical activity

Mind-habit Component
Automatic repeating mental process
that underlies and drives the action-habit

So, to shut down an action-habit, or automatic repeating physical activity, you must shut down the mind-habit, or automatic repeating mental process that's driving the physical activity. Which means, to shut down habit-driven unguided eating you must shut down, or override, the mental process that's causing it. So for most folks the situation is this. The combination of the unguided-eating habit's strength plus lack of understanding of how habits work makes it a major struggle to override the habit of unguided eating for most persons. This, in turn, causes them to eventually give up the battle.

The Solution

So, how does one solve this problem? You involve your *whole* mind, or both conscious and subconscious mind, in your daily pursuit of living in your healthy-weight range. When you do this it brings the faculties of your subconscious mind into your pursuit of healthy-weight living. This results in shutting down, or at least mitigating, the mind-habit component of unguided eating. Which, in turn, results in shutting down or mitigating the action-habit component, or the automatic unguided eating response to the eating triggers of your life. The easiest way to involve your whole mind in your weight success pursuit is do the Weight Success Method.

Coming up is a summary of this chapter in three infographics:

1 – How Overweight Living Comes About

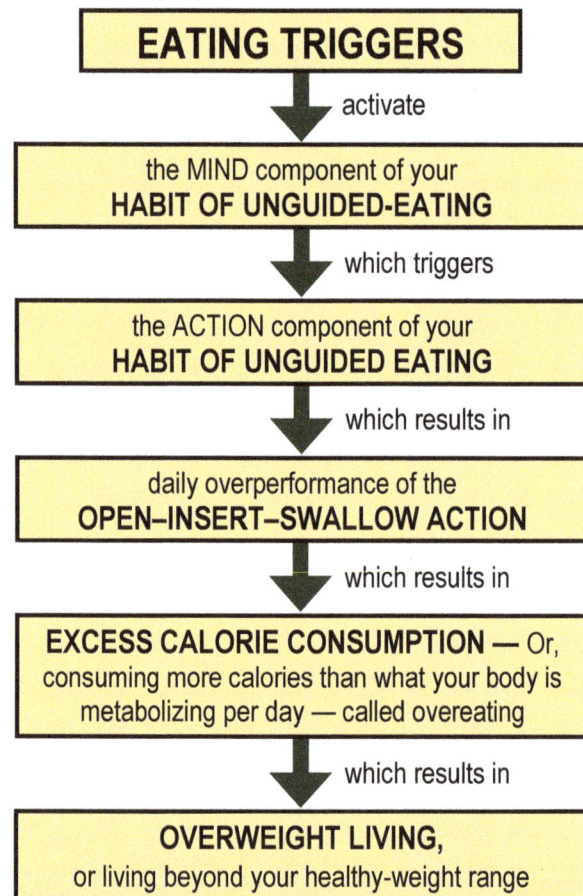

2 – Easiest Way to Beat the Habit of Unguided Eating

3 – The Daily Contest within Your Mind

How Overweight Living Comes About

EATING TRIGGERS

activate

the MIND component of your
HABIT OF UNGUIDED-EATING

which triggers

the ACTION component of your
HABIT OF UNGUIDED EATING

which results in

daily overperformance of the
OPEN–INSERT–SWALLOW ACTION

which results in

EXCESS CALORIE CONSUMPTION — Or, consuming more calories than what your body is metabolizing per day — called overeating

which results in

OVERWEIGHT LIVING,
or living beyond your healthy-weight range

Most people don't realize it, but the process depicted in the above infographic is what makes weight gain happen so easily. It's also what makes weight loss seem so hard. And, lastly, it's what makes weight maintenance, or living in one's healthy-weight range, seem even harder.

But there's a way to break free of this dynamic. It involves something you're already familiar with: the Weight Success Method. Here's the infographic for it, titled "Easiest Way to Beat the Habit of Unguided Eating."

Easiest Way to Beat the Habit of Unguided Eating

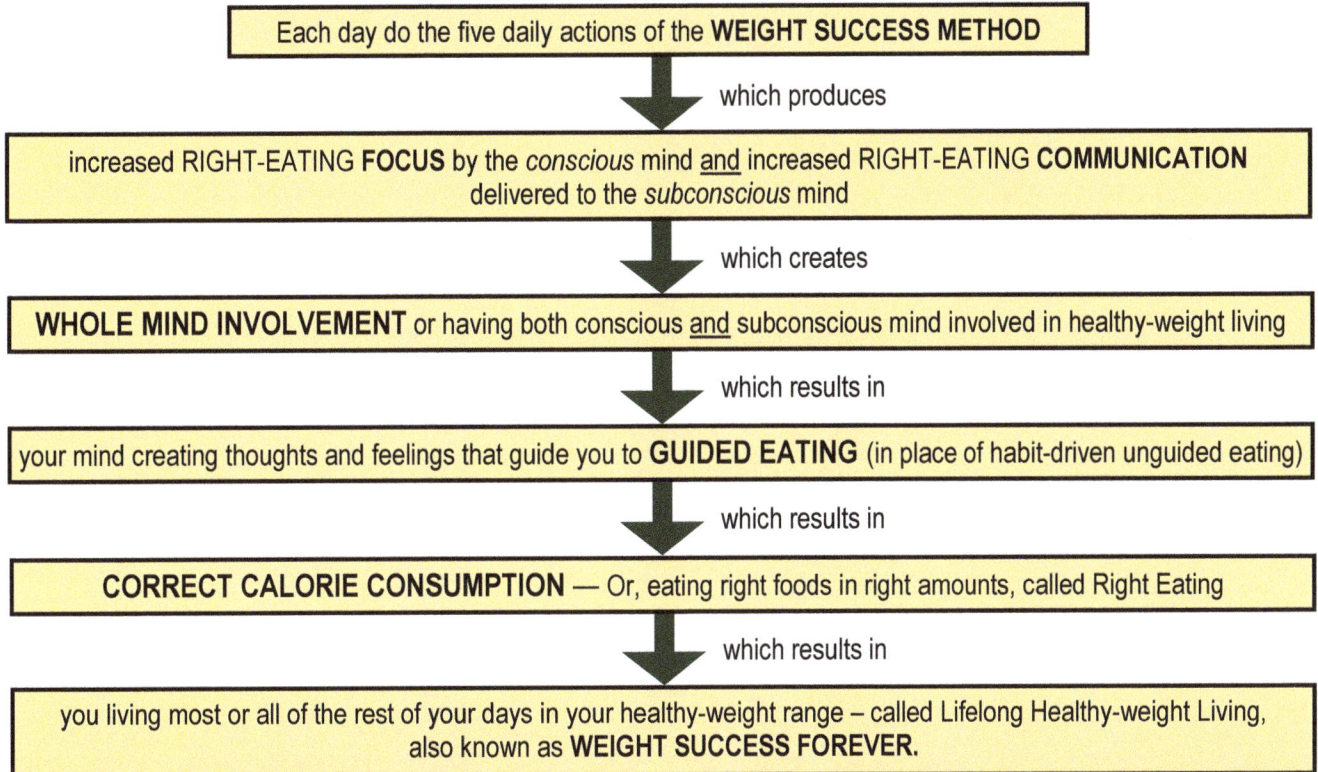

Each day do the five daily actions of the **WEIGHT SUCCESS METHOD**

which produces

increased RIGHT-EATING **FOCUS** by the *conscious* mind and increased RIGHT-EATING **COMMUNICATION** delivered to the *subconscious* mind

which creates

WHOLE MIND INVOLVEMENT or having both conscious and subconscious mind involved in healthy-weight living

which results in

your mind creating thoughts and feelings that guide you to **GUIDED EATING** (in place of habit-driven unguided eating)

which results in

CORRECT CALORIE CONSUMPTION — Or, eating right foods in right amounts, called Right Eating

which results in

you living most or all of the rest of your days in your healthy-weight range – called Lifelong Healthy-weight Living, also known as **WEIGHT SUCCESS FOREVER.**

For an in-depth explanation of how FOCUS and SELF-COMMUNICATION create whole mind involvement, see Ch. **18** at page 109.

Here's a concluding way to view this. Your habit of unguided eating is on a mission to make you overeat. And, as long as you're not doing anything to thwart this mission it will succeed at its mission. Which means, either *you* direct your eating or the *habit of unguided eating* will direct it. And, when the habit of unguided eating is directing it you *will* end up overeating.

In case you might be interested in it, here's the above infographic in a summary sentence: Doing the Weight Success Method each day produces daily Right-eating Focus and Right-eating Communication which, in turn, creates daily Whole Mind Involvement in pursuit of healthy-weight living, which results in daily Right Eating that ultimately results in correct calorie consumption and lifelong Healthy-weight Living.

The Habit vs. You

Here's another way to view it. You and your *Habit of Unguided Eating* are rival contestants in a daily

wrestling match. Each day the Habit shows up for a showdown between it and you. Depending on your resolve, it might be a short match, like, say, 20 seconds, or it might last an entire day. But either way, before day's end one of you will come out on top, dominating the other. When the Habit of Unguided Eating comes out on top, you end up engaging in overeating for the day. When YOU come out on top, you end up doing guided eating, which results in non-overeating for the day.

Now here's the key point. You have a secret weapon that makes the difference: your mind. When you go into the match using only the "conscious half" of your mind you usually lose. But when you involve your whole mind — or both conscious and subconscious mind — you win. This almost always makes it a short contest, with you coming out on top. So each day *you* determine how it will be, and whether the winner will be **IT** (your Habit of Unguided Eating) or **YOU.** We call it "The Daily Contest within Your Mind." Here's the infographic for it.

The Daily Contest within Your Mind

A contest between **IT** (your Habit of Unguided Eating) and *YOU*

IT beats *YOU* when you use "half" your mind.

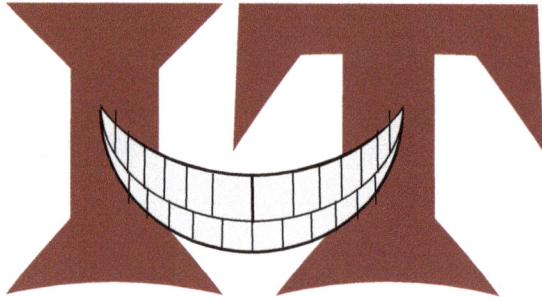

YOU beat **IT** when you use your WHOLE mind.

IT

– beats –

YOU

w/ "half" Your Mind Involved

YOU

w/ WHOLE Mind Involved

– beat –

IT

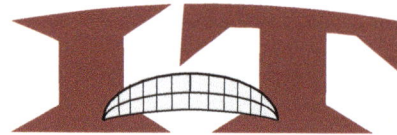

AND, doing Weight Success Actions — such as the five daily actions of the Weight Success Method — every day *greatly assists* you with involving your whole mind — or both conscious <u>and</u> subconscious mind — every day.

For decades now we've been spending thousands of hours and millions of dollars each year searching for the solution to individual and global overweightness. But prior to this book we haven't found it. We haven't found it because we've been assuming it involves anything but what it actually involves, which is each person's **MIND** and the capability of that mind to **SUCCEED** at creating ongoing weight success.

CHAPTER 22: How the Weight Success Method Enhances Your Life Journey

This is how the Weight Success Method makes your weight success journey feel easier and more natural, and also more fulfilling.

THE 19 SUCCESS DRIVERS described in Chapter 19 are outstandingly effective at creating achievement of lifelong healthy-weight living. But upon completing one of the precursor manuscripts for this book I got a suspicion that maybe there was even more going on than that. This prompted some Internet research. I had heard of a relatively new field of psychology called *positive psychology,* but knew nothing about it. So I typed "positive psychology" into my Google search bar and went on a voyage of discovery.

After clicking through a few sites I ended up at one titled authentichappiness.org. This appeared to be the epicenter of the positive psychology movement. I discovered that a founding pioneer in the field is a professor Martin Seligman of University of Pennsylvania — a.k.a. Penn.

At this site I viewed some videos, read some articles, and filled out a couple questionnaires, or tests. I also discovered that Seligman had recently published a book titled *Flourish: A Visionary New Understanding of Happiness and Well-being.* I decided that this is what I needed to be reading. So I ordered a copy from Amazon. I also ordered another book that had been mentioned on the website — a book titled *Flow: The Psychology of Optimal Experience* by a professor Mihaly Csikszentmihalyi of Claremont Graduate University. (Note: Csikszentmihalyi is pronounced CHEEK-sent-me-hi.) And, I ordered a third book — titled *A Primer in Positive Psychology* — by a professor Christopher Peterson of University of Michigan.

In a few days the books arrived. First I read *Flourish,* then *Flow,* then *A Primer in Positive Psychology.* I found each to be interesting and enlightening.

After just a few pages into *Flourish* I came upon a seminal concept. That being, a main tenet of positive psychology is that a person experiences well-being by having five main elements in their life: Positive emotion, Engagement, Relationships (of the positive kind), Meaning, and Accomplishment. The acronym for these five things is PERMA. And the main idea is: The more PERMA — or Positive emotion, Engagement, Relationships, Meaning, and Accomplishment — a person has in their life, the more well-being the person experiences.

I then examined the Weight Success Method in light of the PERMA model. To my astonishment, the Weight Success Method correlated closely with the PERMA model. I discovered that doing the Method results in *expanded actualization* of four of the five elements of the model and, with a little innovation, even all five.

Then a stunning realization hit me. Perhaps this is a reason why creating healthy-weight living with the Weight Success Method seems so easy and natural. It's because gaining healthy-weight living via the Method not only results in creating a "new" physical body it also results in creating expanded psychological well-being, or fulfillment, in a person's life. Or, put another way, it makes one's weight management journey to be an enhancer of the life journey. Which means, it turns weight management from a "life detracting activity" — which is how most view it — into a "life enhancing activity."

Then another realization struck me. Those few people who are seemingly doing right eating easily, enjoyably, and automatically might be doing right eating in a way that results in expanding one or more of the PERMA elements in their life. Conversely, those who are finding right eating to be painful and hard to do might be doing it in a way that results in no expansion, or perhaps even diminishment, of the PERMA elements in their life.

So, I'll now describe each of the five PERMA elements, and explain how doing the Weight Success Method results in expansion of that element. Also, in some cases I'll describe some additional actions a person could take to expand a certain element even further.

Note: In examining the five elements I'm doing it in a slightly different order than the PERMA model. The order I'm using is P-A-R-M-E. I'm doing so because "E" is where I want to end up in the discussion.

Positive Emotion

The first element of the PERMA model is positive emotion. Upon reviewing some literature on the model I soon realized that none of the sources defined the term "positive emotion." What's more, a few didn't even give examples. But some did. Here's a combined list of examples of positive emotions cited in positive psychology literature: pleasure, happiness, joy, satisfaction, gratitude, hope, serenity, kindness, contentment, comfort, interest, pride, excitement, amusement, inspiration, awe, ecstasy, and love.

So, to promote clarity of discussion I now provide this formal definition.

Positive emotion is any harm-free emotion or feeling that one enjoys having.

NOTE: Harm-free = Doesn't derive from doing harm to oneself or others, and doesn't result in harm to oneself or others

So now you likely want to know how the Weight Success Method expands the amount of positive emotion, or enjoyment, in a person's life. Well, you may have already discovered it. The Why the Weight Success Method Is Enjoyable chapter (p. **103**) explains it in detail. It's a full description, based on my personal experiences, of the enjoyment that can be derived from doing the Weight Success Method.

Now here's an important thing to know. Positive emotion, or enjoyment and gratification, that's derived from the Weight Success Method comes two ways: (1) from realizing the desired *outcome*,

or from living in one's healthy-weight range and deriving weight success benefits from it, and (2) from the *process* of creating the outcome. What distinguishes the Weight Success Method from most other weight management programs is Way #2: deriving enjoyment from *the process.*

To illustrate, here's a summation of the enjoyment and gratification I personally derive from doing the Weight Success Method. Some items come from the outcome and some from the process. (Again, for a full discussion go to the Why the Weight Success Method Is Enjoyable chapter, page **103**.)

Enjoyment Derived from the Weight Success Method

Stated in summary, doing the Weight Success Method expands the amount of enjoyment, or positive emotions, in my life because doing the Method results in the following enjoyment-creating experiences: (a) achieving and seeing daily personal progress, (b) delivering and receiving positive self-reinforcement, (c) triumphing over occasional adversity or setbacks, (d) being director of my eating, (e) daily focusing on an exciting ultimate goal, and (f) feeling like a winner by performing daily winning actions.

I also derive enjoyment and satisfaction from (g) succeeding at living in my healthy-weight range, which makes me feel like a high-achiever, (h) realizing exciting weight success benefits from living at my healthy weight, and (i) maintaining awareness of those benefits on a daily basis.

And, finally, I derive enjoyment and gratification from (j) the act of improving my self and my life by pursuing a productive activity in place of a counterproductive one, or by living in my healthy-weight range rather than outside it, and from (k) being a living example that achieving easier healthy-weight living is *doable*, thereby inspiring others to "give it a go."

Items (a) through (f) occur from the *process,* or from performing the actions involved in doing the Weight Success Method. Items (g) through (k) come from the *outcome,* or from having accomplished the desired results connected to the Method.

In short, by doing the Weight Success Method you can *expand* your amount of enjoyment and satisfaction, or the positive emotion element, in your life. This can occur in various ways throughout each day and over your lifetime.

Accomplishment

A look at some positive psychology literature — in particular, Seligman's book *Flourish* (pgs. 18–20) — reveals a clear description of what's involved with the accomplishment element. Deriving from that information I put forth the following definition.

> *Accomplishment is the progressive realization of success, winning, achievement, or mastery in a particular chosen activity or endeavor.*

The literature describes several characteristics pertaining to accomplishment, as follows.

Accomplishment can be for its own sake. That is, for no other purpose than to achieve success, mastery, or a winning position in a particular activity or endeavor. But, in certain cases accomplishment can contribute to expansion of other PERMA elements, such as positive emotion, meaning, or relationships.

Further, it can occur both on-the-job and off-the-job, or at work, home, and in recreational pursuits.

Still further, it can be performed individually or as part of a group.

To create accomplishment with a particular endeavor it helps to apply as many of the 19 Success Drivers as possible. You already know about them; they're described in Chapter 19.

Accomplishment Derived from the Weight Success Method

So how, exactly, does doing the Weight Success Method expand the amount of accomplishment in a person's life? It does it by enabling the person to have these four experiences:

1. Each day, or most days, getting a desired weight reading at the daily weigh-in (Daily Action 1–Weighing);

2. Whenever an undesired weight reading happens, triumphing over adversity, or converting the setback into a progress action (Daily Action 2B–Correction);

3. Acquiring the weight success benefits attached to creating healthy-weight living, and also maintaining a daily awareness of those benefits; and

4. Creating lifelong healthy-weight living, a notable accomplishment, indeed — a feat that proves *mastery* of a special life pursuit and imparts the status of "lifelong healthy-weight winner."

Those are four ways the Weight Success Method can expand the amount of accomplishment in a person's life.

How to Expand Accomplishment Even Further

But, even with all that, it's possible to further expand the accomplishment element in your weight success journey. Here are four ways.

1. *ENHANCE the Weight Success Method.* You can do this by customizing certain parts of the five daily actions. In describing the five daily actions I noted where you might tweak, or customize, an action if you so chose. For example, in doing Daily Action 2A–Reinforcement you might expand on the wording of the Thank You, Keep It Up message. And, in doing Daily Action 3–Benefits Directive you might include various enhancements to the Weight Success Benefits Directive and also apply changes in delivery style (see the "Enhancing the Directive" section and the "Apply Creative Delivery Techniques" section in the Detailed Instructions for the Weight Success Benefits Directive chapter, page **65**). And, in doing Daily Action 4–Goal Statement you might experiment with delivering the Healthy-weight Goal Statement in different ways. Finally, in Daily Action 5–Guided Eating you might use enhanced wording for your guided-eating self-talk. Depending on how you approach it, these enhancement actions can further expand the feeling of accomplishment to be derived from doing the Weight Success Method.

2. *ADD TO the Weight Success Method.* You can do this by including *optional additional* mind motivation actions along with doing the five daily actions. The Six More Mind Motivators chapter (p. **90**) provides six optional additional mind motivators. You can include any one you like. And, you can modify, improvise, or enhance any of them, if you like.

3. *DO the optional Weight Success Actions Scorecard.* This can be a great way to expand the feeling of accomplishment in your weight success journey. If you're one who likes "scoring points," recording what you accomplish, and breaking personal-best records, this is for you. It's in Ch. 27 (p. 154) and also in the Toolkit. Also in Ch. 27 and the Toolkit is the Win-Day Calendar, which is an additional way to expand the feeling of accomplishment. And, finally, if you are presently in weight-reduction mode, doing the Weight-reduction Success Graph, which is in Ch. 27 and the Toolkit, can bring a feeling of accomplishment, too. The Toolkit is at: **correllconcepts.com/toolkit.pdf**

4. *BE CREATIVE in selecting or creating your preferred dietary program.* As you know by now, you have a choice of what dietary program you apply to your weight success journey. It can be one of the established bona fide programs on the market or it can be a program of your own design — your choice. For some people, applying their own custom-designed dietary program might enhance the feeling of accomplishment derived from their weight success journey. For others, going with one of the established bona fide programs is the best, or most productive, way to go. You're the one who determines which is best for you.

In short, by pursuing creation of healthy-weight living via a full, whole-hearted application of the Weight Success Method — plus perhaps taking advantage of the many ways to enhance and add to the Method — you can greatly *expand* the accomplishment element in your life.

Relationships

As with the positive emotions element, I failed to find a tidy definition of the term "positive relationships." So I provide this formal definition.

> A ***positive relationship*** *is a harm-free regularly-occurring interaction between two or more persons, with the interaction mainly involving constructive activity such as mutually enjoyable conversation, meaningful two-way dialogue, inspiring or positively reinforcing words and actions, and the act of treating each other in a thoughtful manner, or in a way you would like to be treated if you were in their place.*

> NOTE: Harm-free = Doesn't result in harm to oneself or others

Of the five PERMA elements, creating positive relationships is the one least impacted by doing the Weight Success Method. This is because the Method has been designed to be a do-it-yourself activity. I made it this way because I don't want your success and my success in the pursuit of healthy-weight living to be dependent on having a certain relationship with others.

But, if you so chose, you could do things that would make performance of the Weight Success Method promote expansion of positive relationships.

Creating Positive Relationships While Doing the Weight Success Method

There are at least two ways a person might expand the relationships element in their life via doing the Weight Success Method.

1. For your preferred dietary program, adopt one of the established dietary programs that includes positive interaction with coaches and co-dieters.

2. Create a "healthy-weight achievement group" consisting of you and one or more others who are pursuing the Weight Success Method, or otherwise pursuing the goal of living in their healthy-weight range.

For either option to qualify as a positive relationship it likely would need to meet the above formal definition of a positive relationship. Meaning, it should include relationship-building activities such as constructive communication, inspiring words or positive reinforcement, sharing of progress actions, ideas, and discoveries, and perhaps even some group exercise activity.

In short, by forming a positive relationship with one or more persons, with one of the goals of the relationship being creation of healthy-weight living, you would *expand* the positive relationships element in your life, and also likely make creating healthy-weight living even easier and more enjoyable.

Meaning

Okay, sounds simple, but what exactly *is* meaning? Like the prior three PERMA elements, a tidy definition is hard to find. In his book *Flow,* Csikszentmihalyi devotes the entire last chapter, titled "The Making of Meaning," to explaining it in detail and depth. In the third paragraph of the chapter it says this:

> "If a person sets out to achieve a difficult enough goal, from which all other goals logically follow, and if he or she invests all energy in developing skills to reach that goal, then actions and feelings will be in harmony, and the separate parts of life will fit together — and each activity will 'make sense' in the present, as well as in view of the past and of the future. In such a way, it is possible to give meaning to one's entire life."

For a shorter definition I turn to Seligman. In his book *Flourish* he defines meaning (by way of a parenthetical phrase) as "belonging to and serving something that you believe is bigger than self."

So that's the long and short of it. For this discussion I split the difference, and do a little paraphrasing and creative adaptation, to derive this formal definition.

***Meaning** is the situation of perceiving one's life as existing for fulfillment of a certain*

worthwhile overriding purpose, or ultimate goal, with that goal being associated with serving or enhancing something bigger than one's self.

So how can a person use the pursuit of healthy-weight living to enhance meaning in their life? Or, put another way, how can they use the pursuit of healthy-weight living to enhance their perspective or belief that their life exists for fulfillment of a certain worthwhile overriding purpose?

Enhancing Life Meaning via Your Pursuit of Healthy-weight Living

From my perspective, the key to making the pursuit of healthy-weight living — or any personal development activity — contribute to enhancement of life meaning is to adopt a life perspective that embraces personal development as an activity that enhances or serves a higher purpose, or "something bigger than oneself."

The easiest, most effective way to explain how one might do this is by citing an example. And the example I know best is me. So here's the approach I personally use for creating overall life meaning and, in particular, for making my pursuit of healthy-weight living contribute to enhancing that meaning. It involves adoption of the following seven assumptions.

1. I assume there's a God. I realize that in the eyes of some this assumption might appear old-fashioned or wrong-headed, but I've found it to be the simplest, most effective starting point for creating and enhancing meaning in my life.

2. I assume that God is a universal spiritual being on an endless journey of conceptualization and actualization, which I call *creation journey* for short. I assume that a result of this creation journey is the evolving universe and everything in it.

3. I assume that part of this creation journey is the creation of life and the evolvement of life forms. I further assume that on planet Earth the present apex of this evolvement of life forms is human beings.

4. I assume that God made this evolvement of human beings to happen for a certain purpose:

specifically, to create beings that can appreciate, contribute to, and be part of his creation journey.

5. I assume that to enable humans to contribute to this journey God made the human species to possess a mini version, or micro extension, of some of God's powers. For reference purpose I call these powers *spiritual powers,* although they could be called spiritual faculties, instead. From my viewpoint, these spiritual powers include (a) the power to deliberately focus, (b) the power to discern, (c) the power to choose, in particular the power to choose what to think, to feel, and to do, (d) the power to depict and describe, (e) the power to create, hold, and act on a belief, including the power to act as-if, (f) the power to appreciate and to express thanks, (g) the power to look toward the future and survey possible outcomes and alternatives, and (h) the power to conceptualize and actualize — a.k.a. the power to achieve and create success — that is, the power to create an actual situation that corresponds to a certain imagined desired situation, or goal.

6. I assume that there are three main ways that each human can contribute to God's creation journey: (1) by performing acts that contribute to them becoming a finer person, (2) by performing acts that contribute to them creating a more beneficial life, and (3) by helping others do the same. I call these three actions God-enhancement Actions 1, 2, and 3.

7. Finally, I assume that the realization of healthy-weight living — or living most or all of our days in our healthy-weight range — is an activity that promotes *all three* of these God-enhancement actions.

In short, adopting the above seven assumptions is how I impart greater meaning to my life. And, it's also how I enhance the meaning of my weight success journey, which, in turn, further expands the meaning element in my life.

Engagement (or Flow)

Upon first encounter, I found engagement — a.k.a. flow — to be the only one of the five PERMA

elements that was confusing. The confusion derived from disparate descriptions of what it is. Here, for example, are seven descriptions, reproduced verbatim, from six pieces of literature.

1. *Engagement = being fully absorbed in activities that use your skills and challenge you.*
2. *Engagement refers to involvement in activities that draw and build upon one's interests. Csikszentmihalyi explains true engagement as flow, a feeling of intensity that leads to a sense of ecstasy and clarity.*
3. *Engagement refers to a deep psychological connection (e.g., being interested, engaged, and absorbed) to a particular activity, organization, or cause.*
4. *Engagement is about being totally absorbed (in a flow) by a present task where time and self-consciousness cease to exist.*
5. *Engagement – being completely absorbed in activities.*
6. *Flow: the psychological state that accompanies highly engaging activities.*
7. *Flow can be described as the experience of working at full capacity.*

Taken in total, this list of descriptions is befuddling. It also seems to indicate that, as a group, positive psychology practitioners seem to lack a unified concept of what engagement is or entails.

So, in an attempt to clarify things I returned to the book *Flow.* Now let me take a second to tell you about this book. If you like easy-reading fluff this book's not your type. It's a densely packed tome. But the good news is: It's a gold mine of intriguing research, insights, observations, and prescriptions. I typically read non-fiction books with pencil in hand so I can mark the occasional good thought or key point. With *Flow,* I found myself seemingly marking entire pages and sections.

So I re-opened *Flow* and leafed through it looking for a tidy definition of flow — a.k.a. engagement. And, guess what, I couldn't find one (which doesn't necessarily mean it's not there but, rather, it could be my old eyes didn't spot it).

So I reconciled myself to constructing a definition based on the information in the book. In Part B, in a section titled "The Elements of Enjoyment," the book describes eight components the author calls "the phenomenology of enjoyment." I then paraphrased and condensed it. What resulted is the following description.

When people reflect on how it feels when their experience is most positive, they mention at least one, and often all, of the following:

1. *it's an activity that's <u>challenging but doable</u>;*

2. *they're able to <u>focus totally</u> on the activity, to the point that doing it becomes spontaneous or automatic;*

3. *the activity has <u>clear goals</u>;*

4. *they get <u>immediate feedback</u> on how they're doing;*

5. *they pursue the activity with a <u>deep, effortless involvement</u> (that excludes everyday worries and concerns);*

6. *they can <u>exercise control</u> over their actions;*

7. *they're <u>free of self-consciousness</u> — that is, thoughts about their self disappear; and*

8. *they're so involved they <u>lose track of time</u>.*

After viewing this paraphrase a realization hit me. When distilled to its essence, what this describes is a situation in which a person has their *whole mind involved* in the performance of a certain activity, or in pursuit of a certain goal. By "whole mind involved" I mean: all the faculties of their mind that contribute to creating optimal performance in that particular activity. This includes both conscious <u>and</u> subconscious mind faculties.

So how does this relate to the prior list of eight factors that constitute the phenomenology of enjoyment? Like this. Items 1, 2, 3, 4, and 6 describe characteristics that foster, or enable, a person to have their whole mind involved in the performance of an activity. Items 5, 7, and 8 describe what a person experiences as a result of having their whole mind involved.

So, from my perspective the situation of engagement, or flow, happens whenever a person has all the performance-enhancing faculties of their

whole mind — that is, both conscious and subconscious mind — involved in a certain activity or in pursuit of a certain goal. As such, this leads me to the following definition.

Engagement *— a.k.a. flow — is the situation of having all the performance-enhancing faculties of one's whole mind involved in optimal performance of a certain activity or in optimal pursuit of a certain goal.*

> NOTE: "all the performance-enhancing faculties of one's whole mind" = all the faculties of one's mind, both conscious and subconscious, that contribute to creating optimal performance of a certain activity or optimal pursuit of a certain goal

So, referring back to the eight elements of "phenomenology of enjoyment," described in the book *Flow,* we could say: For an activity to be optimally conducive to engagement, or optimally conducive to whole mind involvement, that activity should possess the following eight characteristics: (1) be a challenging but doable activity, (2) enable a person to focus totally on its performance, (3) involve clear goals, (4) provide immediate feedback, (5) enable deep, effortless involvement (that excludes everyday worries and concerns), (6) enable self-direction, or the opportunity to exercise control over one's actions, (7) enable non-self-conscious involvement, or doing the activity free of self-consciousness, and (8) allow for uninterrupted performance, or performance that proceeds without interruption by time or any other focus-distracting factor.

Further, Csikszentmihalyi, Seligman, and Peterson, in their respective books *Flow* and *Flourish* and *A Primer in Positive Psychology,* describe a further condition for promoting engagement. They point out that maximal engagement occurs when a person's maximal talents or skills exactly match the challenges presented by the activity.

And why is this match between maximal skills and challenges necessary? Because, when a person's challenge-solving skills greatly exceed the challenges encountered, boredom results. And, when challenge-solving skills are inadequate for resolving the challenges encountered, frustration results. And, when either of these two conditions exists, a person can't get their whole mind involved in performing the activity.

Now here's a key point. Many persons quit the pursuit of weight control due to frustration, or due to a lack of skills that enable them to resolve the challenges they encounter. But the Weight Success Method equips a person with the tools to overcome the challenges involved in this pursuit, thereby removing the frustration and enabling engagement to happen.

> NOTE: As you've seen, the words "engagement" and "flow" are synonyms. Some writers use "engagement," others use "flow." For simplicity, from here on I'm going to use the word **"engagement."** But you should keep in mind that what I'm talking about is what some call "flow."

Engagement and Weight Success Journey

In most cases, when discussing the concept of engagement the writer describes it in the context of a discrete activity — that is, in relation to an activity that has a beginning point and ending point, or involves a distinct period of time that occurs within a certain day. The period of time might be just a few minutes. Or, it might go for a few hours.

But, sometimes a writer implies that the concept also applies to an ongoing activity, or to a pursuit that extends over months, or years, or even a lifetime. For example, in *Flow* Csikszentmihalyi starts by mainly discussing the engagement experience as a discrete activity, such as might occur in activities like rock climbing, chess match, performing a sport, playing music, doing artistic painting, and so forth. But as the book progresses the discussion gradually morphs into focusing more on engagement in *ongoing* activities and eventually ends up discussing engagement in the life journey.

So, this raises a question: Is engagement in an ongoing activity the same as engagement in a discrete activity? My answer would be: Yes and No. In certain basic ways they're alike. Both involve a clear goal, frequent feedback, focus on the task, control over actions, and maximal utilization of

certain skills for resolving challenges and gaining goal achievement. In short, both require a type of whole mind involvement.

But in some peripheral ways they differ. For example, in describing discrete-activity engagement some writers cite the characteristic of time distortion — such as, for example, thinking that only a few minutes have elapsed when actually, say, an hour has gone by. Another thing cited as a characteristic of discrete-activity engagement is loss of self-consciousness. Still another is "merging of action and awareness." None of these things exist as characteristics of ongoing-activity engagement, or at least not to the same extent as with discrete-activity engagement.

With the similarities and differences between discrete-activity engagement and ongoing-activity engagement in mind, I propose that a concept of ongoing-activity engagement can be applied to the pursuit of healthy-weight living. And, I further believe, when one pursues healthy-weight living in a state of ongoing-activity engagement that something good happens: creating healthy-weight living becomes easier and more enjoyable.

So, what are the factors that create, or promote, engagement in the performance of an ongoing activity? You've likely already encountered them. They're the 19 Success Drivers described in Chapter 19. When a person applies these nineteen factors to an important ongoing activity that extends over years or a lifetime, that person becomes engaged with the activity in a way that's absorbing, attention-focusing, performance-enhancing, and gratifying — a situation that I call *ongoing-activity engagement.*

Again, the result of this type of engagement is that performance of the activity and achievement of the desired outcome become easier and more automatic. So, what's the easiest way to involve the 19 success drivers in your pursuit of healthy-weight living? You already know: It's do the Weight Success Method. When you fully apply the Weight Success Method to the pursuit of healthy-weight living, you end up pursuing healthy-weight living with whole mind involvement, or ongoing-activity engagement. Or, put yet another way, you get your conscious mind and subconscious mind synced up and working together in pursuit of achieving the goal of you living the rest of your life in your healthy-weight range.

Summing Up

Briefly put, here's how doing the Weight Success Method expands your amount of well-being. It's based on the PERMA model. First, when you pursue healthy-weight living with the Weight Success Method you end up expanding the amount of enjoyment, or *Positive Emotion,* in your life.

Second, you expand the amount of ongoing-activity *Engagement* in your life. Third, if you apply the Weight Success Method in conjunction with other people you would likely expand the amount of positive *Relationships* in your life. Fourth, if you hold a certain "life meaning paradigm" that embraces personal improvement as a noble activity, then pursuing healthy-weight living via the Weight Success Method could expand the *Meaning* in your life. And, fifth, creating healthy-weight living via doing the Method expands the amount of *Accomplishment* in your life.

Doing the Weight Success Method expands the amount of **PERMA** in your life journey. This, in turn, makes creating healthy-weight living easier, more enjoyable, more automatic, more natural, and more life-enhancing.

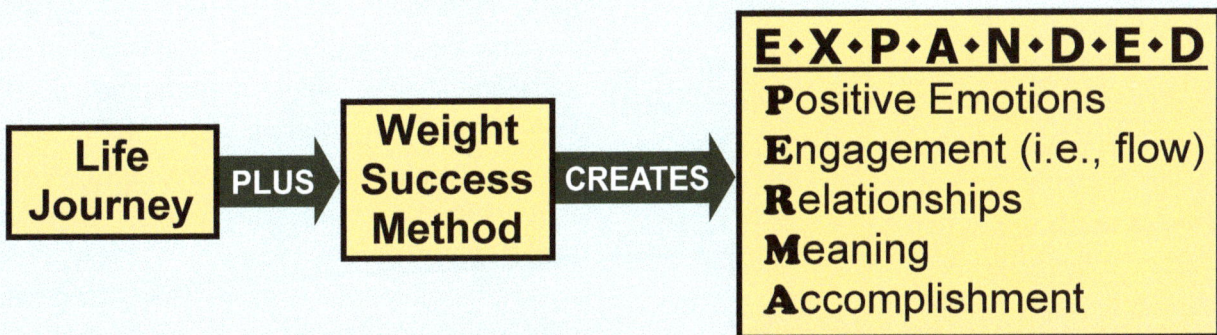

Life Journey PLUS **Weight Success Method** CREATES

E·X·P·A·N·D·E·D
Positive Emotions
Engagement (i.e., flow)
Relationships
Meaning
Accomplishment

Do the **Five Daily Actions** every day . . .
and **Lifelong Weight Success** will be Yours.

Typically takes less than **8** minutes of dedicated time per day.

CHAPTER 23: The No-change Secret of Maintenance Achievement

Here's a little-known type of achievement that enables lifelong healthy weight living and also maximal life journey success.

WHERE I LIVE there's a certain ice cream parlor that's especially popular and successful. It has great product, super service, charming décor, and conscientious staff.

I was there one day enjoying a vanilla malt (they have the best in town) when suddenly the owner came out to clear a couple tables. Often when I have a chance to speak to a business owner I pose a certain question. So I said, "You have an excellent business here. Tell me, if you would, what's the secret to your success?"

There were a couple seconds of silence. Then he gave me an answer I'd never heard before and haven't heard since. He said, "No change."

I must have looked puzzled, so he elaborated. "We have a winning formula here. It has been working year after year since the 1960s. My parents started it and I inherited it. MY JOB is to make sure *nothing changes* ... to make sure we keep doing what we've been doing and to preserve the business the way it is today. Staying the same, or not changing, is the secret to our success."

What makes this perspective unique is that very few businesses — indeed, very few people — have as their goal "staying the same." Instead, whenever the subject of success or achievement comes up it's always defined in terms of *change.* That is, it's described in terms of changing one's self or situation from a present state to some other state. Both individually and societally, we have become "wired" to view success and achievement in terms of how much change we make in going from a present situation to a new situation. Change, or moving from situation A to situation B, is what we think of when we hear the word "achievement." I call this *change achievement.*

But there's another form of achievement, which most folks have no experience with. It's what the ice cream parlor owner described. It's the achievement of staying the same, or continuing to do what

one is presently doing. I call this *maintenance achievement.* It's the opposite of change achievement. With change achievement, success derives from creating certain change; but with maintenance achievement, success derives from creating <u>no</u> change.

Change achievement is imbedded in our culture. We have books, courses, and methodologies that tell us how to create it. So most everyone has at least an inkling of how to create it. But, maintenance achievement is a mystery. Virtually no one knows how to create it. And herein lies a paradox that's driving ultimate weight failure. In weight maintenance mode, the way we succeed is by creating *no-change,* or staying the same. Oddly, most folks think this can be achieved by "non-action" or "doing nothing." But that's incorrect. Staying the same, or creating no-change, requires as much deliberate focus and action as creating the condition of change. I call this the *no-change secret.* Most folks are unaware of it, which is a major reason why most persons are ineffective at creating the no-change situation required for achieving lifelong weight maintenance, otherwise known as "making weight loss stick."

This situation has been causing us to conclude that weight maintenance is tougher than weight reduction. But this is incorrect. Actually, doing weight maintenance is *easier* than doing weight reduction <u>if</u> you know how to succeed at creating weight maintenance. But most folks don't. So we've been achieving a modicum of success at losing weight and failing miserably at keeping it off.

How do we solve this problem? Do the Weight Success Method. It's specially designed to cause you to take the actions that result in you accomplishing *no*-change after you've succeeded at losing weight and entering your healthy-weight range. Or, put another way, it's specially designed for enacting *both* change achievement involved in creating weight loss <u>and</u> maintenance achievement involved in creating lifelong healthy-weight living. As such, it's <u>the</u> tool by which you can more easily get into your desired weight range *and then easily stay there* the rest of your life.

As a people, we applaud persons for the amount of weight they lose. That's fine. But while doing that, we should be giving standing ovations for the number of years a person keeps that weight off. Losing weight is commendable. But *maintaining* one's healthy weight is a truly exceptional accomplishment.

So, allow yourself to have a good feeling from living in your healthy-weight range **every** day you do it.

Do the
Five Daily Actions
<u>eve</u>ry day . . . and
Lifelong Weight Success
will be <u>Yours</u>.

Typically takes <u>less than</u> **8** minutes
of dedicated time per day.

CHAPTER 24: Expanded Weight Success Benefits

Living in your healthy-weight range produces many benefits, which have been previously described. But, amazingly, there are even more benefits to be gained from your weight success journey.

A MAIN RESULT of weight management is a "new" body — specifically, a body that weighs in your desired weight range. This new body and the benefits that come with it are the main outcome of your weight success pursuit.

But, as important as these benefits are, they're not the only possible good outcome to be gained from your weight success journey. There are at least eight possible extra benefits. You might derive one or more — or perhaps all.

1st Possible Extra Benefit: Enhanced Mindset

Along with gaining an enhanced body, you might also gain an enhanced *mindset* — specifically, a mindset having a greater number of success-creating mind elements, or perspectives, feelings, and mind-habits that promote success.

2nd Possible Extra Benefit: Enhanced Self-image

You might gain an enhanced, or more beneficial, self-image. And, along with that, enhanced self-confidence and self-esteem.

3rd Possible Extra Benefit: Success-creation Knowledge

You might gain powerful new success-driving knowledge. While on your weight success journey you might discover, or re-confirm, that most or all of the 19 success drivers that are propelling you to success in your weight success journey can also be used to expedite success in *any other significant endeavor of your life.*

4th Possible Extra Benefit: Mind Awareness

You might discover, or at least become more aware of, the presence, power, and performance of your subconscious mind. And, you might learn of several processes for deliberately communicating with your subconscious mind, thereby giving you the means for deliberately enlisting the performance of your subconscious mind for achieving certain worthwhile ends, any time you desire to do so.

5th Possible Extra Benefit: Daily Good Feeling

You might realize that your weight success journey isn't just some exercise in counting calories and eating certain foods. You might discover that it's actually a special, outstanding accomplishment — an accomplishment worthy of daily recognition and applause, and something you should allow yourself to derive a good feeling from — *every day.*

6th Possible Extra Benefit: Expanded Life Journey

Keep this in mind. Your weight success journey is part of a larger journey, a journey in lifelong personal achievement and fulfillment. As such, you might discover that by succeeding at your weight success journey you're expanding your life journey into something even more beneficial and fulfilling than you previously imagined. This was discussed in the How the Weight Success Method Enhances Your Life Journey chapter (p. **137**).

7th Possible Extra Benefit: Opportunity to Help Others Have a Better Life

Many people cling to the notion that their life impacts only them. Holding this assumption enables them to rationalize that it doesn't matter what they do, or how they live, or what kind of person they decide to be.

But they're wrong. Each person's life *does* impact the life of others — in particular those closest to them, such as parents, spouse, children, grandchildren, siblings, friends, neighbors. Whenever we do something that amounts to us becoming a finer person or creating a more beneficial life it *positively* impacts the lives of those close to us. Conversely, whenever we do something that amounts to us becoming a less-fine person or living a less beneficial life it *negatively* impacts the lives of those close to us. These two things happen regardless of whether we know they're happening and also regardless of whether we want them to happen.

What's more, the impact of some things we do extends beyond us. By a cause-and-effect chain this impact ultimately extends to people we've never met, even to those not yet born.

So how does this pertain to healthy-weight living? In two ways. First, when we make the decision to live the rest of our life in our healthy-weight range, our life becomes a powerful role model for healthy-weight living — a role model that some of those near and dear to us will ultimately emulate. Second, when we live the latter years of our life in our healthy-weight range we reduce the likelihood of contracting a debilitating condition resulting from extended overweight living.

So as a result, two major positive outcomes occur. First, by being a role model for healthy-weight living you (a) inspire and help others to do the same, which (b) makes their life even better, and also (c) makes the world even better, and finally (d) makes your life even more meaningful and beneficial. Second, by reducing the chance of contracting a debilitating condition from overweight living you reduce the chance of someone close to you having to carry the burden of looking after you or taking care of you for years while you're living in an incapacitated state.

8th Possible Extra Benefit: Life Enhancement from Getting Input from God

You might discover and apply throughout your life a simple method for gaining insights from God — these insights enabling you to more readily solve stubborn problems and achieve challenging goals (this method being the Three Steps to Getting and Using Input from God, page **97**).

Contrary to what most people assume, the potential benefits of pursuing and creating lifelong Healthy-weight Living are manifold. Done the right way, it can be one of life's simplest pleasures and also most gratifying accomplishments.

CHAPTER 25: Why Most Persons Never Pursue Weight Control

MOST PERSONS hold numerous misconceptions pertaining to healthy-weight living. These misconceptions cause the majority of people to never make a whole-hearted attempt at creating it. Here are nine common misconceptions that cause people to avoid pursuing healthy-weight living.

Misconception 1: Healthy-weight living is an end-result one must achieve. *The Reality:* Healthy-weight living is an ongoing success-creation <u>process</u> that one sustains by doing simple weight success actions each day.

Misconception 2: Healthy-weight living is a far-off situation. *The Reality:* For most persons it can be attained in a matter of just a few months. Or, if one is a lot overweight, it can be attained in a year or so, which although slightly longer is still a relatively short time.

Misconception 3: Healthy-weight living is hard to accomplish. *The Reality:* If one applies a certain method — namely, the Weight Success Method — healthy-weight living is relatively easy to attain, or at least much easier than most persons imagine.

Misconception 4: Maintaining healthy-weight living is joyless, limiting drudgery that involves much sacrifice. *The Reality:* When pursued a certain way (using the Weight Success Method) healthy-weight living brings more enjoyment, happiness, freedom, and gratification than most persons imagine.

Misconception 5: Certain fat-promoting factors can subvert or prevent healthy-weight living. *The Reality:* There's not a single fat-promoting factor that can prevent a person from creating healthy-weight living.

Misconception 6: Creating healthy-weight living requires special medicine or medical procedure. *The Reality:* Although a medical procedure might be a helpful aid for creating healthy-weight living for a few people, it's likely not a requirement for anyone to create healthy-weight living success.

Misconception 7: Creating healthy-weight living requires daily exercise. *The Reality:* Although exercise can be helpful and beneficial, it's not a requirement for succeeding at creating healthy-weight living for anyone.

Misconception 8: Creating healthy-weight living requires applying a strict dietary regimen or a particular dietary program. *The Reality:* It usually helps to apply a preferred dietary program that fits one's personal preferences, needs, and lifestyle, but there's no one specific dietary program that's a requirement for creating healthy-weight living.

Misconception 9: After healthy-weight living is achieved, it doesn't last for long. *The Reality:* It's true that for the past fifty years or so most persons who have lost weight, or achieved a certain weight goal, have eventually gained back the weight they lost. But, this has happened because most persons haven't applied a method for *maintaining* healthy-weight living once they've achieved it. This book changes that. By applying the Weight Success Method you stay living in your healthy-weight range the rest of your life ... and it likely happens easily and enjoyably, or at least more easily and enjoyably than you likely imagine it to be.

Summation

Misconceptions pertaining to healthy-weight living prevent most persons from ever striving to achieve it, and also work to defeat those persons who do attempt it.

Nine Main <u>Misconceptions</u> Pertaining to Healthy-weight Living are:

1 – It's an end-result that one achieves (as opposed to an activity that one sustains).
2 – It's a far-off situation.
3 – It's hard to accomplish.
4 – Maintaining it involves joyless drudgery and much sacrifice.
5 – Certain fat-promoting factors can subvert or prevent it.

6 – Achieving it requires special medicine or medical procedure.

7 – Achieving it requires daily exercise.

8 – Achieving it requires applying a strict dietary regimen or a particular dietary program.

9 – Once it's achieved it won't last for long.

For more on misconceptions and false assumptions that are sabotaging weight management, go to the 16 False Assumptions that are Sabotaging Us chapter (p. **126**).

Once humankind understands what healthy-weight living really is and the easiest way to create it, the growing global overweightness trend will <u>stop</u> and worldwide healthy-weight living will <u>ascend</u>.

Do the
Five Daily Actions
<u>every</u> day . . . and
Lifelong Weight Success
will be <u>Yours</u>.

Typically takes <u>less than</u> **8** minutes of dedicated time per day.

CHAPTER 26: Message from Healthy-weight Living

Throughout this book, I (the author) have done the talking. So, for some personification fun I'm bringing in *Healthy-weight Living* itself to impart a special message.

Hello, I am Healthy-weight living!
You might think you know me.
> *But most likely you do <u>not</u> know me. I'll explain.*

You think I'm far away and out of reach.
> *But I'm near you this very moment.*

You think I'm hard to get.
> *But I'm so easy to have you don't believe it.*

You think I'm no fun.
> *But I bring more benefits, enjoyment, and gratification than you imagine.*

You think I'm an <u>achievement</u> — a destination or end-result that you arrive at.
> *But, actually, I'm a <u>process</u> — an ongoing **success-creation process** you do each day.*

You think I can be killed by certain fat-promoting factors.
> *But not a one can stop me, not a one can prevent me.*

You think I exist to harass, punish, and limit you.
> *But, in truth, I exist to help you live an easier, happier, freer life.*

You think the way you entice me into your life is to change the way you EAT.
> *But, actually, the way you cause me to join you is to change the way you THINK — in particular, the way you think about your self, your mind, your life, weight management, and <u>me</u> — Healthy-weight Living.*

You think that for me to stick with you you need a special medicine or medical procedure.
> *But — even though a medical procedure might be helpful for some — I don't absolutely require it.*

You think it's required that you exercise each day in order for me to be your friend.
> *But — even though exercise can be helpful and beneficial — I don't require it of anyone.*

You think it's required that you embrace a strict dietary regimen in order for me to accept you.
> *But I don't require that.*

You think it's required that you work hard and sacrifice in order for me to stick around.
> *But I don't require that.*

You think I'm fickle and fleeting.
> *But I'm not. I'll happily stay with you <u>forever</u> IF you treat me a certain way. All I request is that you truly want me to be with you, that you view me in a positive light, that you honor me each day with some whole-mind attention, and that you pursue me as a **daily success-creation process**.*

Yes, I am Healthy-weight living. Know me for what I <u>really</u> am; know how I <u>really</u> work. Then I will become one of your closest, most loyal friends — for life. And, once you and I become friends, please tell your other friends about me. Because I would like to someday be their friend, too. Truth is, I'd like to be a friend of everyone on the planet. But that's not likely to happen today, because most people are confused about me. They think they know who I am and how I work.
> *But, actually, they do not. And, as long as they don't know how I really work, they will be avoiding me, and will be refraining from inviting me into their life.*

Still, it brings me great comfort to realize that YOU now know the truth about me. I trust you'll be putting it to good use ... for the rest of your life.

Weight Success Actions Scorecard™ | Daily Point Calculator

DATE→											
FIVE DAILY ACTIONS of the Weight Success Method											
Did Daily Action 1–Weighing | **50** pts.											
Got a Desired Weight Reading | **100** pts.											
Did Daily Action 2A–Reinforcement **or** Daily Action 2B–Correction | **50** pts.											
Did Daily Action 3–Benefits Directive | **50** pts.											
Did Daily Action 4–Goal Statement | **50** pts.											
Did extra Goal Statement iterations for Daily Action 4 | Score **1** point for each one over 25											
Did Daily Action 5–Guided Eating | **50** pts.											
(A) TOTAL POINTS for doing Daily Actions											
OPTIONAL ACTIONS											
Did my daily exercise | **100** pts.											
Did at least three of the eight eating actions described in Ch. 12 (p. 82) | **30** pts.											
Did Motivator 2: Backup Depiction Statement – Ch. 13 (p. 90) | Score **1** point per iteration											
Did Motivator 3: Upcoming-day Description – Ch. 13 (p. 92) | **30** pts.											
Did Motivator 4: Day-end Thanks – Ch. 13 (p. 94) | **30** pts.											
Did Motivator 5: Benefits Visualization – Ch. 13 (p. 94) | **30** pts.											
Did Motivator 6: Goal Reminders – Ch. 13 (p. 94) | **30** pts											
Applied my preferred dietary program (or did right eating) for the entire day | **100** pts.											
Thanked God for the opportunity to be alive & the power to live my healthy weight | **100** pts.											
Did the setback-reversal process, if needed – Ch. 10 (p. 68) | **100** pts.											
(B) TOTAL POINTS for Optional Actions											
GRAND TOTAL POINTS for the Day (A + B)											

INSTRUCTIONS: In the line near the top, put the date of the day being scored. In the boxes beneath that date, insert the number of points you achieved from doing each of the Actions (both Daily Actions and Optional Actions). Then add up the TOTAL points for the Daily Actions (A) and the TOTAL points for the Optional Actions (B). Finally, add those two totals together for the GRAND TOTAL number of points you achieved for the day. ~ To easily print out this chart, go to: correllconcepts.com/toolkit.pdf

Example of Partial Win-Day Calendar with Some W's Filled In

SUN	MON	TUE	WED	THU	FRI	SAT
1 W	2 W	3 W	4 W	5 W	6 W	7 W
8 W	9 W	10 W	11 W	12	13	14
15	16	17	18	19	20	21

Note: The above graphic was designed to illustrate the W's, which is why there's only a partial month shown.

If you like, also record your daily weight (scale reading) number on the calendar. Write it in the lower right corner of the square for each day.

Making Your Own Calendar

In case you might prefer to make your own calendar instead of buying one, on the next page (**157**) is a blank calendar sheet you can use for any month. Print copies of it for your use. For each month, fill in the appropriate squares with the appropriate date number for each day. Put the date in the upper left corner of the square. Then use the sheet to record your winning days with a "W."

Do the **Five Daily Actions**
<u>every</u> day . . .
and **Lifelong Weight Success**
will be <u>Yours</u>.

Typically takes <u>less than</u> **8** minutes
of dedicated time per day.

Win-Day Calendar™

Month of:					Year:	
SUN	**MON**	**TUE**	**WED**	**THU**	**FRI**	**SAT**

INSTRUCTIONS: Make copies for your use. Fill in the month and year in the line at the top. In the upper left corner of each day box that pertains to that particular month, write in the date of that day. Each day that your daily weight reading is a *desired* reading, write a big "W" in the box. Also, if you like, write in the scale weight reading you got for that day (suggested that you put it in the lower right corner of the box). ~ To easily print out this chart, go to: **correllconcepts.com/toolkit.pdf**

Weight-reduction Success Graph™

Month of: Year:

DAY→ 1 2 3 4 5 6 7 8 9 10 11 12 13 14 15 16 17 18 19 20 21 22 23 24 25 26 27 28 29 30 31

BODY WEIGHT NUMBER – IN EITHER POUNDS OR KILOGRAMS

INSTRUCTIONS: If you happen to presently be in weight-reduction mode, make copies of this graph to record your daily progress. For each month, put your projected declining weight numbers along the left side of the graph. Fill in the month and year at the top. ~ On the next page (**159**) is an example to illustrate how it would work. It's filled in with example pound weight numbers (shown in green) and an example graph line showing a person's body weight for 31 days of that month (in red). ~ To easily print out this graph, go to: **correllconcepts.com/toolkit.pdf**

Weight-reduction Success Graph™

Month of: *AUGUST*   Year: *2018*

EXAMPLE: At the top, fill in the month and year (shown in blue). Fill in the target weight numbers (shown in green). If you weigh in kilograms (as opposed to pounds), it's recommended that your weight numbers be in half-kilogram increments. So, for example, if your present weight were, say, 76 kilograms, the declining weight increments would be: 76, 75.5, 75, 74.5, 74, 73.5, 73 … and so on. If a day's weight turns out to be half way between two weight numbers, then position the dot for that day (shown in red) half way between the two numbers, as done for some days in the above graph. **NOTE:** The above red weight line is a steep line for illustration purposes only. In actuality, your daily weight loss might be much less. Also if you like, for a steeper red line, label the lines in half-pound increments — for example, 168, 167.5, 167, 166.5, 166, 165.5, and so on.

Setting Up a Fail-proof Reminder System

Many persons fail to create healthy-weight living <u>not</u> because they don't know what to do and <u>not</u> because they don't want to do it but, rather, because they *forget* to do it.

Since eating is a daily activity it means that creating healthy-weight living must also be a *daily* activity. The easiest, most effective daily activity for creating healthy-weight living is doing the five daily actions of the Weight Success Method each day.

I know this might sound unbelievable, but a main thing that will stop you from realizing lifelong healthy-weight living is failing to remember to do all five daily actions each day. So, I suggest you set up a fail-proof reminder mechanism that will remind you each day to do these five actions. Here's a sample way to do it.

Print out one or more copies of the rectangle-enclosed messages on the next page (p. **161**). If you need different sizes than these, just put a copy on a copier machine, enlarge or reduce the image to suit your needs, and then print it.

Place copies where you'll see them every day. Possibilities include: (a) in your bedroom, (b) on the refrigerator, (c) in your wallet or purse, (d) in your car, (e) on your computer, and (f) on your exercise equipment.

Plus, also put digital messages on your computer screen, smartphone, and other devices you access every day. For that, go to:

http://correllconcepts.com/wfm-jpg.htm

In short, do whatever it takes to set up a fail-proof reminder system that will remind you each day to do the five daily actions of the Weight Success Method. Installing a daily reminder mechanism is a vital key to more easily living the rest of your life in your healthy-weight range.

It may be that more instances of failure result from **forgetting** to do what one should be doing than from **not knowing** what one should do.

Do the **Five Daily Actions** <u>every</u> day . . . and **Lifelong Weight Success** will be <u>Yours</u>.

Typically takes <u>less than</u> **8** minutes of dedicated time per day.

Weight Success Method

Do it every day. Takes less than eight minutes.

1 – Weighing
2 – Reinforcement or Correction
3 – Benefits Directive
4 – Goal Statement
5 – Guided Eating

(plus Daily Exercise Activity when possible)

Weight Success Method

Do it every day. Takes less than eight minutes.

1 – Weighing
2 – Reinforcement or Correction
3 – Benefits Directive
4 – Goal Statement
5 – Guided Eating

(plus Daily Exercise Activity when possible)

Weight Success Method

Do it every day. Takes less than eight minutes.

1 – Weighing
2 – Reinforcement or Correction
3 – Benefits Directive
4 – Goal Statement
5 – Guided Eating

(plus Daily Exercise Activity when possible)

INSTRUCTIONS: Make one or more copies of this page. If you need different sizes than these, just put a copy on a copier machine, enlarge or reduce the image to suit your needs, and then print it. Cut out the reminder messages and place them where you'll see them every day. ~ To easily print out this page, go to: **correllconcepts.com/toolkit.pdf**

GOING NATIONWIDE

— A How-to Guide for Creating Nationwide Weight Success —

THIS SECTION describes a program that I believe would be the easiest, most effective way to guide the citizenry of a nation to weight success — a.k.a. healthy-weight living. For future reference this program is dubbed *Nationwide Weight Success Initiative,* or NWSI for short.

We define *weight success* as: Living most or all of one's days in one's desired healthy-weight range <u>and</u> deriving benefits, enjoyment, and fulfillment from it. The ultimate goal of the Nationwide Weight Success Initiative is to have nearly everyone in the nation engaged in weight success — or living most or all of their days in their desired healthy-weight range and deriving benefits, enjoyment, and fulfillment from it.

To be effective, any program that aims to motivate an entire nation to pursue healthy-weight living should — or perhaps *must*— include the following eight actions:

1. Identify the misconceptions that exist regarding weight management, right eating, and healthy-weight living;

2. Refute and dispel those misconceptions;

3. Replace the dispelled misconceptions with healthy-weight-promoting conceptions;

4. Describe the possible benefits people can derive from weight success;

5. Explain that the key to creating healthy-weight living is to do Weight Success Actions *every day* — both during pursuit of weight reduction <u>and</u> during pursuit of weight maintenance;

6. Equip people with the wherewithal, including a simple step-by-step weight success program, that makes it easy for them to do Weight Success Actions every day;

7. Provide proof that anyone can easily succeed at healthy-weight living;

8. Make healthy-weight living appear to be, and to actually be, *more rewarding* than non-healthy-weight living, as viewed by the citizenry of the nation.

The above eight actions might not be the only actions that can contribute to creating nationwide healthy-weight living. But they're the essential ones needed for it. I'll now explain each.

ACTION 1: Identify Misconceptions

The starting point to motivating the people of a nation to pursue living their life in their healthy-weight range is to identify the many misconceptions that exist regarding weight management, right eating, and living in one's healthy-weight range. This likely will require broad interviewing and perhaps some psycho-analytical research. Here's the situation.

Most people are carrying in their mind a mountain of weight management misconceptions — including rationalization, self-delusion, and erroneous beliefs. These misconceptions are preventing them from pursuing, or from even considering pursuing, right eating and healthy-weight living. And, for those commendable few who do decide to "give it a try," these misconceptions eventually sabotage their every initiative at doing healthy-weight living, thereby dooming them to being a perpetual yo-yo dieter.

For a starting point in identifying these misconceptions I would suggest referring to (a) the 16 false assumptions listed in the 16 False Assumptions that Are Sabotaging Us chapter (p. **126**) and also (b) the nine misconceptions described in the Why Most Persons Never Pursue Weight Control chapter (p. **150**).

ACTION 2: Refute the Misconceptions

The second action is to line up all the misconceptions — that is, rationalizations, self-delusions, and false assumptions — and shoot 'em dead with refutation. And, then periodically shoot 'em again. This is a situation where beating a dead horse is a *good* thing to be doing, because the horse of weight management misconceptions is big, powerful, and pervasive, and could resurrect any time the refutation stops for long.

This Action Two, and the actions to follow, should be done via a powerful, captivating, broad-based *ongoing* nationwide advertising–communications–publicity campaign constructed to inspire and equip every individual to pursue and create weight success. For future reference I call this campaign the *Weight Success Communication Campaign.*

ACTION 3: Install Healthy-weight-promoting Conceptions

The third action, which would be concurrent with Action Two, is to present the "opposites" of the discredited misconceptions. Or, put another way, in this Action Three we replace the counterproductive rationalizations, self-delusions, and erroneous beliefs — which have been preventing most people from pursuing and succeeding at healthy-weight living — with productive perspectives and beliefs that promote, inspire, and sustain the pursuit and creation of healthy-weight living. This action won't be a one-time occurrence but, instead, along with Action Two, will be ongoing for many years. It would be performed through every communication vehicle available, including the media used in the Weight Success Communication Campaign.

ACTION 4: Describe Weight Success Benefits

The fourth action, which would be concurrent with Action Three, is to describe the many good things that a person can derive from right eating and healthy-weight living — which we call *weight success benefits.* Then, through the Weight Success Communication Campaign, urge each person to identify those benefits that apply specifically to them and their situation. In doing this it's likely that

the weight success benefit that will, or should, receive top billing will be: Maximizing the chance of *living healthier longer* — or maximizing the chance of living free of certain debilitating illnesses and body malfunctions.

ACTION 5: Explain the Key to Healthy-weight Living

The fifth action is to communicate to the entire nation that the key to easier healthy-weight living is: Do Weight Success Actions *every day* — both in the weight-reduction phase and in the weight-maintenance phase. Explain that this can be accomplished by doing the actions prescribed in the Weight Success Method, which causes success drivers to be included in one's weight success pursuit. (An explanation of success drivers is provided in Chapter 19, page 117.) And also, communicate to the nation the *Lifelong Weight Success Dynamic* (p. 45).

ACTION 6: Equip People with the Tools for Easily Doing Weight Success Actions Every Day

The sixth action, which would be concurrent with Action Five, is to equip each person — meaning, the entire nation — with the essential wherewithal they need for easily doing Weight Success Actions every day.

The following six tools, or resources, constitute the essential wherewithal that most persons need in order to easily do Weight Success Actions every day.

Tool 1: A step-by-step healthy-weight living program — a.k.a. weight success methodology — that makes it easy for them to do Weight Success Actions every day — both during weight reduction and during weight maintenance. A recommended program would be the Weight Success Method. All this could be provided on a website set up by the Nationwide Weight Success Initiative, and also made available via a paperback booklet, ebook, and other media forms.

Tool 2: *An accurate bathroom scale,* or daily access to one. Instructions on obtaining a good scale could be provided on a website set up by the Nationwide Weight Success Initiative. Go to the Weighing and Scale Info chapter (p. **62**) for details on scales.

Tool 3: *Knowledge of one's healthy-weight range.* A means for easy automatic ascertainment of one's healthy-weight range could be provided on a website set up by the Nationwide Weight Success Initiative. Also, we must make it possible for a person to make a phone call (in place of accessing a website), give their height, age, gender, and body type information, and receive back their healthy-weight range. This could be handled automatically, as opposed to having an actual person receiving the call. Go to the Healthy-weight Range in Detail chapter (p. **56**) for details on healthy-weight range.

Tool 4: *Recognition of one's weight success benefits* — that is, awareness of the benefits that a person will derive from living in their healthy-weight range. A listing of generic weight success benefits could be provided on a website set up by the Nationwide Weight Success Initiative. Go to the Weight Success Benefits in Detail chapter (p. **60**) for details on weight success benefits.

Tool 5: *Selection of a dietary program or eating strategy,* which could be either an established bona fide dietary program already on the market or a program of a person's own design. This program would be applied in conjunction with the recommended Healthy-weight Living program (Tool 1 above). A sample listing of the many available dietary program choices could be provided on a website set up by the Nationwide Weight Success Initiative. Go to Startup Action 7 in Chapter 1 (p. 19) for details on preferred dietary program.

Tool 6: *A weight success mindset* — that is, a set of perspectives that promotes doing right eating and living in one's healthy-weight range. A description of a sample recommended mindset could be provided on a website set up by the Nationwide Weight Success Initiative. Go to Startup Action 5 (p. 15) for details on weight success mindset.

So, these six resources, or instructions on how to get them, could be provided by the Nationwide Weight Success Initiative via website and also other media.

ACTION 7: Provide Proof that Healthy-weight Living Is Easily Doable

The seventh action is to provide proof that anyone can succeed at living in their healthy-weight range if (a) they make the decision to do so and (b) they get their whole mind involved in the act, which can be accomplished by applying the recommended Healthy-weight Living program (Tool 1 above), and (c) they pursue weight management as a process of doing Weight Success Actions every day.

There are many ways this proof can be provided. One way is to provide explanation of *why* the recommended weight-management method works. (Such an explanation exists in the Why the Weight Success Method Gets Your Whole Mind Involved chapter, page **109**.)

Another way, which likely would be the most convincing, is to provide examples. And, one of the most powerful examples is *demonstration by leaders.* In the case of government-created programs, such as the Nationwide Weight Success Initiative, the leaders are those persons chosen to lead and manage the nation. In the case of the United States, this leadership comprises the key, or high-ranking, persons working in the administration and congressional branches of our government.

So, the most convincing proof that anyone can and should succeed at living in their healthy-weight range would be for the president and his cabinet and also all the senators and representatives of congress to apply the program set forth in the Weight Success Method and, thereby, succeed at living in their healthy-weight range.

This action would be compelling evidence that what the Nationwide Weight Success Initiative is telling the entire nation it should be doing is, in fact, doable, effective, and desirable. Or, put another way, if the several hundred persons who constitute our national leadership do it, then it would be clearly obvious to the entire country that (a) *anyone* can do it and (b) everyone *should be* doing it.

Conversely, if the country's leadership isn't doing what it's telling the citizenry of the nation it should be doing — which is, living in one's healthy-weight range — this would cause many persons to conclude that our leaders are being dishonest and hypocritical. Which would be a significant hindrance to maximizing the success of the Nationwide Weight Success Initiative.

ACTION 8: Make Healthy-weight Living Appear to Be More Rewarding than Non-healthy-weight Living

---

The eighth action is: *Make people realize that healthy-weight living is more rewarding than non-healthy-weight living.* When people view healthy-weight living as being more rewarding (enjoyable, gratifying) than non-healthy-weight living, they choose to pursue healthy-weight living. Conversely, when they view non-healthy-weight living as being more rewarding than healthy-weight living, they choose to pursue non-healthy-weight living.

So, a main aim of the Weight Success Communication Campaign should be to make doing healthy-weight living appear to be, and to actually be, more rewarding than doing non-healthy-weight living, as viewed by the citizenry of the nation. By doing this we motivate people to pursue healthy-weight living and to forego non-healthy-weight living. Expressed in greater detail, this is how we could do it.

Every type of performance, including right eating performance and wrong eating performance, has both an upside and a downside. The upside is whatever a person likes about doing the particular performance. The downside is whatever the person dislikes about doing it. So, the net reward of any particular performance is "the upside minus the downside."

Which means, to expand the net reward that a person derives from doing healthy-weight living we must (a) expand the upside and (b) diminish the

downside of doing healthy-weight living, as viewed by the performer. Conversely, to diminish the net reward that a person derives from doing non-healthy-weight living we must (a) expand the downside and (b) diminish the upside of doing non-healthy-weight living, as viewed by the performer.

What all this comes down to is, the Weight Success Communication Campaign should include messages and programs designed to accomplish these four results.

1. *EXPAND the upside of right eating and healthy-weight living.* ❧ Identify the full upside picture of right eating and healthy-weight living and then project this picture into the minds of the nation.

> NOTE: For a full description of the upside to weight success, see these four chapters: Chapter **7** (p. 60), Chapter **17** (p. 103), Chapter **22** (p. 137), and Chapter **24** (p. 148).

2. *DIMINISH the downside of right eating.* ❧ Identify the aspects of right eating that some people might view as downside and then help them realize that these aspects can be diminished to insignificance. (Note: Part of what the recommended Weight Success Method does is help people reduce to insignificance the imagined downside of right eating.)

3. *EXPAND the downside of wrong eating and non-healthy-weight living.* ❧ Identify the full downside picture of wrong eating and non-healthy-weight living and then project this picture into the minds of the nation.

4. *DIMINISH the upside of wrong eating.* ❧ Identify those aspects of wrong eating, or over-eating, that some people might view as upside and then help them realize that these aspects bring large unintended bad consequences.

Those four results can be summed up by the infographic on the next page.

Conclusion

The most effective way to cause the citizenry of a nation to achieve weight success is to implement a national program that motivates and equips people to do vital weight success actions <u>every day</u> — both while in weight reduction phase <u>and</u> while in weight maintenance phase. The extent to which a program accomplishes this will be the extent to which a nation succeeds in creating nationwide healthy-weight living.

In the MIND of the Citizenry, we must:

EXPAND the **UPSIDE** of Right Eating and also the **DOWNSIDE** of Wrong Eating

&

DIMINISH the **UPSIDE** of Wrong Eating and also the **DOWNSIDE** of Right Eating

With the advent of the Weight Success Method, we now possess the technology for reversing our national trend of growing overweightness. What we need next is for our governmental leadership to step forward and create a Nationwide Weight Success Initiative.

SUMMING UP
For Nationwide Weight Success:

1. Identify misconceptions.

2. Refute misconceptions.

3. Install healthy-weight-promoting conceptions.

4. Describe weight success benefits.

5. Explain the key to healthy-weight living.

6. Equip people with the tools for easily doing Weight Success Actions every day.

7. Provide proof that healthy-weight living is easily doable.

8. Make healthy-weight living appear to be, and to actually be, more rewarding than non-healthy-weight living.

If we as a nation do those eight actions overweight living will decline and healthy-weight living will ascend. Or, put another way, most of the people in the nation will achieve lifelong *weight success* — that is, they will live most or all of their days in their desired healthy-weight range <u>and</u> derive benefits, enjoyment, and fulfillment from it.

WEIGHT SUCCESS
——— is the GOAL ———

WEIGHT SUCCESS METHOD™
——— is the MEANS ———

Goal+Means+<u>Action</u>=WEIGHT SUCCESS™

WEIGHT SUCCESS = Living most or all of one's days
in one's desired healthy-weight range AND
deriving benefits, enjoyment, and
fulfillment from it.

GLOSSARY OF TERMS
GLOSSARY OF TERMS
The Lexicon of Weight Success

Accomplishment: A desired situation, or goal, that has been realized

Achievement (a.k.a. achieving): The act of creating a certain desired situation, or the act of achieving a certain goal

Achievement Action (a.k.a. achieving action): An action that contributes to achieving a certain desired situation or goal

Achievement Activity (a.k.a. achieving activity): An activity that contributes to achieving a certain desired situation or goal

Achievement Pursuit: A pursuit that's conceived and executed in a way that involves performing ongoing achievement actions, or performing actions that foster achievement of a certain desired situation or goal

Achieving (a.k.a. achievement): The act of creating a certain desired situation, or the act of achieving a certain goal

Acting As-if: (1) The act of holding in mind an assumption that a particular situation presently exists or is in the process of coming about, *and then conducting one's thinking, feelings, and actions in accordance with that assumption.* (2) A real-life role-play of a situation one wants to exist or have happen.

Actualization (a.k.a. actualizing, actualization process): The act of creating an actual situation that corresponds to a certain imagined situation, such as a goal

Automatic Eating: (See Unguided Eating)

Belief: Assumption

Believing: The act of assuming that a particular situation exists

Calorie (a.k.a. food calorie): A measure of energy that a food or beverage provides. Note: In this book when the term *calorie* is used it's referring to "metabolizable calories," or calories that the human body is capable of metabolizing, or converting into energy.

Causal-factor Eradication: An approach to creating life enhancement that involves eradicating a particular factor that's causing a problem at the present time

C-B-A Process: A three-step process consisting of Communicating, Believing, and Appreciating. It's a key process of the Weight Success Method, specifically used in the Guided Eating Process of Daily Action 5.

Daily Achievement Action (a.k.a. daily success action): (1) An action that's performed every day or most days for the duration of a particular pursuit, and which contributes to achieving a certain desired situation or goal.

Daily Reminder Mechanism: A tool or means used for reminding you each day to do the five daily actions of the Weight Success Method

Daily Success Action (a.k.a. daily winning action): A success action that's performed every day or most days for the duration of a particular life-enhancing pursuit

Daily Weighing Hour: The set 60-minute period in which you weigh yourself each day

Daily Weight Success Action: A weight success action that's performed every day or most days for the duration of a weight success pursuit

Depiction Statement (a.k.a. verbal depiction): A verbal or word description of a situation. Typically the situation being depicted is either (a) an imagined desired situation you want to actualize, or make real or (b) a desirable present situation you want to perpetuate. The Healthy-weight Goal Statement is the primary depiction statement used in the Weight Success Method. Optional backup depiction statements are also verbal depiction statements.

Desired Weight Reading: (a) When in weight reduction pursuit, a desired weight reading would be a scale reading that shows a weight loss from the prior day. (b) When in weight maintenance pursuit, a desired weight reading would be any scale reading that's within your healthy-weight range

Directive: An instruction, order, or request delivered to your mind for the purpose of motivating it to perform a certain action or create a certain result

Don't-eat-it Signal: (See Stop-eating Signal)

During-eating Self-talk: Guided-eating self-talk that's delivered while *in the process* of eating

Easiest Way to Realize Healthy-weight Living: The Weight Success Method, which makes each day be a Weight Success Day

Eating: The act of consuming food, including liquid food (a.k.a. beverage)

Fat-promoting Factors: Factors that promote overeating or fat gain, or make it easier for a person to overeat or gain weight (but which do not cause overeating or fat gain)

Food: Any solid or liquid nutritive substance consumed by humans

Full-stomach Feeling: A feeling that your stomach is filled with food. It typically includes a feeling of pressure or tightening at the top of your stomach, or where your stomach joins your throat. This feeling can come even when your stomach isn't completely full.

Goal-achieving Action (a.k.a. *achieving action*): An action that contributes to achieving a certain goal

Goal-achieving Day: A day in which one does certain goal-achieving actions. In one's weight success pursuit, a goal-achieving day is sometimes called a Weight Success Day

Goal-promoting Belief: A belief that promotes actualization of a certain goal

Goal-promoting Communication: A communication that tells your mind what it should be doing in way of assisting with achieving a certain goal

Goal-realization Action: A daily action that leads to attainment or realization of a desired situation or goal

Guided Eating (a.k.a. *controlled eating, directed eating*): Eating activity that's guided by the eater, typically for the purpose of curtailing overeating and, thereby, creating right eating and living at one's desired weight

Guided Eating Process: A three-step process involving Communicating, Believing, and Appreciating, and which is used for creating guided eating

Guided-eating Self-talk: Any message delivered to your self — or your mind — while eating, for the purpose of causing your mind to guide you away from wrong eating and toward right eating, or away from overeating and toward non-overeating

Habit: An automatic frequently-repeated behavior or activity. A habit consists of two components: a physical component and a mental component. The physical component, which we call *action-habit,* is an automatic repeating physical activity. The mental component, which we call *mind-habit,* is an automatic repeating mental process. The mind-habit underlies and drives the action-habit.

Healthy Eating (a.k.a. *healthy-weight eating, right eating*): (1) Eating that promotes good health and living in your healthy-weight range. (2) Eating right foods in right amounts and in a way that creates right eating enjoyment.

Healthy Weight (a.k.a. *right weight*): Every weight that's in your healthy-weight range is regarded as being a healthy weight for you

Healthy-eating Day (a.k.a. *right-eating day*): A day in which your overall eating for the day amounts to right eating and non-overeating

Healthy-weight Achievement Scorecard™ (See Weight Success Actions Scorecard)

Healthy-weight Achievement: The repeated daily act of creating an actual body weight that's within a certain desired healthy-weight range

Healthy-weight Action (a.k.a. *healthy-weight achieving action, healthy-weight-creating action*): (See Weight Success Action)

Healthy-weight Calorie Allotment (a.k.a. daily calorie allotment): The amount of daily calories that maintains your body weight within your healthy-weight range

Healthy-weight Daily Method: (See Weight Success Method)

Healthy-weight Eating (a.k.a. healthy eating, right eating): (1) Eating that promotes good health and living in your healthy-weight range. (2) Eating right foods in right amounts and in a way that creates right eating enjoyment.

Healthy-weight Eating Actions (a.k.a. right-eating actions): Eating actions that result in living in one's healthy-weight range

Healthy-weight Goal Statement (a.k.a. healthy-weight focus statement): A word depiction of the ultimate goal, or desired ultimate outcome, of one's weight success endeavor — specifically: "I am the person of my healthy weight. I am healthy, happy, and doing great."

Healthy-weight Living Success: (See Weight Success)

Healthy-weight Living: Living most or all of one's days in one's healthy-weight range

Healthy-weight Method: (See Weight Success Method)

Healthy-weight Mindset (a.k.a. right-eating mindset): (See Weight Success Mindset)

Healthy-weight Prayer: A prayer expressing thanks to God, including thanks for the opportunity to easily live in one's healthy-weight range

Healthy-weight Range: The weight range that maximizes the likelihood of you living in optimal health. Every weight within your healthy-weight range is regarded as being a healthy weight for you.

Healthy-weight Success: (See Weight Success)

Healthy-weight Success Action: (See Weight Success Action)

Healthy-weight Winner (a.k.a. weight winner): A person who's in process of creating weight success

Healthy-Weight Success Day: (See Weight Success Day)

Healthy-weight-creating (a.k.a. healthy-weight-promoting): Creating or promoting the creation of healthy-weight living; used, for example, in the context of healthy-weight-creating thoughts, feelings, decisions, actions, communications, foods

Healthy-weight-promoting Action: (See Weight Success Action)

High-power Eat-right Solution: A multi-action procedure for ending recurring overeating and creeping weight gain, used in Optional Action 7 of the setback-reversal process.

Ideal Weight: (1) A body weight that's considered to be ideal for you. (2) A body weight that's most apt to promote good health for you. (3) A body weight number produced by any of the ideal weight formulas that exist in the medical field (ex., the Robinson formula).

Life-enhancing Situation: A new situation that's an improvement over a present situation

Lifelong Weight Success Dynamic: A dynamic in which doing the Weight Success Method each day installs and maintains success drivers in one's weight success pursuit which, in turn, results in experiencing weight success which, in turn, fosters continuation of doing the Weight Success Method

Maintenance Achievement: The act of applying success drivers, or success methodology, for the purpose of maintaining a certain situation, or for "staying the same"

Maintenance Eating: Consuming an amount of calories nearly equal to what your body is metabolizing, or "burning up," per day — typically done to maintain yourself in your healthy-weight range

Mealtime Gluttony-eating: (1) Eating until you're stuffed or until your stomach can't hold any more. (2) Overeating at mealtime.

Mind Actions: Actions that occur in one's mind — e.g., thoughts, feelings, and decisions are mind actions

Mind-motivation Action: A daily action that motivates a person to perform the goal-realization actions necessary for attaining or realizing a certain desired situation or goal

New-situation Creation: An approach to creating life enhancement that involves creating a desired *new* situation that, when actualized, automatically replaces a non-desired present situation

Non-healthy Eating (*a.k.a. wrong eating, unhealthy eating*): Any eating that hinders good health or hinders living in your healthy-weight range — typically, overeating

Open–Insert–Swallow Action (*a.k.a. Open–Insert–Swallow Process*): The three-action process of opening one's mouth, inserting food into one's mouth, and swallowing the food

Overeating: Consuming more calories than what your body is metabolizing, or "burning up," per day. Note: In this book when the term calorie is used it's referring to "metabolizable calories," or calories that the human body is capable of metabolizing, or converting into energy.

Overeating-reversal: The act of replacing recurring overeating and weight gain with right eating and healthy-weight living

Over-snacking: Snacking to the point where it results in overeating for the day

Overweight Body Weight: A body weight that's above your healthy-weight range. An *underweight body weight* would be a weight that's below your healthy-weight range.

Pleasure-priority Eating: Eating that has eating pleasure maximization as its top priority or focus

Preferred Dietary Program (*a.k.a. preferred dietary strategy, preferred eating strategy*): A set of eating guidelines and eating practices you prefer to follow and which, when followed, cause you to realize good health and healthy-weight living

Preferred Eating Strategy: (See Preferred Dietary Program)

Reinforcement (a.k.a. positive reinforcement): The act of giving someone something they like as a response or consequence for performing a certain action or creating a certain result

Right Amount of Food: (1) An amount of food that promotes living in your healthy-weight range. (2) An amount of food prescribed by your preferred dietary program.

Right Eating (a.k.a. healthy-weight eating, healthy eating): (1) Eating that promotes good health and living in your healthy-weight range. (2) Eating right foods in right amounts and in a way that creates right eating enjoyment. (3) Eating prescribed by your dietary program.

Right Food (*a.k.a. right type of food*): (1) Food that promotes good health and healthy weight. (2) Food prescribed by your dietary program.

Right Type of Food (*a.k.a. right food*): (1) A type of food that promotes good health and living in your healthy-weight range. (2) A type of food promoted or prescribed by your preferred dietary program.

Right Weight (*a.k.a. healthy weight*): Every weight that's in your healthy-weight range is regarded as being a right weight for you

Right-eating Communication (*a.k.a. right-eating-creating communication, right-eating-promoting communication, healthy-weight communication*): Communication that tells yourself — or your mind — to steer you toward right eating and healthy-weight living

Right-eating Day (*a.k.a. healthy-eating day*): A day in which your overall eating for the day amounts to right eating or non-overeating

Right-eating Focus (*a.k.a. healthy-eating focus*): (1) Time spent thinking about, talking about, pursuing, and/or enjoyably doing right eating and healthy-weight living. (2) Focus on right eating and healthy-weight living

Right-eating Mindset (*a.k.a. healthy-weight mindset*): A set of perspectives and feelings that steers a person toward achievement of right eating

Right-weight-promoting: Promoting living at one's right weight, or in one's healthy-weight range; used, for example, in the context of right-weight-promoting thoughts, feelings, decisions, actions, communications, foods

Self-reinforcement: The act of delivering reinforcement to oneself or to one's mind

Setback Reversal: The process of creating a progress action out of a misstep or a progress lapse

Startup Action: An action that's performed at the startup of a particular pursuit, and which installs into that pursuit one or more vital success drivers

Stop-eating Signal (a.k.a. don't-eat-it signal): A signal from your subconscious mind that it's time to stop eating (for that eating session or meal). Most likely the most common, or #1, stop-eating signal is the full-stomach feeling.

Subby: (1) A nickname for the subconscious mind. (2) The nickname John Correll uses for his subconscious mind.

Subconscious Mind: (1) The part of the mind that is not the conscious mind. (2) The part of the mind that operates "behind the scene" or "in the background."

Succeeding Activity (a.k.a. success activity): An activity that contributes to creating a certain desired life-enhancing situation

Succeeding Day (a.k.a. success day, winning day): A day that contributes to creating a certain desired life-enhancing situation

Success : The act of creating a desired life-enhancing situation <u>and</u> deriving benefits, enjoyment, and fulfillment from it

Success Action (a.k.a. winning action): An action that contributes to creating a certain desired life-enhancing situation

Success Activity: An activity that contributes to creating a certain desired life-enhancing situation

Success Day (a.k.a. winning day): A day that contributes to creating a certain desired life-enhancing situation

Success Driver (a.k.a. success factor, achievement driver): A condition or activity that, when present, increases the likelihood of a person succeeding at a certain pursuit — or, more specifically, increases the likelihood of a person performing actions that contribute to creating a certain desired situation or outcome associated with the pursuit

Success Killer (a.k.a. fail factor): A condition that, when present, increases the likelihood of a person failing at a certain pursuit, or causes the person to experience needless hassle and difficulty in succeeding at the pursuit. Basically, any particular

success killer is "the opposite" of a certain success driver.

Success Methodology (a.k.a. achievement methodology): An action plan that pertains to a certain pursuit and consists of specific actions that, when performed by a person, cause a maximal number of success drivers to be included in that pursuit, thereby resulting in easiest possible creation of the desired situation or outcome associated with the pursuit.

Success Process: An ongoing series of success actions aimed at creation of a common goal

Success Pursuit: A pursuit involving an ongoing series of success actions aimed at creating a certain desired life-enhancing situation or outcome

Success-creating Action: (See Success Action)

Success-creation Process: An ongoing series of actions all aimed at creating a certain desired life-enhancing situation

Success-creation: The process of creating success

Thank You, Keep It Up message: A special type of message delivered as a reinforcing response to someone who performed a desired action or created a desired result. This "someone" can be you (or your mind), another person, or God.

Under-eating: Consuming fewer calories than what your body is metabolizing, or "burning up," per day

Underweight Body Weight: A body weight that's below your healthy-weight range. An *overweight body weight* would be a weight that's above your healthy-weight range.

Undesired Weight Reading: (a) When in weight <u>reduction</u> pursuit, an undesired weight reading would be a scale reading that shows a weight <u>gain</u> over the prior day. (b) When in weight <u>maintenance</u> pursuit, an undesired weight reading would be a scale reading that's <u>outside</u> your healthy-weight range — typically a reading that's <u>above</u> your healthy-weight range.

Unguided Eating (a.k.a. non-controlled eating, undirected eating, automatic eating): Eating activity that's not guided by the eater, or eating that's done automatically and without conscious deliberation

Unhealthy Eating (a.k.a. wrong eating, non-healthy eating): Any eating that hinders good health or hinders living in your healthy-weight range — typically, overeating

Weight Control (a.k.a. weight management): (1) The act of creating an actual body weight that corresponds to one's desired body weight (a.k.a. healthy-weight goal). (2) The act of regulating one's amount of body fat for maintaining one's weight in a certain weight range

Weight Correction Day: A day in which you take immediate action to correct an undesired weight reading that occurred in a daily weighing. This action typically involves under-eating (total fasting or semi-fasting) for a 24 to 48 hour period.

Weight Failure (a.k.a. non-healthy-weight living): Living most or all of your days outside your healthy-weight range

Weight Freedom Method: (See Weight Success Method)

Weight Freedom: (See Weight Success)

Weight Maintenance: The act of maintaining one's body weight in one's desired weight range

Weight Management (a.k.a. weight control): (1) The act of creating an actual body weight that corresponds to one's desired body weight (a.k.a. healthy-weight goal). (2) The act of regulating one's amount of body fat for maintaining one's weight in a certain weight range

Weight Winner (a.k.a. healthy-weight winner): A person who's in process of creating weight success

Weight Success (a.k.a. healthy-weight success): Living most or all of one's days in one's desired healthy-weight range <u>and</u> deriving benefits, enjoyment, and fulfillment from it

Weight Success Action (a.k.a. weight winning action): An action that contributes to creating weight success. Examples of weight success actions include: the ten Startup Actions, the five Daily Actions, the actions described in the Weight Success Benefits Directive, and any of the actions prescribed in Ch. 2–27 of this book.

Weight Success Actions Scorecard™: A score-card for recording and scoring one's daily Weight Success Actions

Weight Success Benefits (a.k.a. healthy-weight benefits): The good things you derive from your weight success pursuit, or from living in your desired healthy-weight range

Weight Success Benefits Directive (a.k.a. healthy-weight benefits directive): (1) A directive that's delivered to your mind, and which describes certain weight success actions to be performed by your mind, including subconscious mind. (2) A directive delivered for the purpose of instructing your mind to perform certain weight success actions

Weight Success Day (a.k.a. weight winning day): A day that contributes to creating weight success

Weight Success Dynamic: A dynamic in which doing the Weight Success Method each day installs success drivers into one's weight success pursuit which, in turn, results in experiencing weight success (see also Lifelong Weight Success Dynamic)

Weight Success Empowerment: (1) Power or ability to create weight success. (2) The empowering of humans to create weight success.

Weight Success Forever: Living in a state of weight success for the rest of one's life.

Weight Success Methodology: An action plan that consists of specific weight success actions that, when performed by a person, cause a maximal number of success drivers to be included in a weight success pursuit, thereby resulting in easiest possible creation of weight success

Weight Success Method™ *(a.k.a. healthy-weight method, weight freedom method):* A particular success methodology for weight management, this methodology involving a certain set of ten startup actions and also a set of five daily actions consisting of weighing, reinforcement or correction, benefits directive, goal statement, and guided eating

Weight Success Mindset (a.k.a. healthy-weight mindset): A set of perspectives and feelings that steers a person toward achievement of weight success

Weight Success Pursuit: A pursuit involving an ongoing series of weight success actions

Weight Success Secret™ *:* To succeed at lifelong healthy-weight living, do Weight Success Actions every day.

Weight Winning Action (a.k.a. weight success action): An action that contributes to creating weight success.

Weight Winning Day (a.k.a. weight success day): A day that contributes to creating weight success

Weight Winning Pursuit: A pursuit involving an ongoing series of weight winning actions

Weight-reduction Success Graph™: A graph for tracking daily success in weight reduction.

Weight-success-creating (a.k.a. healthy-weight-promoting): Creating or promoting achievement of weight success; used, for example, in the context of weight-success-creating thoughts, feelings, decisions, actions, communications, foods

Weight-success-creating action: (See Weight Success Action)

Whole-mind Dynamic of Healthy-weight Living: A dynamic involving applying one's whole mind (both conscious and subconscious) in the pursuit of healthy-weight living

Win-Day Calendar™: A calendar for keeping track of the healthy-weight success days, or weight success days, in each month.

Winning Action (a.k.a. success action): An action that contributes to creating a certain desired life-enhancing situation

World Weight Success Empowerment Series™: A collection of publications containing information that empowers people to achieve weight success

Wrong Amount of Food: (1) An amount of food that hinders living in your healthy-weight range. (2) An amount of food prohibited by your preferred dietary program.

Wrong Eating (a.k.a. unhealthy eating, non-healthy eating): (1) Eating that hinders good health or hinders living in your healthy-weight range — typically, overeating. (2) Eating prohibited by your dietary program.

Wrong Food (a.k.a. wrong type of food): (1) Food that hinders good health or hinders living in your healthy-weight range. (2) A food discouraged or prohibited by your preferred dietary program.

Wrong Type of Food (a.k.a. wrong food): (1) A type of food that hinders good health or hinders living in your healthy-weight range. (2) A type of food discouraged or prohibited by your preferred dietary program.

Yo-yo Dieting: (1) Ongoing alternating periods of dieting and non-dieting. (2) Ongoing alternating periods of weight loss and weight gain.

INDEX OF SUBJECTS

Where to Go for What You're Seeking about Weight Success

success driver #19, 121
  what it is, what it does, 121
Whole-mind Dynamic of Healthy-weight Living, 122
Win-Day Calendar, 154

y

Yo-yo dieting
  the cause of, 122

Do the **Five Daily Actions**
<u>every</u> day . . .
and **Lifelong Weight Success**
will be <u>Yours</u>.

Typically takes <u>less than</u> **8** minutes
of dedicated time per day.

— Weight Success Benefits Directive —

INSTRUCTIONS: Use this Directive for Daily Action 3. ● Where there's a dotted line (...........), say the name you use when speaking of or to your subconscious mind. ● Read this directive aloud <u>and</u> say it with some emotional intensity. (Reading aloud is best, but when you can't do that, whisper it to yourself.) When reading it, **strongly desire** for the actions it describes to be realized. And, **hold the belief** and act as-if what's described in this statement is *in the process of happening.* After reading the list of weight success benefits, for at least 30 seconds **visualize** at least one of the benefits as an accomplished fact. As you go through the day, *continue* believing and acting as-if what's described in this directive is in the process of happening. ● For set-up, insert your healthy-weight range and preferred dietary program into the blanks. For the "pounds–kilos" phrase, draw a line through the word that doesn't apply. List your weight success benefits on the lines at the end. Hint: Use pencil, not pen. Or, type it up and tape it in. (For more, see Ch. **9** at page 65.)

*   *   *

..........................., today and *every* day for the rest of my life, do these five very important actions.

1 – Guide me to *easily* living in my **healthy-weight range,** which right now is
_____ to _____ pounds–kilos.

2 – Guide me to *fully* doing my **preferred dietary program**, which right now is the
_____ program.

3 – When I say my Healthy-weight Goal Statement while eating, automatically create thoughts and feelings that guide me to Right Eating, that guide me to eating the *types* of food and the *amount* of food that results in me living in my healthy-weight range.

4 – Whenever I make a decision to stop eating, make the urge to eat *immediately* begin to fade away for that eating session. And, if anytime I happen to accidentally overeat, create an uncomfortable bloated feeling that lasts for a short time.

5 – Whenever I say my Healthy-weight Goal Statement, bring to mind a thought of at least one of my weight success benefits. And, then, create within me a *happy, positive feeling.*

The Weight Success Benefits I gain from living in my healthy-weight range include:
1. A greater chance of *living healthier longer* — or greater chance of living free of debilitating accidents, illnesses, diseases, and bodily malfunction.

_____

_____

_____

_____

_____

_____

_____

_____

_____

_____

_____

_____

_____

_____

_____

_____

_____

_____

_____

_____

_____

_____

_____

_____

I thank you, God, for the opportunity to live my life this way.

......................., please do *everything you can* to assist me in creating lifelong healthy-weight living in a positive, pleasurable way. This benefits me *greatly.* I realize you're now doing it, and I thank you for it.

Living in my healthy-weight range is a *mandatory,* <u>must</u>-have feature of my existence. I am doing it *now* and for the rest of my life — and doing it *easily* <u>and</u> *enjoyably.* Yes! Yes! YES!

*   *   *

NOTE: After delivering the directive, close your eyes and say your Healthy-weight Goal Statement <u>three</u> times. Do it with intensity. ~ Plus, each day allow yourself to get a *good feeling* from making your weight losses stick and from having realized healthy-weight living. You deserve it. It's a substantial praiseworthy achievement.

> The **Weight Success Benefits Directive** is an important message for your mind, especially your subconscious mind. Deliver it like it is and your subconscious mind will act accordingly.

Messengers
of Disaster

Raphael Lemkin, Jan Karski, and
Twentieth-Century Genocides

A N N E T T E B E C K E R

Translated by Käthe Roth

THE UNIVERSITY OF WISCONSIN PRESS

Publication of this book has been made possible, in part,
through support from the George L. Mosse Program in History at the University of
Wisconsin–Madison and the Hebrew University of Jerusalem.

GL M
GEORGE L.
MOSSE
PROGRAM IN HISTORY

The University of Wisconsin Press
728 State Street, Suite 443
Madison, Wisconsin 53706
uwpress.wisc.edu

Gray's Inn House, 127 Clerkenwell Road
London EC1R 5DB, United Kingdom
eurospanbookstore.com

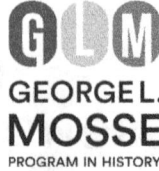

Originally published in French as *Messagers du désastre: Raphael Lemkin,
Jan Karski et les génocides*, copyright © 2018 by Librairie Arthème Fayard
Translation copyright © 2021 by the Board of Regents of the University of Wisconsin System
The Board of Regents of the University of Wisconsin System
All rights reserved. Except in the case of brief quotations embedded in critical
articles and reviews, no part of this publication may be reproduced, stored in a retrieval
system, transmitted in any format or by any means—digital, electronic, mechanical,
photocopying, recording, or otherwise—or conveyed via the Internet
or a website without written permission of the University of Wisconsin Press.
Rights inquiries should be directed to rights@uwpress.wisc.edu.

Printed in the United States of America
This book may be available in a digital edition.

Library of Congress Cataloging-in-Publication Data
Names: Becker, Annette, author. | Roth, Käthe, translator.
Title: Messengers of disaster : Raphael Lemkin, Jan Karski, and twentieth-century genocides
/ Annette Becker ; translated by Käthe Roth.
Other titles: Messagers du désastre. English | George L. Mosse series in the history of
European culture, sexuality, and ideas.
Description: Madison, Wisconsin : The University of Wisconsin Press, [2021] |
Series: George L. Mosse series in the history of European culture, sexuality, and ideas |
Originally published in French as: Messagers du désastre : Raphael Lemkin,
Jan Karski et les génocides. | Includes bibliographical references and index.
Identifiers: LCCN 2021008855 | ISBN 9780299333201 (cloth)
Subjects: LCSH: Lemkin, Raphael, 1900–1959. | Karski, Jan, 1914–2000. |
Genocide—History—20th century. | Genocide—Europe—History—20th century. |
Genocide—Armenia—History—20th century. | World War, 1914–1918—Atrocities. |
World War, 1939–1945—Atrocities.
Classification: LCC HV6322.7 .B43513 2021 | DDC 940.53/180922—dc23
LC record available at https://lccn.loc.gov/2021008855

To the next generation: to Sarah

To Colombe and her baby Siné/Alexandra,
and to Sandrine, Cynthia, and Laurie, who adopted me
as a grandmother in their country, Rwanda

To Philippe

To Jan

Everything occurred as if most people were turning half-closed eyes on the surroundings of an exterior world that they disdained to notice.

—MARC BLOCH, "Reflections of a Historian on the False News of the War," trans. James P. Holoka, *Michigan War Studies Review*, 2013

CONTENTS

Messengers
of Disaster

Introduction

The Unnamable Is Unnamable

"So much cruelty." In July 2016, in Auschwitz, Pope Francis stood alone at the foot of the gate whose arch is inscribed with the words *Arbeit Macht Frei*. He expressed his sense of bewilderment in the camp's guest book in a way that conflated the tortures inflicted on the Polish coreligionists of his predecessor, John Paul II, in the concentration camp with the killings of Jews deported from Poland and occupied Europe at the extermination site in Birkenau. If this speaks volumes about the difficulty today of differentiating the Nazi oppression that fell upon everyone from the singular fate of the Jews, one can imagine how such a distinction was even more unthinkable between 1939 and 1945.

Yet, in 1941 and 1942, a handful of men recognized the specificity of the extermination of Jews amid the chaos of World War II. Among them were two Poles: a Jewish lawyer who had fled the Nazis and a Catholic student who had joined his country's resistance. The traces left by Raphael Lemkin and Jan Karski in the gigantic war-torn world and the reactions of their interlocutors both anonymous and well known open a window on one of the mysteries of recent history: how could it be that only a tiny number of people "saw" while others denied the knowledge of what was in front of their eyes? These messengers wanted to open people's eyes, to offer what they had seen and understood about the truth of the disaster, in the spirit of Charles Péguy's injunction "We must always tell what we see. Above all, and this is more difficult, we must always see what we see."[1]

❡

January 1945. The *Polish Review*, a New York journal linked to the Polish government in exile in London, published parts of the "spy novel" that was Jan Karski's memoir, *Story of a Secret State*,[2] as well as excerpts from Lemkin's *Axis Rule in Occupied Europe*, which was published in the fall of 1944; the preface was written in 1943, and chapter 9 is titled "Genocide."[3]

The hero of the resistance and the activist lawyer, neither of them well known at the time, accomplished their mission: to tell about what they had themselves witnessed in Europe—up to the winter of 1941 for Lemkin and up to October 1942 for Karski. The *Polish Review* was glowing in its praise of Karski's work: "This book is a cry from the abyss. Much more than that, it keeps the flame alive . . . in the diabolical world of the Nazis." But no details were provided about the nature of this "diabolical world." Nor was it mentioned that Lemkin was Jewish; the crime of "destruction of a people" was noted in passing but without specifying that its goal was the extermination of Jews, even though the mass murder was extensively documented in its pages after 1943. Lemkin and Karski were among the first links in a chain of public testimony about the extermination. Starting in 1939–40, and especially between 1941 and 1943, they took on the task of transmitting what they knew about persecution of Jews to readers in France, then in Great Britain and the United States. Although some disseminated their ideas, while also gleaning information from other sources, most did not listen to, or did not hear, them.

"I know humanity, I know man, no, no, it's impossible." This cry of rejection was uttered in 1943 by Supreme Court justice Felix Frankfurter, himself Jewish and kept informed of all the dispatches on a daily basis. When Professor Karski was reminded of it in 1978, he answered, "I think he believed me, of course; I have no doubt he did his best, whatever he could have done. . . . Probably he wanted to show me that the world is unprepared, this is an unprecedented problem, a horrible problem."[4] The question therefore has to be shifted from "Who knew what?" or "Who denied what?" to "Why did no one believe what was said by those who took so many risks to spread the message?" Raymond Aron expressed it well: "The gas chambers, the industrial killings of human beings, no, I admit, I did not imagine them, and because I couldn't imagine them, I didn't see them."[5] The "engaged spectator" disengaged himself; he was neither the sole resister nor the only

Jew in London, in the United States, or in the world at war to refuse to believe the "vision" offered by the messengers of mass death who had come from Eastern Europe.[6]

I have always been struck by the impossibility of apprehending the extermination of Jews at the time that it was taking place, between 1941 and 1945. It seemed to me, as a historian of memories and repressions of World War I, that the rumors—especially those related to the German, Russian, and Ottoman atrocities—made the crimes of the following war, which was, in many respects, the first war's extension, opaque, from the atrocities of the invasions and occupations to the extermination of Armenians and the civil wars. Lemkin, born earlier, in 1900, and Karski, born in 1922, were also faced with the epistemological obstacle engendered by the preceding war and its perpetuation into the 1920s, but they broke through it.

In the 1920s, Lemkin had written a great deal about the tragedies of the Great War; he knew that the horrors of World War II were not without precedent in the recent past but that forgetfulness or alterations of memory could make knowledge of the crimes inaccessible. But how could those who felt that they had been duped by various false atrocity stories during World War I and had long forgotten the fate of the Armenians be made to believe in the specificity of the extermination? In this book, I answer that question.

A paradox remains: although the mental universe resulting from World War I and the 1920s and 1930s impeded, in most cases, comprehension of the specific fate of the Jews, it enhanced the precocious lucidity of those few who were conveying the indescribable. Lemkin and Karski were eyewitnesses who became moral witnesses, ready to take every risk to make their message heard.[7] Dante, whom they quoted often, wrote that hope comes to one man because another man brings the message.

The diplomat Varian Fry and the authors Franz Werfel, Arthur Koestler, and George Orwell also transmitted the scope and nature of the disaster that was raining down upon Jews in Europe; they drew upon their experiences of 1914–18 and between 1917 and 1938 in the Russian revolutions and the Spanish Civil War.[8] Aware that civilians were suffering, they described the hardships and deaths of families in great detail and tried to reconstruct the tragedy of persecution and then extermination. They chose to name the unnamable; few heard or understood them.

In this book, I retrace their paths through texts and images from British, American, French, Israeli, and Polish public and private archives, as well as those of the International Committee of the Red Cross in Geneva and the International Tracing Service in Bad Arolsen. Completing the picture are the accounts of historian-victims such as Simon Dubnow and Emanuel Ringelblum and of the Soviet war reporter Vassili Grossman, who was among those who discovered Treblinka.

Most of these sources were transmitted, verified, and cross-checked in real time in the offices of the Foreign Office in London, the State Department in Washington, DC, and the foreign affairs offices of the Polish and Czech governments in exile in London, as well as in the heart of liberated France and by Jewish organizations, and even in Mandatory Palestine. Articles, photographs, and drawings were published by the clandestine press, by newspapers, and in Jewish, British, American, Swiss, and other organs. Even given the war censorship in democratic countries, these documents were not confined to the circles of power, or at least not always; most of the information was within the reach of the general public. Who was reading, watching, listening; who might have known that an "ethnic and religious group"—a people—was being wiped out?[9]

Convinced that his personal grief would be possible only if it was borne by all of humanity, Lemkin applied his original thinking to the crimes against the Armenians and the Roma. The life of Karski, the resister, was thrown into upheaval by his discovery of the extermination of the Jews. A fervent Catholic, he related how his "self-Judaization" started after he donned, fraudulently, the uniform of a Ukrainian reservist. He felt his body and soul being defiled by what he saw, smelled, and heard in Izbica, not far from Belzec: the cries and atrocious deaths of human beings crammed into wagons into which quicklime had been poured.[10]

Karski was not able to return to Poland after his last mission in 1942–43. Like Lemkin, he took refuge in the United States. Both were refugees with the message of barbarism. Whereas Karski "made his report," Lemkin was simultaneously the "alarm" for the fire and its theoretician. He invented the term "genocide" and, in December 1948, was instrumental in getting the General Assembly of the United Nations to adopt the Convention on the

Prevention and Punishment of the Crime of Genocide—almost a miracle as the Cold War was dawning.

Lemkin always presented himself as a man who had had the premonition of a disastrous genocide (even before the word existed) when he was a child. He set to work in the 1920s, and the intellectual formulation to which he was committed was illustrated in 1941 and 1942 by the murder of his own family. After enduring all kinds of abuse in their shtetl of Volkovysk, which became a ghetto, his parents were gassed at Treblinka. We may accuse Lemkin of using tautology in his reconstruction of facts in order to prove his visionary foresight,[11] but we must acknowledge that he was one of the few to think the unthinkable: that during his lifetime, two peoples, the Armenians and the Jews, had been intentionally condemned to extermination.

Karski fought against the Nazis in the military; Lemkin conceived the "crime of crimes" as a legal scholar. Both men came from a Poland in which the relationships with power, territory, the nation, and minorities were different from those in Western Europe. When they arrived in England and the United States, they were faced with incomprehension. Messengers with an inaudible message, they perceived great resentment about it. But from the point of view of the Allies, didn't the extermination of the Jews, in 1944 and 1945, seem secondary, both in public opinion and in the view of the governments struggling against the Axis: shouldn't they first win the war and then punish those responsible for the crimes?

This book does not stop in 1945–46. It does not end in Nuremberg, where Lemkin was very disappointed that the concept of "genocide" was not integrated into international law, or in Washington, DC, where Karski returned to his studies while continuing his fight for a free and independent Poland. Although Lemkin died early, in 1959, his work continued thanks to the legacy of the 1948 convention, even when it became mined territory during the Cold War: some consigned "genocide" to the Nazi past, whereas others broadened it to other populations, following Lemkin's opinion. Unfortunately, the future bore out his vision, and so this book concludes with the genocide of the Tutsi in Rwanda.

Jan Karski, who became "Righteous Among the Nations" and an honorary citizen of Israel, continued his fight until his death, in 2000. Elie Wiesel and Claude Lanzmann brought him back into the public light; he was featured in Lanzmann's film *Shoah*, released in 1985. As a fictional character in Yannick Haenel's novel *Jan Karski*, published in 2009, even in posterity he revisited the question of true and false. And the debates that then arose around what had been known about the extermination of the Jews joined in an endless cycle with what I could read at the same time in the archives: starting in 1941 and 1942, eyewitnesses to the Nazi atrocities had crossed the Channel and the Atlantic, their reports had been analyzed, and they were not believed.

"Even words fail."[12] Samuel Beckett gave up on naming the unnamable, but Raphael Lemkin and Jan Karski did not.

1

Karski the Soldier, Lemkin the Lawyer

1939–40

This war was waged by the Nazis not only for frontiers, but for the alteration of the human element within these frontiers.

—Raphael Lemkin

In September 1939, certain Poles reacted to the defeat of their country with extraordinary courage and decisiveness. Among them were two men who had very little in common: Jan Kozielewski and Raphael Lemkin. The former, a young man, chose military action; the latter found a way to continue his work as a legal scholar.

Kozielewski, a Catholic student, was mobilized in eastern Poland, soon to be occupied by the Soviets following the signing of the Nazi-Soviet Pact. His determination to return to his homeland to fight saved him from probable death when he exchanged his officer's uniform for that of a simple soldier, as the Soviets were executing the elite of the Polish army in Katyn.[1] At the same time, Lemkin was trying to travel from Warsaw to the town of Volkovysk (near Bialystok), in the eastern part of the country, where his parents lived, and convince them to follow him out of their homeland. He, too, had to take on a different identity. He had been warned that his hands, the pale hands of an intellectual, would likely betray him—the lot of many Polish officers who tried to pass for peasants in order to escape captivity. These two men would come to resemble each other in two ways: both refused to hide reality, and both had to disguise their true identities in order to survive and fight.

Meeting up with the embryonic Polish resistance was not difficult for Kozielewski; his older brother, Marian, had been kept on as chief of the Polish police when Warsaw surrendered, on September 28, 1939. A World War I veteran who had fought in the Pilsudski Legion, Marian was in contact with the Polish government in exile in France and quickly converted his office into a headquarters for the early resistance. Created on September 30 and led by General Władysław Sikorski, the Polish government in exile was based in Paris and Angers and then, after the defeat of France, in London. It was to these three cities that Jan Kozielewski, who now called himself Karski, went on two courier missions. The first lasted from late 1939 to early 1940, after which he returned to the Polish resistance. The second took place in fall 1942 and was extended by an unplanned detour to the United States in 1943. Because this mission became public knowledge, Karski could no longer return to Poland.

When Poland surrendered, Lemkin, a thirty-nine-year-old Jewish lawyer, decided to leave for the Baltic states, which were not yet occupied, as a stepping-off point for Belgium. His ultimate destination was to be the United States, where he had long cultivated professional contacts. In Vilnius, Lithuania, and Riga, Latvia, he shared the fate of members of the Polish Jewish intellectual, religious, community, and professional elite, who had lost everything when they fled and now depended on charity. "Maybe I will be luckier now, as a nomad, than I was as a member of a sedentary society," Lemkin wrote in the notes that would later become his autobiography.[2] A fugitive in his own country, then a refugee, he had quickly realized that for him, an ambitious lawyer in Warsaw, and for his parents, shopkeepers in eastern Poland now under Soviet rule, life as they had known it was gone forever. His parents declined to follow him but supported his plans. As he was leaving Europe, he expressed his last qualms: "As long as I was in Europe, I had felt that I was watching over them. But it was only a geographical illusion. . . . When I was on the constant run, escaping from actual dangers, I called myself an escapee. But now that direct and immediate danger of losing life and liberty did not threaten me, I became a refugee. Now I was threatened with the disintegration of my personality through idleness, apathy, loss of self-esteem and assertiveness."[3] Taking inspiration from the poetry of Dante, also a fugitive, Lemkin wrote a detailed account of this time of wandering in search of a visa—the curse of refugees. Although he took an ironic tone, he was not unaware that most of those whose paths he crossed had been moved into ghettos, put into forced labor, mistreated in every conceivable way, murdered.

> A consulate at that time was the god and the supreme ruler of the race of refugees. They studied their gods, whose idiosyncrasies and habits of conversation they had learned from people who had already been received by them. The waiting rooms of the consulates were social meeting places for refugees. People would go there just out of habit. From there they would go to another meeting place . . . where they would report to their friends that they had just come from the consulate and that their visas had not yet arrived. For a long time the real relationship between a refugee and a consulate was just waiting.[4]

As he traveled from Poland to the Baltic states and Sweden, Lemkin met with many people and scoured libraries; he brought to bear in the struggle against "Axis domination" his knowledge about war and crimes against humanity garnered from his analyses conducted during the 1920s and 1930s and from what he had learned since the beginning of the war. His mission: to convince the world of the significance of the new territory being mapped out by the Nazis—or, at least, that is how he reconstructed it later: "This war was being waged by the Nazis not only for frontiers but for the alteration of the human element within these frontiers. This alteration meant that certain people were to be annihilated and supplanted by Germans. Their destruction would be irrevocable and their cultures erased forever."[5]

Lemkin, or the Weapons of the Intellect

The man who had fought briefly in the Russo-Polish War in 1920 now found himself banned from his homeland, Poland—a stateless Jew. The situation was paradoxical for a tireless legal scholar who had helped to write the Polish criminal code, as well as those of the Soviet Union and Italy. Just as ironic was that his major opus, *The Regulation of International Payments*, a study of the trade systems of fifty-four countries, was being published in Paris at that very time.[6] Lemkin was also interested in recent history: the disasters of World War I and the Russian Civil War, the conflicts that had crushed the Jews of Russia and Galicia—his people—and the Armenians. Fascinated by the rich Jewish cultural life in 1930s Poland, expressed in Yiddish and

Hebrew despite growing state persecution, he compared it to that of the Armenians: "These wretched and insecure people had a unique capacity to absorb and digest culture. It went straight into their bloodstream. In their cultural ability and receptivity there was also a great deal of resemblance between the Jews and the Armenians, who, in 1915, lost more than a million people by genocide in Turkey."[7]

"There is nothing new in the sufferings of Jews, especially in time of war"[8]

During his difficult crossing of a Poland defeated and occupied by the Nazis and the Soviets in the fall of 1939, Lemkin found refuge among his fellow Jews, who reflected all the complex facets of Judaism at the time—observant and secular, socialists of all types, leftwing and rightwing Zionists. Some, like him, had quickly realized that flight was the only solution in the face of imminent Nazi persecution. Yet, this remained to be achieved. Different, and even opposing, encounters, each of which revealed the state of Polish Jewish society at the time, touched him deeply. For, to start with, the Jews themselves had to be convinced.

In Dubno, Lemkin was given warm hospitality by his host, a strictly observant baker. The baker felt that Hitler and the new war would change nothing for the Jews, who had endured adversity for generations: "My grandfather used to tell me stories about pogroms by Kosaks. . . . In the last war, 1915–1918, we lived three years under the Germans. It was never good, but somehow we survived. I sold bread to the Germans; we baked for them from their flour. We Jews are an eternal people, we cannot be destroyed. We can only suffer." Lemkin attended Shabbat services in the shtetl, and he gave a sensitive description of his hosts' faith. Although he no longer shared it, as a former student in a *heder* (Jewish school), he understood it intimately: "This was where my host changed from a poor baker into a king." Recounting this episode often after he arrived in the United States, he spoke of it as both the culmination of his knowledge of Polish Judaism and the beginning of his mission; he apparently shared his vision of "genocide" with the incredulous baker: "He could not believe the reality of genocide [of course, the word did not exist in 1939] because it went against nature, against logic, against life itself. . . . There was not much sense in disturbing or confusing him with facts. He had already made up his mind. He had a private, bilateral covenant with

God. When born this contract devolved on him from his father. He was ready to take his punishment if he were to violate this covenant . . . he would not complain about it."[9]

The baker was living in the time of God; Lemkin was living in the historical present. He tried to bring the two together to convince his hosts that the Nazi aggression was something new: "It is not a war to grab territory so much as to destroy whole peoples and replace them with Germans. It is like Assur, which you remember from the Bible, who destroyed many nations and settled their lands with its allies."[10] The baker seemed unwilling to accept this comparison, even reinforced by the Bible, because he knew well that ever since the biblical confrontation between Jacob and Esau, the survival of the Jewish people had been guaranteed by scattering—and, above all, by faith.

An Orthodox Jew from the Warsaw ghetto responded similarly to the socialist Zionist historian Emanuel Ringelblum, who wished to amass as many documents as possible to archive the lives of Jews in Poland before they disappeared: "Jews have no history, all of it is only myth. . . . Only a myth will remain of the present time. Will it be the myth of Sodom or the myth of Abraham's charity?"[11]

Lemkin was both moved by such firmness and fervor and despairing about what he sensed was coming. In this, he shared the view of the historian Simon Dubnow, whom he met in Riga. As an intellectual, Lemkin had probably read the new edition of Dubnow's *Histoire moderne du peuple juif*, published in 1938, in which he took stock of the danger with remarkable prescience: "We are living at a turning point in world history, and this turning point, at present, is leading us toward the worst, toward the worst centuries in human history. . . . The theory of racism leads from humanity to bestiality."[12] However, Lemkin certainly had not read the article that Dubnow had sent to the editors of a Yiddish journal founded in Paris after the Munich Agreement and the failure of the Evian Conference. In his article, Dubnow observed that democracies had no intention of helping persecuted Jews by accepting more refugees and loosening immigration quotas: not the British in Palestine, nor the United States, nor Switzerland, nor Australia, nor France.

Dubnow referred not to Assur but to Haman and the Book of Esther: "And the letters were sent by posts into all the king's provinces, to destroy, to kill, and to cause to perish all Jews, both young and old, little children and women, in one day."[13] In 1939, Dubnow was eighty years old, and he knew Jewish history better than anyone else. He had grasped the uniqueness of what Hitler and the Nazis thought and planned to undertake: "We are witnessing the beginning of the obliteration of European Judaism. . . . The hegemonic center of our people will have to be transplanted beyond the seas—to America or Asia." Dubnow used the word *khurbn*, "total destruction," reserved up to then for the destruction of the temple in Jerusalem—a word that would come to mean, in the following months and years, "extermination system" and "expulsion from Germany" of Jews by the Nazis— expressions that he was already using. Dubnow concluded, still in 1939, "It is their bodies that must be saved. First the Jews—and then the entire Yiddish way of life.[14] We must fight against the scourge of anti-Jewish hate in its Nazi form and against the plans to organize new expulsions and persecutions in eastern Europe."[15] Lemkin was obviously impressed with the elderly historian during their sole meeting; when he related their dialogue, he had found refuge in Washington, DC, and was aware that Dubnow had been murdered, along with all the Jews in the largest ghetto in Latvia, in the Rumbula forest in 1941. "In the city of Riga, Latvia, 8,000 Jews were killed in a single night. A week later 16,000 more were led into a woods, stripped and machine-gunned."[16] In just a few weeks, Latvia was rendered *judenfrei*.

"How can we comprehend this hate that rises from the abyss?" (Franz Werfel)

Other Jewish intellectuals, such as Franz Werfel, faced similar challenges and tried to analyze them. Born in Prague and having fought on the Russian front during World War I, Werfel, who wrote in German, had enjoyed some celebrity before the publication, in 1933, of *The Forty Days of Musa Dagh*, a novel about what was not yet being called the Armenian genocide. In 1932, he toured Germany reading excerpts of the forthcoming book. At that time he made public two chapters in which he reproduced excerpts of an interview conducted by Johannes Lepsius, a German Orientalist theologian who had taken the side of the Armenians, with one of the three people responsible for the genocide, Enver Pasha:[17] "'In our very own time, one of the oldest and most venerable peoples of the world has been destroyed, murdered, almost exterminated—and not by warlike enemies but by their own countrymen.'"[18] In chapter 5, the comparison between Armenians and Jews is more pointed. Lepsius observes that a great deal of information on the deportations of the Armenians was available in 1915 thanks to reports by Christian missionaries and Henry Morgenthau Sr., ambassador from the United States, which was still neutral, to the Ottoman Empire. "'Mr. Morgenthau,' said Enver brightly, 'is a Jew. And Jews are always fanatically on the side of minorities.'"[19]

In his talks, Werfel explained that in Germany in 1932, the SA and the SS were taking part in demonstrations during which they shouted the same kind of hate. He nevertheless thought that Hitler had no political future and was convinced that his book, in which he attacked what he called national fanaticism, would be very important in the struggle: "My book may be read symbolically, outside of time, because of current events: oppression and destruction of minorities by nationalism."[20] Werfel was naive: he believed, in 1933, that he could retain his membership in the literary section of the Prussian Academy, and he expressed the conviction that Roosevelt and the pope would ultimately get rid of Hitler. Culturally assimilated, he apparently thought that the Nazis had banned his book on the massacre of the Armenians because he was making a barely veiled attack against them by equating them with the Ottomans. In fact, his book was burned because he was Jewish.

In 1936, Werfel, basking in the success of his book, received a standing ovation in New York from three hundred members of the Armenian community during a gala dinner attended by Henry Morgenthau Sr., former US ambassador to Turkey. After the Anschluss, Werfel had to flee Austria, where he had been living, and he took refuge in France. And then 1940 came: "We're trapped," he admitted to other immigrants who hoped that his celebrity could be of use to them.[21] It was thanks to assistance from the Emergency Rescue Committee in Marseille, organized by the American writer Varian Fry, that he was able to reach Spain, accompanied by Heinrich, Nelly, and Golo Mann, via an exhausting march across the Pyrenees to Portbou.[22] He finally reached Portugal, then left for the United States. "Exile is a terrible disease," wrote his wife, Alma Schindler (who had previously been married to Gustav Mahler and Walter Gropius).[23] Meanwhile, Werfel's parents were unable to leave Marseille. His father died there; at the last minute his mother, again thanks to Fry's team, was able to join him in the United States.

When Werfel arrived in New York in late 1940, he was physically and mentally exhausted. Having meditated and written on the extermination of the Armenians, he found himself gripped by the situation, both similar and different, that Jews were facing. He wrote a remarkable essay, published in a German émigré journal, in which he explored the recent sufferings of Jews in the light of world history, religion, and human nature:

> How are we to comprehend this hatred from the abyss, which is massing more horrifyingly than ever around an ethnic group that has preserved its existence among the nations for several millennia now? . . . In earlier times, hatred of Jews was always parochial, limited in scope. Today, in our technical age, it is global. . . . It is the most monumental religious war of all time, a war that the human race is waging against the two-thousand-year-old paradox, against the spirit of Israel, the biblical spirit in all its manifestations. . . . But if Israel's God and spirit are to vanish from this planet, the physical vehicle of this spirit— the Jewish people—must first be annihilated, down to the very last man.

Werfel was even more despairing when he looked beyond Nazism: he was convinced that humanity was entering a new age that he called the "motorized golem" that "dreams with strange fanaticism of a value-free, spiritless, and soulless world that resembles a technically elaborate frozen hell."

As 1940 drew to a close, only the British were waging war in Europe; would the Americans join the fight? Werfel was increasingly prophetic as he took stock of the catastrophe: "We Jews are fighting today for more than the continued existence of our communities in the Diaspora, for more than the development work in Palestine, yes, for more than our lives. We are engaged in God's struggle for the salvation of the entire world."[24]

Some had read *Mein Kampf* and listened closely to the speeches given by Hitler and his henchmen, and they sounded the alarm. Others had closed their eyes to the whole thing. All had been massacred. Lemkin had had conversations with an erudite historian and a devout baker. One might say that he and Dubnow were intentionalists ahead of their time, but that would be to grant too much significance to references that no longer made much sense. In light of what they had perceived, they agreed with the most innovative present-day historians of the extermination of the Jews, such as Omer

Bartov and Peter Longerich: from the start, anti-Jewish policies had been the tie that bound the Nazi racial community together, and the transition from rhetoric to implementation of the extermination was inherent to Germany's will to transform the demography in the eastern territories that it now occupied.[25]

In the 1950s, Lemkin instrumentalized Dubnow's moral and intellectual unction: he had likely told Dubnow in 1939 about the great work that he was planning. Dubnow acknowledged that it was "strange how initiatives taken by dictators fascinate and even paralyze statesmen of democratic nations, and how easily they let them get away with such bold actions." Lemkin then told him about his plan "to outlaw the destruction of peoples." Dubnow's "reaction was vivid: 'The basic value of your plan lives in the criminal character of the act,' he said. 'Obviously if killing one man is a crime, killing of entire races and peoples must be an even greater one.'" Lemkin responded, "'Murder of a whole people must be recognized as an international crime, which should concern not just one nation but the entire world.'"[26]

Was this really the content of their dialogue? Did Dubnow really say this in 1939? He suffered to the end for being an intellectual—his library was confiscated when he was confined to the Riga ghetto—and would have encouraged survivors to write history. And this was true up to his last breath: during the *Aktion* of December 1941, he was killed by a bullet probably fired by a Latvian militiaman. He supposedly called out, as he lay dying, "'Write it down, write it down!' It was a historian's testament."[27]

Like Ringelblum, who took inspiration from him when he created the Oyneg Shabes archivists' group in the Warsaw ghetto in 1941, Dubnow had felt since the late nineteenth century that history was the means by which the Jewish people would resist and survive.[28]

Fleeing, Making History

Lemkin wanted to make history. That is why he sought exile in the United States: there, it would be possible to work toward punishing mass murderers. But how would he reach North America?

In the 1930s, Western democracies, jointly and separately, closed their borders. For Poland, the war and the double occupation made the situation catastrophic. Anti-Semitism was nothing new; the rebirth of Poland in 1918 had been accompanied by a nationalism that took an aggressive stance toward the "Jewish problem"—a minority seen as too large. Especially after the death of Marshal Pilsudski in 1935, the country instituted a state policy of anti-Semitism: bans on professionals—of which Lemkin was a victim in 1933—quotas or even outright bans on students, separate seats for those still taking courses, boycotts of Jewish businesses, expulsions. The Catholic Church expressed full-throated support for the ideology of exclusion promulgated by nationalist political parties that used anti-Semitism as both program and strategy.

Edward Raczynski, the Polish ambassador to London and a future minister of foreign affairs for the government in exile, stated in January 1939, "There exist in Poland great numbers of Jews who far exceed the power of economic absorption of that country and whose rapid rate of natural increase has already for many years past subjected them to a necessity growing ever more urgent of considerable and continuous emigration."[29] Both hard-line and moderate anti-Semites agreed with the Zionists' solution: emigration. Yet, "emigration" meant "Palestine," and Palestine was under British mandate. Not only were the British limiting the number of Jewish immigrants to Palestine, but they preferred the persecuted German Jews who had been seeking refuge since 1933, who were deemed more assimilated and therefore more assimilable. The British concurred with the Poles' attitude toward "their" Jews.

Starting in the summer of 1939, Polish Jews found themselves in the same predicament as German Jews—or worse. There was no longer any question of emigrating; they had to find refuge from horrible persecution at a time when the world war was further restricting border crossings. And yet, the government in exile and the British authorities were always thinking about the future in terms of emigration, one result of which was this surreal note written by Frank Roberts, one of the Foreign Office diplomats in touch with Karski in London, on May 13, 1941:

> Since there are some three million Jews in Poland (ten per cent of the population of prewar Poland) and many of these are not very well assimilated, any Polish government must inevitably aim at finding some solution of this problem by emigration. Since, however, no other country is willing to accept Polish Jews, and the absorptive capacity of Palestine is strictly limited, it is not in the interest of H.M. Government to encourage such a policy on the part of

the Poles. All we can do is express the pious hope that the Poles will in fact do their best to assimilate the Jews.[30]

In June 1941, Operation Barbarossa and then the mass extermination of the Jews in Eastern Europe obviated any political move by the Polish, British, and other governments. There would soon be no more Polish Jews.

The British, dogged by the Palestine question, nevertheless continued to reflect upon refuge as a solution. The Home Office, Aliens Department, met with the High Commissioner of the Refugee Bureau of the League of Nations on January 6, 1942. What would the refugees—and, in particular, the most numerous among them, the Jews—choose to do after the war? There had to be agreement on acceptable guarantees for them in their countries of origin so that they could return to them. Otherwise, "the long-term refugee pb [problem] would then become insoluble."[31] The solution to the "Jewish problem" devised by the Nazis was called death.

Karski Encounters Poland's "Jewish Problem"

As Raphael Lemkin was fleeing east through Poland, passing through his hometown of Volkovysk, Jan Karski was starting his first mission in that part of Poland. The young activist had been dispatched by his brother, Marian, and his resistance organization to convince the various underground movements to unite—a mission made trickier because Poland was occupied by the Nazis to the west and the Soviets to the east. Sent to Lvov in the fall of 1939, Karski entered the Soviet zone with help from someone in the Jewish resistance who smuggled people in when they were convinced that they would be safer there than in the Nazi-controlled zone.

In early 1940, Karski traveled to France to give an account of what he had seen. He was physically strong, spoke many languages, and proved to be dependable, accurate, and discreet. He relied for the first time on what he would later call his "photographic memory." His debriefing dealt essentially with the conditions under which the resistance was operating in the two occupation zones, which were of particular interest to the government in exile: what was really going on in Poland? Karski's report took another form when the minister of the interior, Stanislaw Kot, asked him to put down in writing everything he had seen, listing the different themes—military, political, social—that should be discussed; a secretary would encrypt his

notes to guarantee his safety and that of people whom he might quote. Did
Kot choose the theme of the "Jewish problem," or was it Karski's initiative?
Karski barely mentions the report in his memoir. Yet, in 1940, he wrote
some ten detailed pages on the situation of the Jews. The ardent young
patriot had eyes only for Poland and for the men, like his brother, who had
made it possible for Poland to be resurrected after World War I and who
had immediately committed themselves to ensuring that it would not disappear again. Although the fate of the Polish Jews was a secondary concern,
his report nevertheless included a remarkably pointed analysis.

The historian David Engel unearthed the report in the archives of the
Polish government in exile at Stanford University's Hoover Institution. He
asked Karski about it, and Karski confirmed its provenance in 1982. Engel
then translated and published it in 1983.[32]

This fascinating ten-page document describes the discovery by the Polish
Catholic majority of the tragedies of the occupation; Karski took exception
to certain discriminatory measures that most people considered legitimate,
at least in 1936, when they oppressed the Jewish minority. In the view of the
core members organizing the underground state, the nation now needed
everyone, Jews included, at a time when defeat had exacerbated nationalism. How were things going in the field? Karski described the "Jewish Question ... in the homeland," a homeland now divided into three zones: the
regions annexed by the Reich; the Generalgouvernement, in which Warsaw
was situated; and the territories occupied by the USSR. He noted that he
had not written about the Nazi-occupied regions because "the situation of
the Jews in these territories is clear, uncomplicated, easy to understand." They
were officially destined, "through the use of force, law, and propaganda, for
destruction or removal. . . . The intent is toward the complete cleansing of
this area of the Jewish element. . . . The tendency is toward a resettlement
of all Jews from the annexed territories to the Generalgouvernement."[33] In the
Germans' view, these territories, "essentially German but disgracefully Juda-
ized by the Poles," had to be re-Germanized—that is, populated with *Volks-
deutsche* (ethnic Germans), Germans of the Reich, and wiped clean of their
Jews. In the majority "Polish" zone, now designated the Generalgouvernement, there was "the impression that the Germans would like to create . . .
something along the lines of a *Jewish reservation*" (emphasis in original). In
particular, Jews expelled from the annexed territories were resettled in the

Lublin region and "all wear stars or patches . . . which indicate that they are Jews." For "in the territory of the Generalgouvernement . . . 1) there are more Jews here; 2) Jews cannot be sent farther away from there. . . . The Germans nevertheless are attempting suitably to 'organize' the Jews here, 'to teach them [how to] work,' 'hygiene,' and 'respect for Nordics and Aryans in general,' to ruin them materially and to limit their life to an extremely narrow range." Karski sanitized his description of public sessions of torture and humiliation, speaking instead of forced gymnastic exercises and the cutting of beards of observant men. "Forced physical labor for Jews is organized on a large scale—mainly for the purpose of 'cleansing' Warsaw and other cities of garbage."[34] Well aware of how the Nazis reified the Jews— they had become malodorous trash that had to be disposed of by the master race—he wrote, "The 'Master Race' is really a nation of madmen, of brutal haters and heartless beings."[35] He carefully distinguished between the "legal" violence inflicted on Jews and the cruelties superimposed on this violence to increase their suffering and the enjoyment of their torturers.[36]

Although the first few pages of the report give a glimpse of Karski's compassion for the Jews persecuted in the Nazi zone, the tone changed when he described the Soviet zone. There, Jews "do not experience humiliations or persecutions," as the occupiers made "no distinctions . . . among nationalities or religious groups." Not only did Jews feel "at home" there because of their "ability to adapt," but they became members of political cells and took over "the most critical political-administrative positions." Because of his anti-Sovietism, understandable in a young soldier who had just escaped from Soviet prison camps and had been instructed on Judeo-Bolshevism through an atavistic anti-Semitic lens—he noted without batting an eye their supposed power over money and sex—Karski did not hide his disgust for Polish Jews who adapted to the Soviet system and who "are involved in loan-sharking and profiteering, in illegal trade, contraband, foreign currency exchange, liquor, immoral interests, pimping, and procurement."[37]

Karski knew that the zone annexed by the Soviets presented a complicated situation. First, he adopted the Polish doxa that likened the Jews there to communists who had betrayed their homeland by welcoming the occupiers with "baskets of red roses," but he nevertheless made "certain distinctions." The Jewish proletariat saw its situation improve "*structurally*": its members had "formerly been exposed primarily to oppression, dignities, excesses, etc., from the Polish element," and the fact that they "responded positively, if not enthusiastically, to the new regime" seemed, to Karski, "quite understandable."[38]

Karski began to use the first-person voice at this point in his text. In giving his opinion, he no doubt came to conclusions that went far beyond what his interlocutors could have imagined. For, in his view, if Jewish communists had frequently betrayed the Poles, other Jews, among the intelligentsia and the well-to-do, were persecuted by the Soviets to the point of undergoing "collective liquidation"[39] and had proved loyal to the homeland. They wanted to revive a democratic and independent Poland within which they would be welcomed. Karski was speaking here of Jews to whom he felt socially and politically close, even though he used the usual anti-Semitic slurs: "Of course, a certain calculation of self-interest is involved in all this."[40] It went without saying, in Karski's view, that the Jews, including the most respectable, "counted" everything, which included weighing the value of supporting the homeland. They would have no one to blame but themselves if their "devotion" to the Bolsheviks brought upon them the vengeance of the Poles!

Testimonials by Jews confirmed and fleshed out Karski's portrait. With the Soviets, Jews may have felt that they had escaped not only the Nazi horror but also Polish anti-Semitism. This was the sense in Volkovysk, Lemkin's native shtetl, where many members of his family still lived; they did not want to exaggerate the Soviet danger when he suggested that they flee with him. His father told him, "I have been living in retirement for more than ten years because of my sickness. I am not a capitalist. The Russians will not bother me." His brother added, "I gave up my store and registered as an employee before it was taken over by the new government. They will not touch me either."[41] The *Volkovysk Memorial Book* includes accounts of the long history of terrible relations between Polish and Jewish communities, which were made worse by the war. When the Polish army withdrew before the Soviet advances in this region, some residents, assisted by soldiers, organized a pogrom during which they pillaged, robbed, and murdered people, including Jewish fighters. "Who knows what cruelties the Poles might have accomplished? The Soviets entered the town and ended the anti-Semitic depredations. . . . The Jews began to breathe again. Many, such as the old shoemaker who climbed on a Red Army tank crying victory, even greeted the Soviets with great joy." The *Memorial Book* then related how the man was "rewarded": the "anti-Semite who had led the pogrom" had him arrested by the Soviets, who shot him dead.[42]

When the Soviet troops entered Luck, the Zionist Moshe Kleinbaum saw some young communist Jews applauding them. Such gestures could not hide the convoluted emotions experienced by everyone: "'We were condemned to death, but our sentence has been commuted to life-long imprisonment.' The Nazi danger meant the death penalty for the Jews. The Red Army came and rescued a million and a half Jews from a sure physical and civil death, but the Red Army rescued no more than the bare lives of Jews. . . . Life continues, but with nothing more than black bread and water, and people are no longer free. . . . At least 80 percent of the Jews think that way, and . . . they accepted Soviet rule first with a sigh of relief, because of the weeks of anxiety regarding the threat of Nazi invasion, and then with a sigh of deep concern: What will the morrow bring us?"[43]

In Otwock, near Warsaw, Calel Perechodnik expressed this stark lack of options even more directly: death for some, a gagged life for others. "Although I had been against communism throughout my life," he wrote, "now I begged God that the Bolsheviks would occupy the area up to the Vistula. I was ready to lose [everything] in order to be able to live as a free man, without any racial restrictions. Still, I did not jump for joy at the sight of Soviet tanks."[44]

Indeed, the Soviets were still Soviets. In Volkovysk, citizenship was offered to residents and many refugees from Nazified Poland; those who refused were sent to Siberia. And yet, the *Memorial Book* ends, in 1946, with, "Ultimately, this decree was a godsend for thousands of Jews from Poland and Lithuania. It saved their lives."[45]

"Repayment in blood"

Karski's handlers were keenly interested in what Poles thought about the fate of the Jews during the early months of the double occupation. The question turned out to be so complex that Karski rewrote his account three times, either on his own or according to requirements. The text was no doubt intended for the Allies: after the German-Soviet Pact was signed, they were eager for any criticism of the "Bolsheviks." And yet, Karski did not hesitate to expose Poles' mistrust of Jews, who apparently did not resist the Germans' orders but seemed capable of fleeing to the Soviet zone at any instant: "The Jew here would rather commit suicide than resist the Germans."[46]

In the first version of the report, Karski noted, "It would be advisable were there to prevail in the attitude of the Poles . . . the understanding that in the end both peoples are being unjustly persecuted by the same enemy." This was no doubt his own position, and he was aware that it was the exception: "Such an understanding does not exist among the broad masses of the Polish populace. Their attitude toward the Jews is overwhelmingly severe, often without pity. A large percentage of them are benefiting from the rights [over the Jews] that the new situation gives them. They frequently exploit these rights, and even abuse them. This brings them, to a certain extent, nearer to the Germans."[47] It is understandable why a different version of this paragraph was written—one in which the Poles were presented as being in the process of changing "under the influence of what is happening" and discovering "visible sympathy" for the Jews "given the unbounded bestiality of the Germans."[48] If the original version were to fall into the hands of the British and French allies—this was in February 1940—it might have a terrible effect: how could it be stated so plainly that the defeated Poles found a certain satisfaction in seeing Jews mistreated and hoped to profit from it? For, Karski specified, the Germans not only mistreated the Jews but hoped to use their anti-Jewish policy to "win over the Polish masses." The persecution by the Poles was intended, in part, to extort as much as possible from the Jews, as one way to "solv[e] the Jewish Question in the Generalgouvernement . . . [and] it must be admitted that they are succeeding in this. . . . The Polish peasant[s] . . . proclaim: 'Now then, they are finally teaching them a lesson.'—'We should learn from them.'—'The end has come for the Jews.'— 'Whatever happens, we should thank God that the Germans came and took hold of the Jews.'"[49] As might be expected, this section also had a different version: "[The Germans] are attempting to play upon as many and various conflicts as possible within Polish society . . . probably not assuming the fact that the mass of Polish society is not anti-Semitic. . . . But the Polish populace more and more frequently [is] thinking out loud: 'This is already too much.'—'These are not people.'—'This must end with some horrible punishment for the Germans.'"[50]

Karski understood the trap that Germany had laid for the Poles: to play on their visceral anti-Semitism in order to encourage them to collaborate by hunting down Jews and pillaging their goods, after which it would turn against them. Although his new version softened the wording, it was clear to Karski that Germany's perfidious solution took advantage of Polish anti-Semitism.

The government in exile, which was trying to unify the early resistance, faced a dilemma: given the active anti-Semitism of some of its own members, could showing any compassion, however minimal, toward Jews victimized by the Nazis alienate the Poles who might win the nation's cause?[51] Karski would be confronted with this predicament in all of his missions: to say or do something for the Jews always carried the risk of seeming to transform the war being waged by the Poles, the British, the Americans, the free French, and the rest into a war for the Jews; this was the basis of the propaganda put out by the Nazis and the collaborationists in occupied Europe. George Orwell made this bitter observation in an article written in April 1945: "It so happens that the war has encouraged the growth of anti-Semitism and even, in the eyes of many ordinary people, given some justification for it. To begin with, the Jews are one people of whom it can be said with complete certainty that they will benefit by an Allied victory. Consequently, the theory that 'this is a Jewish war' has a certain plausibility, all the more so because the Jewish war effort seldom gets its fair share of recognition."[52]

In 1940, Karski's conclusion to his report was categorical: in the annexed zone, "Virtually all Poles are bitter and disappointed in relation to the Jews; the overwhelming majority (first among them of course the youth) literally look forward to an opportunity for 'repayment in blood.'"[53] Karski was, in a way, clairvoyant. There were some cases of Polish participation in extermination of Jews, starting with the massacre in Jedwabne, for which historian Jan Gross forged the concept of "neighbors."[54] This episode of "repayment by blood" took place on July 10, 1941, barely three weeks after the Nazis invaded the Soviet zone.

When Karski wrote his memoir in 1944, however, he made no mention of what he had so subtly perceived in 1939–40. Throughout his account of the birth of the underground, he talked only about the Soviets and the Polish resisters whom he had secretly encountered. The only Jews he mentioned were those fleeing Nazi-held territory with whom he sneaked across the border to Lvov. "I could see that there were many of all ages, old men and women, two women with babies in their arms, and a few young men and girls. They were all escaping Jews. It seemed as if they sensed what the future held in store for them, that soon the pitiless extermination of the Jews would start."[55]

By 1944, Karski knew just about everything about the extermination of Polish Jews by the Nazis. But those who reached the Soviet zone in 1939 could not have known. Couriers had a tendency to exaggerate their premonitions, even though the reports that reached the provisional government at the time confirmed Karski's observations about the Poles and the Nazis: "The Jews persecuted the Poles so horribly . . . that at the first opportunity all the Poles—here, from old people to women and children—took a revenge so terrible upon the Jews that no anti-Semite would have thought it possible . . . the choice was no longer between Zionism and the previous state of affairs; rather, it was between Zionism and extermination."[56]

This was why Lemkin was trying to flee not just Poland but also Europe.

New York, Emergency Committee in Aid of Displaced Foreign Scholars, Box 87, File 39, Raphael Lemkin: Rejected[57]

Lemkin wanted to keep working. His odyssey took him across Poland, Lithuania, and Latvia to Sweden, where he was hoping to obtain a visa for the United States through his prewar academic contacts. He and a law professor at Duke University, Malcolm McDermott, had in fact translated the 1932 Polish Criminal Code into English. McDermott responded to his appeal and contacted the Emergency Committee in Aid of Displaced Foreign Scholars. The letters, phone calls, and telegrams back and forth between the committee, located in New York, and McDermott, in South Carolina, and the appeals made to the National Refugee Service, also in New York, by Lemkin, immobilized in Sweden, are poignant. There were no fewer than twenty-four exchanges between May 27 and July 31, 1940. Those involved in the effort alternated between hope and despair, including Betty Drury, the Emergency Committee's secretary, who responded with the same cordiality to all demands and tried to find solutions; without a financial guarantee, no visa would be granted: "Mr. Henry Bane, attorney at law, tells us that according to Prof. McDermott, Dr. Lemkin is a most inspiring and brilliant man and would be a credit to any institution. McDermott is ready to take him into his own home, but a stipend will be needed" (June 4, 1940). Lemkin had naively assumed that his impressive curriculum vitae, his participation in numerous international judicial conferences, the list of his publications in multiple languages, and the assurance from Duke University that it would find a teaching position for him would easily swing open the doors to the United States.

Lemkin was not taking into account the drastic quotas and the extreme competition for visas by "displaced academics"—"displaced" being a euphemism for "fleeing, hunted, persecuted." It went without saying that although the word "Jew" was not used, it applied to most of the "displaced" people. Before the war, they had been Germans, Austrians, and Czechoslovaks; now they were Poles. After two months of correspondence, Lemkin became increasingly uneasy. He saw the war setting Europe ablaze: Belgium—where he had been promised a position—Holland, and France were defeated. He had spent two months stuck in Stockholm; soon it would no longer be possible to leave. But his American friends could not find the money necessary. At Duke, his application was rejected: "The financial limit here has been reached in the employment of refugee professors." McDermott, pressed by Lemkin, pressed the committee: "In a recent letter Dr. Lemkin informs me that after the month of June he would not be permitted to pass through Finland. He indicates that every day will make it more difficult for him to get out of Sweden. If your committee finds it possible to supply the necessary funds in aid of this brilliant Polish legal scholar, I suggest that you act promptly, for time is of the essence in this matter" (June 18, 1940). Lemkin also contacted Jewish organizations, but it was the fact that he was a lawyer that was emphasized: "I'm familiar with his scholarly work and with the remarkably high reputation for scholarship and general intellectual achievement which he enjoys with the world of learning and letters. I should like to express my own ardent hope that your esteemed committee will find it possible to contribute to the rescue of this brilliant and worthy man."[58]

Once again, letters, telegrams, and telephone calls followed until the decision—rejection—was made known: "The European crisis has brought so many urgent applications for funds and the C[ommittee] was obliged to try to stretch its limited resources to take care of as many scholars as possible. Preference was given to those scholars who were technically eligible for our support. As a former attorney, Dr. L[emkin's] case did not come within the scope of our work. . . . Then, too, the C[ommittee] preferred not to use its funds for scholars who were still in Europe."[59] This was the twenty-first letter. The committee knew all about Lemkin's double career as a lawyer and researcher and about his impressive bibliography. One can imagine his disappointment when he heard the news. And then, a dramatic turn of events: his persistence paid off as he found distant relatives living in New York who offered the required $1,200 to Duke; he could finally proceed with his visa application. Ms. Drury spread the news: "It is not very often that cases of this sort turn out so happily" (July 31, 1940).

"Okay, boy, you're in"[60]

Over nine months, Lemkin crossed the Soviet Union on the Trans-Siberian—it is difficult to understand how he was able to do this—reached Japan, then took a ship to Seattle. He was finally in the United States. He remembered his arrival, in April 1941, as if he were in a dream: the American customs agents, rude and punctilious, nevertheless seemed very friendly and welcoming to him. At least, that is how he reconstructed it later, out of his desire to portray himself as an exemplary future American citizen. He hurried to Duke to get to work, accomplish his mission, bring sight to the "blind world." Lemkin, a typical Central European intellectual, planned to fight against barbarism by putting his legal expertise to work to create new laws.[61] "I realized that the real issue at stake in the war was civilization not as a weapon of propaganda or a slogan but as a palpable reality."[62]

2

$$\infty\!\infty\!\infty$$

Karski Discovers the
Annihilation of Lemkin's World

1941–42

The Germans are not trying to enslave us as they have other people; we are being systematically murdered. That is the difference. That is what people do not understand. That is what is so difficult to make clear. Over in London, Washington or New York, they undoubtedly believe that the Jews are exaggerating, that they're hysterical. . . . Our entire people will be destroyed. A few may be saved, perhaps, but three million Polish Jews are doomed. As well as others, brought from all over Europe.

—Karski reporting what his guide in the Warsaw ghetto said, summer 1942

"A crime without a name" (Winston Churchill)

After the defeat of France in June 1940, the Polish government in exile moved from Angers to London. In June 1941, the Nazi invasion of the Soviet Union opened a new phase of the war. Many members of the Polish underground state were tortured and murdered, particularly in the horrible Pawiak prison in Warsaw. Large numbers of Poles were deported to the concentration camp in Oswiecim (Auschwitz), including Marian Kozielewski, Jan Karski's brother, who was later released thanks to the intervention of his wife, a German-born Pole.[1] This, however, was no act of mercy. The Oswiecim concentration camp was being used as a site of terror against the Poles, and the few releases were employed mainly as a means of pressuring families.[2] Karski always kept in his archives a book translated into English from a 1943 Polish resistance booklet on the atrocities at Oswiecim, *The Camp of Disappearing Men*.[3] The book's protagonist is a fictional Christian resister,

Jan, who suffers many kinds of mistreatment: he must perform "gymnastics" in bare feet on sharp pebbles and is put to work exhuming the bodies of five hundred Soviet prisoners from a cave where they had just been tortured to death: "Jan discovered the secret of Purgatory and of five hundred dead Russians. He had a corpse by the arm and suddenly he stopped and stared into its face. 'My God!' he screamed. . . . Years ago—in 1917—he had seen that same spectral appearance when he came across a dead soldier in an abandoned trench. It was the mark of poison gas."[4] Jan, who has seen everything, borne everything—even the unbearable—finally throws himself against the electrified fencing. In a remarkable illustration by John Groth, the *Chicago Sun* war correspondent, the barbed wire forms a crown of thorns around his head; like so many Poles, Jan has met the "Golgotha of Oswiecim." There is no mention of Jews in the original Polish-language booklet; the American version contains a final note: "According to information from the Polish underground, up to July 1942 94,000 people were executed in Oswiecim. The death toll rose to 667,161 for the period between September 1942 and August 1943. According to a report by the Very Reverend Paul Vogt, of the Swiss refugee organization the Fluchtlingshilfe, the execution of Jews in Oswiecim amounted to 1,715,000 during the two years ended April 15, 1944, as reported in the *New York Times*, July 6, 1944."[5] The explicit listing of precise numbers of dead at Oswiecim was inversely proportional to the silence regarding the mass extermination still under way at Birkenau, the name of which wasn't even mentioned.

Executions of Polish Jews, and then Russian Jews, started in June 1941; most were shot by mobile killing teams until gas began to be used. In the former case, the murderers traveled to their victims; in the latter, the victims were transported to stationary death facilities. In 1940, Auschwitz had become the seventh concentration camp in the Reich's territory; in 1942, the sixth site for killing Jews was created at Birkenau—after Chelmno, Belzec, Sobibor, Treblinka, and Majdanek, all situated in the zone of the Polish Generalgouvernement.

The Nazis used trucks, then trains, to deport Polish Jews the short and medium distances from the ghettos and work camps to which they had been confined since October 1940; in 1942, the operation was extended throughout occupied Europe. The two forms of murder coexisted. Mobile killing teams operated up to the end of 1944, in parallel with the gas chambers at the largest extermination center, Birkenau, which received its first Jews on March 26–27, 1942, from Poprad, Slovakia, and from the Bourget-Drancy and Compiègne train stations, the origins of the first convoy from France. (My own great-uncle, Pierre Ignace, was in that convoy.)

But we must not let what we can reconstruct with some accuracy, eighty years later, hide the incredible chaos that was experienced in these places, and in the rest of the world, when the Nazis transitioned from active persecution of Jews to their extermination. On August 24, 1941, Winston Churchill, who had met with President Roosevelt on August 14—the United States was not yet in the war—gave an overview of the situation in Europe and Asia in a radio address:

> Since the Mongol invasions . . . there has never been methodical, merciless butchery on such a scale. . . . And this is but the beginning. Famine and pestilence have yet to follow in the bloody ruts of Hitler's tanks. . . . [The aggressor behaves with] the most frightful cruelties. As his armies advance, whole districts are being exterminated. . . . Literally scores of thousands of executions in cold blood are being perpetrated by the German police troops. . . . We are in the presence of a crime without a name.[6]

Did Raphael Lemkin, who had arrived in the United States in April 1941, listen to this address, broadcast around the globe, as he was already devoting himself to giving this crime a name? His relatives and friends in Poland were suffering through confinement in ghettos, forced labor, torture, and, finally, death. Churchill obviously had highly specific information on what Jews in Poland, the Baltic nations, Ukraine, and Belarus were living through, as the British had broken the Enigma Code in July 1941 and read the reports of killings carried out by the Einsatzgruppen. But he did not utter the word "Jew." As a politician and author, he chose his words carefully. He named all of Eastern Europe as the victim of these "frightful cruelties." The terms "execution" and "extermination" did not refer to a particular situation, and all the peoples under occupation were named one by one, except the Jews. In the summer of 1941, the mingling of war crimes and crimes against Jews was complete . . . or being maintained.

Of course, neither Churchill nor the governments in exile in London could have known what the Nazis had not anticipated. Although many Jews were killed as the troops passed, no general, global extermination plan had yet been established. During the winter of 1942, however, the increasingly detailed radio reports and information from couriers, including photographs, left no doubt: Jews were now the target of a massive, unprecedented extermination. While killings by shooting continued in the Soviet Union and in Lithuania and Latvia, which were very quickly rendered *Judenfrei*, the death centers were receiving more and more convoys. Most of the Jews in the Warsaw ghetto were murdered in Treblinka starting in summer 1942. It was at this time that Karski was brought into the ghetto as a resister, before leaving for London.

"A bestial policy of extermination, committed with sang-froid" (December 1942 memorandum addressed to President Roosevelt)

The information arriving in London was piecemeal and incoherent; it was often difficult to decipher, and what was known differed from what was believed or understood. The archives for the summer and fall of 1942, just before and during Karski's stay in London, offer a cruel demonstration of this. Day after day, documents arrived at the Foreign Office from occupied or neutral European countries and from Palestine. This information was cross-checked against that held by the Polish government in exile and by representatives of Polish Jewish organizations and the World Jewish Congress. Gerhart Riegner, a representative of the Congress in Switzerland, warned his counterparts in London in the summer of 1942 that 3.5 million European Jews were to be deported to the east and murdered with prussic acid. It was by this channel that Rabbi Steven Wise, president of the American Jewish Congress, directly received information that he agreed not to make public at the request of Secretary of State Sumner Welles. When Wise met with Karski several months later, he did not hear much that he did not already know.[7]

On December 8, 1942, the Americans—and, most significantly, President Roosevelt—received an extremely detailed nine-page memorandum on the extermination of the Jews, sent by a Polish resistance courier who had recently arrived in London: Karski.[8] By the time Roosevelt met with Karski six months later, in June 1943, he had read his report, along with dozens of others. Information was therefore circulating widely on both sides of the Atlantic. Proof of this is that the *New York Times* published, on the very day it was issued, the declaration regarding the "bestial policy of cold-blooded extermination" of Jews proclaimed jointly in London, Moscow, and Washington on December 17, 1942.[9]

Yet, far from being considered unique in the annals of war cruelties, the extermination of Jews was generally perceived as one atrocity among others. The information accumulated, but very few, including Jews, were capable of appreciating it—whence the despair of those who, through pessimism or lucidity, realized what was happening.

"Warning: Some images may cause distress"

One section in the British National Archives was titled "German Atrocities in Poland." It covered the entire country, and it contained much material. The rapacity had grown since the beginning of 1942: "It is clear that the terror campaign against the Poles in the annexed territories and the Gouvernementgeneral intensified in the period from January to March 1942; there have been more arrests and executions. It seems that the regime in the camp at Oswiecim has become even stricter in recent months. The Poles see this terror with their own eyes and suffer it in their own bodies"[10] No mention of Jews. On the other hand, the Polish point of view prevailed—a first draft of what the Allies would constantly repeat by rote: it was difficult, even impossible, to act at the moment, but once the war was won the German torturers would be punished.

Yet, in spring 1942, some interlocutors brought up the scope of the extermination. For instance, Ignacy Schwarzbart, one of the Jewish representatives (with Shmuel Zygielbojm, of the Bund) to the Polish National Council in London, wrote to the Foreign Office, "Please read this document with the greatest discretion: Statement on German Crimes Committed against the Jewish Population in Poland. These crimes form part of the atrocities committed against the population of Poland as a whole. The numbers speak for themselves."[11]

> The specific aspect of the catastrophe of European Judaism lies in the fact that contemporary Germany under Hitler's leadership is aiming at the complete destruction and annihilation of Jewry, its biological destruction. . . . Hitler, the killer, is achieving this aim by converting areas of suffering Poland into mass graves for Jewry. . . . What is not accomplished by famine, disease, or natural death is organized by the murder of Polish Jews and Jews from other

countries deported by Hitler to Poland . . . This surpasses the worst examples of barbarism in history. . . . All nations under Hitler's domination are experiencing terrible trials, but the Jewish nation is the greatest victim. We must do everything in our power to keep the population of Poland from being annihilated, especially the Jewish population, which is threatened with complete extermination, now. Only immediate action will keep Hitler from completing his criminal action.[12]

Words, numbers, photographs. Frank Savery, formerly the British consul in Warsaw and the Poland expert at the Foreign Office, complained about the reluctance of the cabinet of the Polish prime minister in exile, Stanislaw Mikolajczyk, to send him photographs that had been brought to England on microfilm by an underground courier in March 1942: "I had to remind him at least four times." Finally, the British had these thirty-eight photographs in their hands. The images were so dreadful that archivists attached a label to the file when they were declassified: "Warning: some images may cause distress."[13] By 1972, archivists and historians were well aware of the traumatic effects of images of the opening of concentration camps, of extermination sites, and of other Nazi and post-Nazi cruelties.

The photographs were in two series: Soviet prisoners of war in "occupied Poland" and "ghetto scenes." The diplomats called them "abominable" or "horrific." One of them wrote in the margin, "We don't want to see them again!" Is this why these pictures weren't distributed at the time? Or was there a more political reason? In the first series, prisoners of war have been killed "during escape attempts"—a body caught in barbed wire, a woman hanged—or "for guerrilla activity." In the second series, bodies of children and adults are seen in ghettos; these piles of skeletal corpses prove that civilians died of hunger or deprivation-induced disease. The diplomats were interested in the prisoners of war and wrote captions, in Polish and English, for these pictures. No explanatory details, however, were added to the ghetto pictures.

"No action seems necessary"
(Foreign Office memorandum, September 1942)

Were the "ghetto scenes" destined to remain hidden from the public? They were not; people in the British services were not the only ones to have seen them or to have read descriptions in the secret diplomatic telegrams and courier debriefings.[14] Representatives of Jewish organizations in London had received the same microfilm strips and published them in leaflets that were sold openly in order to make the public aware of the specific crimes against Jews. They also "illustrated" speeches given during public protests. On July 22, 1942, a first demonstration by Labour supporters was held to protest against the "Nazi atrocities in Poland and Czechoslovakia." It was known that liquidation of the Warsaw ghetto was in the process of being completed and that the trains had begun to roll from occupied Europe to the extermination centers. Shmuel Zygielbojm described things as follows:

> The Germans have chosen Poland for the place of execution of Jews of all the occupied countries, as well as Germany herself. . . . The fate of the remaining Jews in the ghettoes awaiting their doom, is much worse than the fate of those who have already been murdered. As a representative of those masses, I echo their outcry of pain and protest, and their appeal to mankind that means should be found to stop the greatest crime in history![15]

In London, meetings, declarations, and demonstrations succeeded each other throughout 1942. People spoke out constantly to keep the fate of the Jews in public view. For instance, General Władysław Sikorski, chief of the Polish armed forces and prime minister of the Polish government in exile, stated in a radio address, "The Jewish population of Poland is condemned to extermination in compliance with the principle that all Jews must be massacred, whatever the outcome of the war."[16] Nevertheless, in the six pages that he read into the microphone, Sikorski devoted only one short paragraph to the Jews and insisted that the "greatest crime" of the German Reich had been to force Poles to join its army.

Like Churchill and Roosevelt, Sikorski argued that, given that Goebbels and Nazi propaganda claimed that the war had been wanted and fomented by Jews, it would fit with their racist ideology to differentiate the suffering inflicted. As to the figure of seven hundred thousand exterminated, it was deemed highly unreliable. Even the idea that the Warsaw ghetto had been liquidated left diplomats skeptical. They attributed the suicide of the "mayor," Adam Czerniaków, and three other leaders of the Judenrat to their refusal to "see 100,000 Jews deported from the ghetto. . . . As regards the mass killings we have no very precise evidence although it seems likely that they have taken place on a large scale. *No action seems necessary,*" as a highly placed member of the Foreign Office put it.[17] Civil servants in the British government and the Polish government in exile were not the only ones to doubt the reality of the extermination; community leaders in the British Jewish community feared that publication of this information would sow panic among Jews with family in Eastern Europe.[18]

Conversely, the two Jewish members of the Polish National Council of London felt that it was crucial to point out what was happening to their people amid the catastrophes raining down on Europe.[19] In the leaflet *Stop Them Now: German Mass Murder of Jews in Poland*, Zygielbojm repeated the words of Nazi leaders—"Rid the world of the Jewish Pest . . . Exterminate the Jews"—and concluded, "It is evident that the policy of the Germans is to wipe out entirely, not only the Jews in Poland but the Jewish population of the whole of Europe."[20] "It *is* true," he insisted—and he repeated it over and over. Zygielbojm was well informed, but no more so than the authorities in London. Nevertheless, he quickly put words to the facts in the leaflet subtitles—"Mass murder by poison gas," "Gas chambers," "The dead desecrated"[21]—and publicized the testimonials of victims, such as a letter written by a woman to her sister, "one of the many thousands of letters travelling between the ghettoes of Poland": "'My dear, my hands shake so that I cannot write. It is very bad here. Our hours are numbered. God alone knows if we shall ever see one another again. I write and weep and my children are in despair. We want so much to live. We all take leave of you and kiss you. If you do not get another letter from me very soon, we shall be no more.'" Zygielbojm finishes her story: "The woman who wrote this letter and her children have since died. They were killed by poison gas."[22]

As desperate as he was, Zygielbojm wanted to continue to believe in his compatriots laboring in the resistance: "The walls of the ghetto have not really separated the Jewish population from the Poles. The Polish and the Jewish working masses continue to fight together for common aims, just as they have fought for so many years in the past."[23] Was this a fervent wish, an ideological conviction, or prudence on the part of this Bund member isolated in London? His family had remained in the Warsaw ghetto, and he opposed Zionists and other Bundists who did not share his views.

Zygielbojm pleaded stridently with his readers: "Will the world allow it? Will YOU allow it? Means must be found to prevent it. STOP THE GER-MANS NOW"![24] Convinced that the disaster would have to be seen to be believed, he published three photographs from the Foreign Office series and captioned them. Under a pile of utterly emaciated bodies: "Not an illus-tration from Dante's 'Inferno,' but a real photograph of a mass grave of mas-sacred Jews in Central Poland."[25] He may have thought that this was a ditch that the victims had dug together before being shot. In a reframing of the negatives, uniformed gravediggers can be seen, indicating that these were pictures taken, no doubt, in late 1941 or early 1942 at the Warsaw ghetto ceme-tery. These men, women, and children had died of hunger, deprivation, or ill treatment, as the captions make explicit. "Starvation" is the caption for the photograph of a man wearing a kippah who holds a horrifyingly thin dead child.[26] In a fourth picture, the bodies of four naked children have been tossed on the ground. The gravediggers, members of the Chevra Kadisha, are almost as thin as the people they are leading to their graves. Another picture is captioned "The tally of the dead": in front of the morgue door, a ghetto official fills out papers beside a small cart piled with corpses—human remains of bone and skin.[27] During his trip into the ghetto in the summer of 1942, Karski was stunned to see corpses lying in the streets. "'When a Jew dies,'" his guide told him, "'his family removes his clothing and throws his body in the street. If not, they have to pay the Germans to have the body buried. They have instituted a burial tax which practically no one here can afford. Besides, this saves clothing. Here, every rag counts.'"[28]

If Zygielbojm decided to publish these pictures, it was because he thought that they would allow people to see, and thus to "know," as much as—or even more than—the texts would tell them. Like many well-educated observ-ers, he evoked Dante's imaginary "inferno,"[29] also used, later, by the Italian author Primo Levi. The author Marcel Cohen has remarked, however, that we always forget that Dante's inferno contained the guilty, not the innocent.[30]

Photographic evidence can be found, as we know, in the British National Archives, including the details of the liquidation *Aktion* in the Warsaw ghetto, which began on July 22, 1942. Although some information had arrived ear-lier, well before the summer, it had not been decrypted. Was this due to politi-cal calculation? Military choice? Indifference? Anti-Semitism? Because it was impossible to believe such aberrations? Or for all of these reasons?

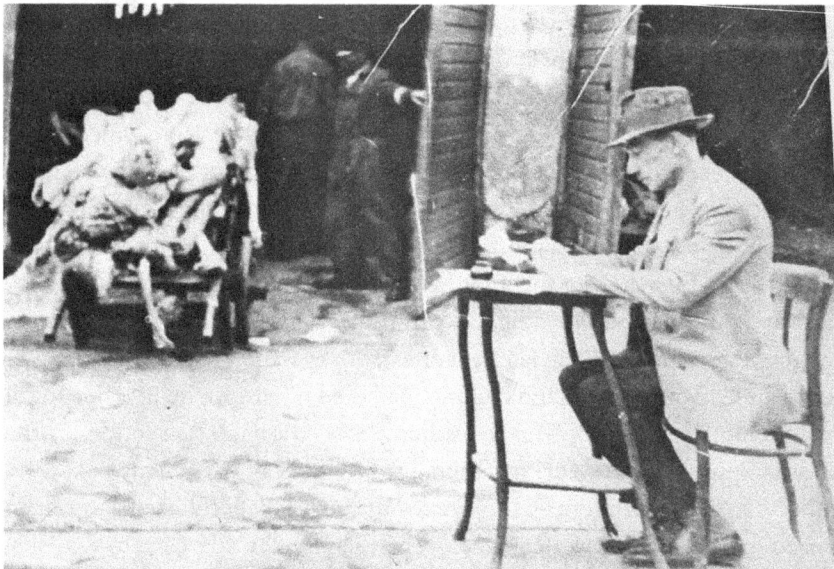

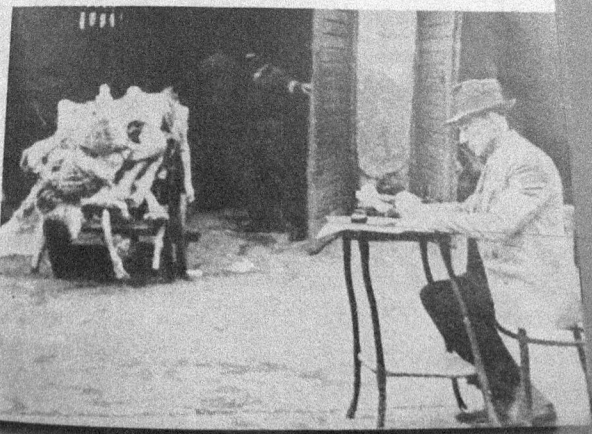

Archival photograph sent to the Foreign Office and distributed in Shmuel Zygielbojm's leaflet *Stop Them Now: German Mass Murder of Jews in Poland*, p. 9, with the caption "The Tally of the Dead." In the BNA, photograph FO 371 31097. Kew National Archives.

Nevertheless, on June 26, 1942, Emanuel Ringelblum, the historian confined to the Warsaw ghetto, noted with relief the content broadcast in a BBC program:

> For long months we had been suffering because the world was deaf and dumb to our unparalleled tragedy. We complained about Polish public opinion, about the liaison men in contact with the Polish government-in-exile. Why weren't they reporting to the world the story of the slaughter of Polish Jewry? We accused the Polish liaison men of deliberately keeping our tragedy quiet, so that *their* tragedy might not be thrown into the shade. But now it seems that all our interventions have finally achieved their purpose. There have been regular broadcasts over the English radio the last few weeks, treating of the cruelties perpetrated on the Polish Jews: Belzec and the like. Today there was a broadcast summarizing the situation: 700,000 the number of Jews killed in Poland, was mentioned. At the same time, the broadcast vowed revenge, a final accounting for all these crimes. . . . Now for the first time we understood why they kept silent. London simply didn't know what was happening in detail; hence the silence. But another question [suggests itself]: Having their own radio station, how could the Polish government-in-exile not have known what was happening? Why did they know in London the very next day about 100 persons—political prisoners—executed in the Pawiak Street jail, but months passed before London found out about the hundreds of thousands of murdered Jews? This is a problem that no solution can satisfy.[31]

Ringelblum found it difficult to understand the time lag between the receipt of the information and its dissemination—between knowledge and action. He managed to persuade himself, however, that the message had finally gotten through. He even mentioned the "joy" that people in the ghetto felt when they realized that the world was better informed than they had presumed about the particular tragedy of the Jews within the tragedy of the war.

> "For us, it was war and occupation.
> For them, it was the end of the world." (Jan Karski)[32]

In his piece for the BBC on December 12, 1942, George Orwell cited part of the memorandum sent two days earlier by the Republic of Poland in Exile to governments at the United Nations:[33]

It is absolutely not propaganda and has been confirmed by various sources, starting with the statements by the Nazi leaders themselves. For example, in March, Himmler, head of the Gestapo, promulgated a decree requiring the "liquidation"—don't forget that in totalitarian language, liquidation is an elegant euphemism for murder—of 50 percent of the Polish Jews who survived the pogroms. . . . Out of slightly more than three million, one third, a million human beings, have been killed in cold blood or have died of hunger and physical misery. Many thousands of them, men, women, and children, were deported to Russia, crammed into cattle cars, without water or food, in which they traveled sometimes for weeks; by the time they reached their destination, half of the occupants of these cars had succumbed. If I mention this persecution of Jews, it is not solely to report atrocity stories; it is because this sort of cold and methodical cruelty, totally different from the violence that goes hand in hand with war, is proof of the true nature of the fascism against which we are fighting.[34]

Orwell acknowledged that "even after three years of war, during which sensibilities have been numbed, this news has provoked horror and deep emotion the world over." His faith was returning, especially because he believed that the Allies were finally ready to take action.[35]

Yet, although the suffering of the Jews was not glossed over, it continued to be generally thought of as confined to the occupation of Poland. This interpretation was perpetuated throughout the duration of the war, including in the French underground press. *Les Cahiers du Témoignage chrétien*, which devoted a full issue to Poland in early 1943, did not omit to mention the situation of the Jews—and in this respect it was unusual—but allotted it just a few lines, which was completely inadequate given the spectacular nature of the information:

Finally, it must be mentioned that the Gouvernementgeneral has become a ghetto in which all the Jews in Poland and Germany have been gathered and to which all Jews from all occupied countries are currently being brought. They are interned in ghettos established in large cities. Anyone who leaves the ghetto is shot. Exhaustion due to labor, hunger, cold, and disease deliver a rich harvest to death. Sometimes the Gestapo enters and conducts massacres. Mass shootings and gas poisonings are on the agenda. . . . *In total, more than seven hundred thousand Jews have been murdered in Poland, and there is no doubt concerning Hitler's plan to completely exterminate the Jews on the continent of Europe.*[36]

Both in official and public circles in England and in some underground press outlets in occupied countries, the specific situation of the Jews was indeed brought up. But what was the author of the piece in *Les Cahiers* thinking when he wrote, "There is no doubt concerning Hitler's plan to completely exterminate the Jews on the continent of Europe"? What did his readers make of this statement? *Completely exterminate*: words that were read, reread, repeated—words that made no sense, as they were senseless.

This was what so troubled the two activists who hoped to meet with Karski in Warsaw before he left for London. They were a Zionist and a Bundist—the same political configuration as that of the two Jewish members of the Polish government in exile, Schwarzbart and Zygielbojm. Karski, resister in the field, was now being asked to serve as eyewitness. His direct account would play the same role as photographs or reports, now so numerous that they had become illegible, incomprehensible. In fact, Leon Feiner, the underground Bundist called upon to guide Karski in the ghetto, had sent a first report on the massacres of Jews throughout Poland to London in May 1942 and a second one in late August. He also used the figure of seven hundred thousand exterminated, stated that at this pace there would soon remain not a single Jew in the country, and advocated for reprisals against German civilians. He wrote, furthermore, that the war had been started by Hitler to exterminate Jews; even if the Germans, in the end, were defeated, the primary goal—the only goal?—would have been achieved: "We are stunned and petrified at the scope of this murder, its massive nature, its cruel and sophisticated methods of killing."[37] Karski noted Feiner's extreme agitation and sense of absolute urgency. They no doubt met on August 31, 1942, just after Feiner sent this second missive.[38]

Feiner and his companion knew that the reports were reaching their addressees, that they would be published and debated but would remain incomprehensible, and so they once again described the senseless: "The Germans are not trying to enslave us as they have other people; we are being systematically murdered. That is the difference. That is what people do not understand. That is what is difficult to make clear. Over in London, Washington, or New York, they undoubtedly believe that the Jews are exaggerating, that they're hysterical. . . . Our entire people will be destroyed. A few may be saved, perhaps, but three million Polish Jews are doomed. As well as others, brought in from all over Europe."³⁹ Karski was now charged with their mission: "This was the solemn message I carried to the world. They impressed it upon me so that it could not be forgotten. They added to it, for they saw their position with the clarity of despair. At this time, more than 1,850,000 Jews had been murdered."⁴⁰ Although the constantly repeated figure of seven hundred thousand was one of the reasons for incredulity in 1942 and 1943, the figure put forward by Karski was much closer to reality—but a reality still not being heard in 1944, when he was writing his memoir.

Why Karski?

Given the information available in London when Karski arrived there in November 1942, why were the Polish Jews there, increasingly feeling abandoned, convinced of his specific importance, and how did the government in exile decide to send him to testify in the United States? The day after he met with Karski, on December 5, 1942, Ignacy Schwarzbart sent a telegram to the World Jewish Congress in New York: "Special envoy gentile . . . arrived here left capital this October saw Warsaw ghetto or last August and September witnessed mass murder of one transport six thousand Jews at Belzec . . . confirm all most horrible mass atrocities still living all remnants of Jews facing death. Brought desperate appeal of this remnant to world Jewry . . . details shortly."⁴¹ Zygielbojm also returned to the subject in a telegram sent to Churchill several days after he spoke with Karski: "Last desperate appeal . . . the entire Jewish population of Poland, women, children, men, is disappearing."⁴²

December 1942 was particularly crucial. Karski was far from the only one to testify to this. Abraham Stupp, a Galician who had studied in Lvov—as had Karski and Lemkin—and immigrated to Mandatory Palestine in 1939, sent a telegram from Tel Aviv to the World Jewish Congress on December 4, 1942:

Some Polish with visas they report deportations started April after Himmlers visit first case Lublin 70000 deported out [of] those 7000 sent camps Majdany [Majdanek, several miles from Lublin] 63000 no trace left presumably murdered stop Krakow in May only 6000 Jews remained others deported unknown direction presumably murdered Tarnow deported 10000 7000 shot railway station stop Warsaw deportations since 22 June 7000 daily once 20000 stop By October 36000 remained stop Deported carried Treblinka there everey [*sic*] day trainloads Jews arrive they are stripped naked clothes given tailors be cut through search jewellery heaps clothes lie about then Jews taken socalled bathhouse hermetically closed chamber air pumped away people suffocate other reports say Jews killed poison gas.[43]

Other reports arriving from Poland, the Yishuv, Sweden, and Switzerland were full of similar information during the fall and early winter of 1942. But Karski's words touched his interlocutors, at least, and ultimately those who knew already. His meeting with Zygielbojm was an example. All his life, Karski felt a form of guilt over Zygielbojm's suicide a few months later. He remembered it even during the shooting of *Shoah* in 1978, as the rushes show:

KARSKI: I saw in Zigelboim a man—with this kind of man I had no dealings, frankly, very much, either in my underground activities or before the war. . . . Very Jewish. . . . I had before me a proletarian.
CLAUDE LANZMANN: Did he have a Yiddish accent when he spoke Polish? . . . And he looked very Jewish?
K: He looked Jewish. He had rough hands, you know . . . nothing refined about Zigelboim. . . . Nervous. Agitated. . . . Most of the time he was pacing the room. . . . On numerous occasions I would stop. He said [Karski faces the camera and shouts], "Why don't you talk! Talk! You came here to talk!" From the very beginning we didn't start well. . . . He asked me in a rather sarcastic way Mr emissary I was told you want to see me. What do you want?[44]

Karski didn't realize—he had been in London for only a few days—how much information on the extermination had preceded him; at first, Zygielbojm "was not impressed." But when he realized that this non-Jew had actually entered the Warsaw ghetto—to which his own family was confined—and visited what they believed in 1942 was Belzec, Zygielbojm seemed increasingly desperate: "Aggressive, unfriendly . . . something like disintegrating." Karski reconstructed Zygielbojm's words:

к: He says: "So, what can I do! What can I do that I am not doing? I do everything! I do everything possible." So then I also half in anger at that time, I
gave it to him. I closed my eyes. [which Karski also does in this 1978 inter-
view] . . . "Jews are dying. There will be no Jews. What is the use of having
Jewish leaders? Let the Jews go to the most important officers, Allied officers. Let them demand. If they are refused, let them go out. Let them stay
outside. Let them refuse drink. Let them refuse food. Let them die. Let
them die a slow death. Let humanity see it. Perhaps it will move humanity."
And then he jumps [Karski, as Zygielbojm, jumps to his feet and spins in
the room]: "Madness! Madness! They are mad! The whole world is mad!
They do not understand anything! They will not let me die! They will send
two policemen, they will arrest me! They will take me to an asylum! . . .
Everybody is mad! So I have to do something? I don't know what!"

cl: Do you think he was already in complete desperation?

к: He is not mad, he is totally normal. I did not attempt any kind of what
today we call psychiatry. He was a leader, only he was lost in helplessness.[45]

Playing on the contradiction between his modesty and his heroic strength,
Karski was able to maintain his resister's image between 1942 and 1944, particularly by writing his memoir and giving a series of talks across the United
States. But the celebrity that he acquired in the 1980s should create no illu-
sions in retrospect, for his mission had concerned essentially the Polish
underground, not knowledge about extermination of the Jews. Why did his
different missions make him much more than a simple courier?

On the one hand, when he was arrested during one of his missions to
Poland, his courage while being tortured and his spectacular escape made
him a symbol of the resistance. On the other hand, the fact that he was a
practicing Catholic forestalled any suspicion that he had a special interest
in the Jewish cause, even though he was accused of exaggerating, spreading
rumors, or lying by those most determined to ignore the reality of the extermination. It was because he was not Jewish—he also undoubtedly evinced
a certain anti-Semitism that was unremarkable for Poland—that Karski
could speak of the fate of the Jews. But this was also true of other couriers,
such as Jan Nowak. When they went together to Westminster, they were
allotted only ten minutes to talk about the Polish resistance. Elsewhere,
both talked also about the Jews to people such as Anthony Eden.[46]

§

In London and then in Washington, Karski was at the service above all of the Polish clandestine state, as the title chosen for his memoir, *Story of a Secret State*, makes clear.[47] There were "us," the Poles, and "them," the Jews. However, Karski forcefully explained during a BBC program broadcast in early 1943, during his stay in London, why it was his "duty" (a key word for him) to take an interest in the fate of the Jews.[48]

> I was a member of the Polish Underground Movement. It was my duty to keep in touch with all underground parties, including the "Bund." . . . Among my other duties, I collected matter on the Jewish mass-extermination. . . . I am not a Jew myself, and before the war I had very little contact with Jews; in fact, I knew practically nothing about them. But, at present, the extermination of the Jews has a special significance. The sufferings of my own Polish compatriots are terrible, and they are, of course, nearer to my heart; but the methods employed by the enemy against Poles and against Jews are different. Us, the Poles, they try to reduce to a mediaeval race of serfs. They want to deprive us of our cultural standards, of our traditions, of our education, and reduce us to a state of robots.[49]

Robots. Karski was appealing to history, in this complex dichotomy of Nazi anomie—or, rather, surnomie—between a return to barbarism and sophisticated modernity. Carel Capek coined the word "robot" in Czech in 1924 for his science-fiction play *Rossum's Universal Robots*. The word is derived from *robota*, "forced labor," "work party." Karski used it in this sense when he described the passing of a brigade of forced laborers, haggard with fatigue, in the Warsaw ghetto. Writing this word of Czech origin at a time when the Nazis were doing their best to make Slav cultures disappear was deliberately ironic. He continued, "But the policy towards the Jews is different. It is not a policy of subjugation and oppression, but of cold and systematic extermination. It is the first example in modern history that a whole nation (not 10, 20 or 30, but 100 percent of them) are meant to disappear from this earth." Karski emphasized both the historical continuity of the persecutions and the Nazi rupture: "I know history. I have learned a great deal about the evolution of nations, political systems, social doctrines, methods of conquest, persecution, and extermination, and I know, too, that never in the history of mankind, never anywhere in the realm of human relations did anything occur to compare with what was inflicted on the Jewish population of Poland."[50]

As a witness to the crime, Karski had to pass on what he had seen, but he was also entangled in the contradictory requirements of his sponsors. In late December 1943, knowing that he could no longer return to Poland because he had been too exposed, Karski submitted a report on the Polish underground state to the Ministry of Information in exile, written for the first time under his own resister's name. It would serve as the source for his memoir, published barely a year later, in which the paragraph titles would become chapter titles.[51] Yet, in this text, not a word on the Jews.

However, chapters 29 and 30 of the memoir were about his two "visits" into death zones: the Warsaw ghetto and "The final step" / "To die in agony," Belzec/Izbica. The Catholic resister deemed it necessary to combine in the last two chapters of his 1944 book the disaster experienced by Poles in general and that experienced by Polish and European Jews. In these passages, which represent less than 10 percent of his book, Karski returns to his previous accounts, including those that had been published by some underground newspapers in occupied countries. For instance, in September 1943 the French newspaper *Fraternité* translated from English what he had written in July; here we see the transfer of information from Polish to English, from English to French:

> I must, I think, explain why we were so interested in Jewish questions. I am not Jewish, and, before the war, I knew very little about Jews. I was even very ignorant about the subject. But at this time, the massacres of Jews are taking on special significance. . . . For them, it is a policy not of oppression and enslavement but simply of coldblooded and systematic extermination. It is the first time, in modern history, that an entire people . . . has been condemned in this way to disappear completely from the face of Earth.[52]

In 1942, depending on those he met with, Karski separated his accounts on the Poles and the Jews. In 1944, he added "Jewish" chapters to his final account, forming a sort of coda. Also in 1944, the *Polish Review* devoted much more space to the fate of Polish Jews. But, in 1944, there was no longer anyone to save. This was not the case in 1942, when Karski was preparing for his mission.

"The methods of this process are known to a certain extent, but the details are not"

Karski had seen. He gave details: "The method is, as you know, to collect the Jews from all over Europe, to dispatch them to the Ghettos of Warsaw, Lwev and Soon, where they stay for a certain time. From the ghettos they are 'taken East' as the official term goes, that is, to the extermination camps, of Belzec, Treblinka and Sobibor. In these camps they are killed in batches of 1,000 to 6,000, by various methods, including gas, burning by steam, mass electrocution, and finally, by the method of the so-called 'death train.'"[53] None of this information was new in London in fall 1942. It was also known that adjacent to the Oswiecim–Auschwitz concentration camp the Nazis had erected gas chambers at Birkenau to murder Jews swept up from throughout Europe. Those who were deported from France, Belgium, Slovakia, and Holland no longer transited through ghettos and work camps in the east. Starting in summer 1941, German and Czech Jews were deported to Riga, Krakow, Lublin, and smaller "transit" centers such as Izbica, from which they were deported again, to the first extermination sites.

The first stationary killing center, in Belzec, was designed and run by technical, medical, and police personnel, who had killed those who were supposedly mentally or physically handicapped and other "asocial" people in hospitals transformed into execution centers in Germany during *Aktion* T4. The code name came from the address of the Berlin headquarters for "euthanasia" operations, Tiergartenstrasse 4. It was ironic that this street was named after a zoo, as the Nazis were killing those whom they had condemned as bestial and monstrous.[54] Lorenz Hackenholt, driver and gravedigger at T4, played a major role in construction of the gas chamber at Belzec, under the leadership of Dr. Christian Wirth, one of the initiators of the T4 program. Wirth was made manager of Belzec, then inspector of the three main Reinhard *Aktion* killing centers, Reinhard Heydrich having been the supervisor of killings by the Einsatzgruppen since summer 1941.

Although most Jews were killed by blows or bullets, subjected to starvation and torture, or burned alive, some were temporarily kept alive for forced labor. Near the extermination centers, the inhabitants of small towns such as Volkovysk mingled with those who arrived by train from the huge ghettos in Poland, Lublin and Warsaw, and from Germany and Czechoslovakia.

Indeed, European Jews received differentiated "treatment." To the east, in occupied Poland and the occupied Soviet Union, the Nazis and their auxiliaries practiced cruelty over the long term: extermination by bullets or poison gas was preceded by weeks, months, or even years of confinement to ghettos, persecution, robberies, rapes, manhunts, arrests, forced labor, famine, torture, and the murder of sons and daughters, parents, spouses, cousins. Jews from Western Europe and, later, Hungary were destined for factory-style murder and killed much more quickly; from the roundup to the transit camp and the gas chamber took only a few days or weeks.

How Were the Jews of Volkovysk, Lemkin's Shtetl, Exterminated?

When Karski went to eastern Poland upon the request of two Jews he met in the Warsaw ghetto, he "saw" the destruction of Lemkin's family and the world of his youth. The "I" of the witness crossed paths with the "I" of the victim, now confronted with the death of his people—Jews killed because they were Jews. Indeed, Lemkin discovered, from the United States, the reality behind the concept that he had been trying to put forward since the 1920s:

> When I first conceived the idea of a law to make genocide illegal, how could I have imagined that I would be directly affected? During the war, forty-nine members of my family died in the genocide, including my parents. Suddenly I felt that the earth was crumbling before me, that the meaning of life was disappearing. . . . I decided to find strength in this law, to alleviate my sorrow by doing this work.[55]

It is very likely that Lemkin had read *The Volkovysk Memorial Book*, published in New York in Yiddish in 1949.[56] By adding the archives of the International Tracing Service and a few accounts by survivors, we can reconstruct the steps from the persecution to the extermination of the Jews of Volkovysk, his people.

Volkovysk had a population of seven thousand Jews out of a total of seventeen thousand in 1939. After the Soviet occupation started, about three thousand flowed in from the Nazi-occupied zone. The town was retaken by the Wehrmacht on June 28, 1941, six days after German troops entered Soviet-occupied Poland. Now, a descent into death began, in terror and abominable physical and mental suffering.

Ten thousand Jews were no doubt living in Volkovysk at the time, minus the approximately fifteen hundred killed in the Luftwaffe bombings during preceding days. They had to wear a yellow star on the front and back of their clothing, and their houses—or what remained of them—were marked with a yellow circle; they were forbidden to walk on the sidewalks and had to raise their hats when a German passed by; these were ordinary humiliations. Above all, the soldiers stole and killed. Then the members of the Einsatzkommando 8, seconded to Einsatzgruppe B, came to execute Jews who had been denounced by Polish informers for collaboration with the communists.

A cascade of guilty verdicts would attribute responsibility for these initiatives during postwar trials. Otto Bradfisch, leader of Einsatzkommando 8, testified in detail on the operations against "Communist subversion and looting" in the Bialystok region. Arthur Nebe, leader of Einsatzgruppe B, had not given the specific order to "annihilate the Jewish population of a town or area solely on the grounds of their racial identity," but in reality "every Jew was to be seen as a danger to combat troops and therefore liquidated."[57] In his turn, Nebe took shelter behind his hierarchy: he claimed that Himmler, visiting Bialystok on July 8, 1941, told him that "as a matter of principle any Jew was to be regarded as a partisan."[58] Nebe apparently interpreted his orders as "In some places and districts all Jews were to be exterminated irrespective of age or sex."[59] Battalion 322 of Einsatzgruppe B performed a "demonstration exercise" for Himmler that consisted of searching for partisans with the Wermacht, the police, and the Sicherheitsdienst (the information service of the SS) in attendance.[60] The partisans caught and killed were exclusively Jews, including women and children. After this conclusive exercise, all Jews "encountered" were killed, which explains the triumphant statistics of Einsatzkommando 8. From Himmler to Nebe, senior officials attended all of these *Aktionen*. In most cases, the massacres began with men; the extermination of women and children intensified only in September. Einsatzkommando 8, however, had anticipated Himmler's instructions: to empty the area of Jews. Volkovysk was situated in the unit's murderous path. At the same time, other SS units liquidated handicapped people in compliance with the T4 program; one of them was Hannah, a blind Jewish child in the village.

As chief of the Reich's criminal police, the Kripo, Nebe was involved with the T4 program and then became head of its Institute for Criminal Biology. The Reich's central security office did not take "biological" prevention and repression principles lightly. Nebe was very familiar with one of the techniques used since summer 1941 to kill mentally ill Poles in this region: gas canisters placed in trucks. Why not further simplify the procedure: route the exhaust pipe into the truck to make it into a transportable gas chamber? By early December, such trucks were in operation in the Soviet zone, and they were in Chelmno on December 8.

Although he did not know all of these details, Karski reported to his interlocutors in London on the scope of these killings and Himmler's role in the process. This information was reproduced in the note by the Polish government in exile on December 10, 1942, and in the joint declaration of the seventeenth.

In Volkovysk, the bombardments of June 1941 had been so violent that it was difficult to form a real ghetto in the ruins. In one photograph, a column of Jewish forced laborers crosses the village accompanied by guards—an armed Ukrainian (perhaps) and a member of the Judenrat recognizable by his armband—as non-Jewish people seem to go about their daily business, without glancing. Starting in spring 1942, hundreds of men and women were compelled to work for the municipal administration and the German Red Cross, erecting a rest center for the soldiers. The village, like Bialystok, the nearby large town, was within the borders of the Reich.

Some, such as "Lemkin's son, the blacksmith" (Raphael's cousin), joined the Soviet partisans. Doctors and radio technicians were tortured, then executed, for this, along with several hundred hostages. As usual, they were forced to dig their "trench grave," which was subsequently covered with earth and replanted so that the mass execution site would be hidden. According to one survivor, when they left the area, "the forced gravediggers suddenly saw the ground rise. They had to hit the ground until everything was still."[61]

Grueling labor, lack of food—much of it was rotten—and drinking water, heat or cold, and disease killed dozens, or even hundreds, of people. The living took possession of the clothing of the dead; some went mad beside the corpses of their loved ones. The guards sometimes shot randomly into crowds; bodies piled up, decomposing, or were carried to common trenches and thrown into them like animal carcasses.

The first "ghetto" liquidation *Aktion* took place on November 2, 1942. It was similar to the one that had taken place on October 5 in Dubno, the hometown of the Orthodox baker whom Lemkin had met on his exodus across Poland in fall 1939:

> The people who had got off the trucks, men, women, and children of all ages, had to undress upon the orders of an SS man, who carried a riding or dog whip.... Without screaming or crying, these people undressed, stood around by families, kissed each other, said farewells, and waited for the command of another SS man who stood near the excavation also with a whip in his hand.... At that moment the SS man at the excavation called something to his comrade. The latter counted off twenty persons, and instructed them to walk behind the earth mound.... I walked around the mound and stood in front of a tremendous grave; closely pressed together, the people were lying on top of each other so that only their heads were visible. The excavation was already two-thirds full; I estimated that it contained about a thousand people.... Now already the next group approached, descended into the excavation, lined themselves up against the previous victims and were shot.[62]

There were many Jews in Volkovysk, and the *Aktion* lasted a long time. The Nazis and their Polish and Ukrainian auxiliaries took sadistic pleasure in their unlimited power over life and death. They promised work farther east, saving a life—for two hours, or three days—for a fortune: a piece of moldy bread. Fathers were killed in front of their sons; children were torn from their mothers, who were executed in front of them. Lemkin's cousin was taken and killed as his parents watched.

The guards were insatiably corrupt. Indeed, one might wonder, given the general state of the town in 1942, what else could be found to offer in exchange for a life. On the slightest pretext, human beings were tortured, as Goldberg relates: "The Germans were beating Mr. Galin fiercefully, vehemently and without any mercy. ... Then we heard two gunshots and the Germans left. We came out and found the body of Mr. Galin. He could not be recognized. It was a mass of bloody, contused and crushed meat. It was a terrible scene. It made a very depressing impression, even on us, who were accustomed to Nazi cruelty."[63]

From Einsatzkommando 8 to Treblinka

Now, the Jews of Volkovysk were confined and kept under guard, along with all those gathered from the region, including Bialystok. Volkovysk became the camp for this area, and no doubt twenty thousand people transited through the town on their way to the gas chambers at Treblinka. Vassili Grossman, war correspondent, gave an account of the arrival of Soviet troops in Treblinka:

> As a final way of tricking the people arriving from Europe, the bay platform itself at the death camp was made to look like a passenger station. At the platform, where the next twenty cars in line were being unloaded, they had erected a railway building with ticket offices, luggage storage, a restaurant with a dining area, and signs all over the place with arrows: "Board for Bialystok," "To Baranovichi," "Board for Wolkowysk," and so on. . . . There was something threatening and terrifying about this square, trampled on and leveled by millions of human feet. People's sharpened gazes quickly grasped the threatening details—on the ground, hastily swept probably just a few minutes before, discarded objects could be seen: a bundle of clothes, opened suitcases, shaving brushes, enamel pots. How did these items get there? And why did the railroad end immediately after the station platform, and beyond it there was only yellow grass and a three-meter fence? Where were the tracks to Bialystok, Siedlce, Warsaw, Wolkowysk?[64]

In the bunkers in Volkovysk, which had served as stalls for Polish army horses until 1939, several thousand people awaited transport toward what they were told were labor camps, but now, in late 1942, everybody knew better. Families were separated, with nothing or little to eat, in the cold, with the stenches and the diseases, including a violent typhus epidemic as well as tuberculosis, typhoid fever, and skin rashes:

> People walked around like shadows. They stopped talking to each other. What was the use? They died like flies. Every morning the ground in front of

the clinic was piled with dead people. Their bodies lying one near the other. Their faces seemed to be directed toward the skies and asking the eternal question, "Why, what did we do, to deserve such a miserable death." No answer! Quiet all around.[65]

The Judenrat was supposed to prepare lists for the "labor camps to the east." No one was fooled; everyone now knew how the story would end. Some preferred to die right away: mothers committed suicide, taking their children with them. Others were willing to do anything not to appear on the lists. Still others tried to flee: "If we're going to die, we'll die together." In the end, the lists were unnecessary: most of the Jews in Volkovysk were transported to Treblinka, where they were killed, between late November and December 1942.

Grossman continued his account:

The process of murdering in the chambers took from ten to twenty-five minutes. Initially, when the new chambers had just been put into operation and the executioners hadn't immediately figured out the gas supply and were conducting experiments to determine the dosage of various killing agents, the victims were subjected to terrible torments, taking two to three hours to die. In the first few days, the delivery and exhaust systems worked poorly, so the torments of the victims were prolonged, lasting for nine to ten hours. . . .

Residents of the village closest to Treblinka, Wólka, tell how sometimes the cries of the women being murdered were so awful that all the villagers, going out of their minds, ran into the distant forest just to get away from those earsplitting cries, cries that drill through logs, sky, and earth. Then the cries would suddenly stop, only to start up again later just as suddenly, the same awful, earsplitting cries, drilling through bones, skulls, souls. . . . This happened three or four times a day.

I asked S., one of the captured executioners, about these cries. He explained that the women cried out when the dogs were unleashed and the whole crowd of the condemned was herded into the house of death: "They saw death. Moreover, it was very crowded in there, and the *Wachmänner* beat them savagely, the dogs ripped at them."

The sudden silence descended when the gas chamber doors were closed. The cries of the women started up again when a new group was brought to the gas chamber. This happened two, three, four, sometimes even five times a day. The Treblinka slaughterhouse was no ordinary executioner's block. It was a conveyor belt of execution, organized in the flow method, borrowed from modern, large-scale industrial production.[66]

Were Lemkin's parents, Joseph and Bella, killed at Treblinka? As they were elderly, they may have been murdered by gas right in Volkovysk. The Nazis squeezed the last eighty ill and elderly people into an airtight cellar and pumped in sulfur dioxide. "The cellar was opened two days later and the bodies were found in all sorts of positions, distorted, the slow agony inscribed on the faces. The eyes of the dead were wide open, staring."[67]

The healthiest, who were still able to hide or to pay guards to escape Treblinka, were caught and sent to Birkenau; in both cases, they died in the gas chambers.

The hellish fire, extending its tongues like open arms, snatches the body. . . . The hair is the first to catch fire. The skin, immersed in flames, catches in a few seconds. Now the arms and legs begin to rise—expanding blood vessels cause this movement of the limbs. The entire body is now burning fiercely; the skin has been consumed and fat drips and hisses in the flames. One can no longer make out a corpse—only a room filled with hellish fire that holds something in its midst. The belly goes. Bowels and entrails are quickly consumed, and within minutes there is no trace of them. The head takes the longest to burn; two little blue flames flicker from the eyeholes—these are the eyes burning with the brain, while from the mouth the tongue also continues to burn. The entire process lasts twenty minutes—and a human being, a world, has been turned to ashes.[68]

In January 1943, Volkovysk and environs were finally declared "free of Jews," and neighboring regions also profited into the bargain. Karski had noted this in his 1939 report; Poles' hatred of Jews, particularly in the Soviet zone, did not escape survivors, who spoke of "pogromchiks," "organized anti-Semites,"[69] "Polish, Russian, or Ukrainian collaborators," denouncers of Jews, and partisans who "jeered" or "sneered" as they watched the forced marches of groups of deportees. During the winter of 1943, after the killings and the deportations to Treblinka and then Birkenau had come to an end, "the best items were sent to Germany for the 'German War Fund,' and the rest was sold to the local Polish population, which had long awaited the chance to do such good business."[70]

As of May 1945, seventy Jews in Volkovysk had survived six years of terror, committed mostly by Nazis but also, for those who had been sent to the gulag, by communists. Others, conversely—like Elias Lemkin, Raphael's brother—owed their survival to having gone over to the Soviet side while there was still time. What Raphael Lemkin discovered only between 1945 and 1949, Jan Karski, the non-Jew, had seen in 1942.

"The Spectacle of a People Dying": Karski in Warsaw and Izbica

"The cemetery is in Belzec in the exact same way as in Chelmno. . . . Chilling here is the same as in Chelmno. Our turn is approaching! . . . [It is] chilling the villages I mentioned in my letter."[71] In the winter of 1942, the historian of the Warsaw ghetto Emanuel Ringelblum was receiving letters like this, situating the Belzec extermination center near Zamosc and giving coded reports on the killings. He published these accounts of poisoning by carbon monoxide in Chelmno and by gas at Treblinka and Belzec in his underground archives, the Oyneg Shabes. This information, written in Yiddish, was also sent to all the underground Jewish and Polish broadsheets and reached the Polish government in exile in London.[72] In June 1942, the first real-time synthesis of the plan for total extermination of the Jews was published. "With the German attack on the Soviet Union a new, most horrible link has been added to the chain of unending Jewish suffering—Ausrottung, the physical extermination of the Jews, whom the Germans hold responsible for the outbreak of a war whose intensity has dwarfed all previous conflicts."[73] In the field, the different strata of murders could be easily grasped—the massacres by bullets in summer 1941, by gas in the fall—as the carnage by the killing squads continued. The liquidation of the Warsaw ghetto began in July 1942. This is where Karski's account begins.

To cover his tracks and protect himself and his informants, Karski said that he went to the Warsaw ghetto and to Belzec in July or September 1942. His account does not inform us of the number of daily killings. When he arrived in London, on November 25, 1942, it was more the way in which he reported the information than the information itself that would strike those who really wanted to hear him.

Karski had been able to observe the fate reserved for Jews in the Warsaw ghetto and in what he believed was Belzec. This location was in fact the transit station in Izbica-Lubelska, situated on the Lublin–Lvov railroad axis, near Zamosc, some fifty miles from Belzec. Izbica was the site of the final spoliation, where the fiction of deportation to a labor camp came to an end. Karski called it "some sort of transitional camp."[74] When there was congestion in Belzec, the trains were held at a stop until there was room in the gas chambers. In these few hours or days, the torture and killing took place in other ways.

In 1940, Karski had traveled with Jews passing through the Soviet occupation zone. He had left them on the way to accomplish his first resister's mission. After he saw the Warsaw ghetto and Izbica, his accounts differed radically from his 1940 report, that of a patriotic Catholic law student, little affected by the persecution and dispossession suffered by the Jewish minority. Now, he internalized the dehumanization that he beheld, as his ghetto guides had foreseen—and hoped: "They warned me that if I accepted their offer I would have to risk my life to carry it out. They told me, too, that as long as I lived I would be haunted by the memory of the ghastly scenes I would witness."[75]

Karski remained in the ghetto for only a few hours, however, and in Izbica for one day. In both cases, he disguised himself to pass unnoticed. In Warsaw, he was a Jew wearing a yellow star; in Izbica, he was a guard, in Latvian or Estonian uniform depending on the report version, but in reality he was dressed as a Ukrainian. And so, he passed as a victim in Warsaw, as an executioner in Izbica. The witness camouflaged himself to uncover the most extraordinary camouflage in history. In his accounts of late 1942, published in London and New York in 1943, and in his 1944 memoir, he wrote that the change in appearance gradually began to affect the witness's soul. He was no longer content with looking but began to engage more physically, with his senses.

Thus, Karski was adopting the strategy of his two Jewish guides who came and went under different identities and accoutrements on either side of the ghetto wall like performers in a laborious "farce." Their Judaism was literally stuck to their skin; their "Jewish features [were] difficult to . . . disguise."[76] And the moral spy serving the Polish cause, who was he?

"To pass that wall was to enter into a new world utterly unlike anything that had ever been imagined"

"Is it still necessary to describe the Warsaw ghetto? . . . There have been so many accounts by unimpeachable witnesses."[77] In his memoir, Karski minimized his personal testimony. Indeed, in 1944, one year after the revolt in the ghetto was quashed and the ghetto itself was destroyed, what he had seen in 1942 no longer existed. Nevertheless, he chose the chapter "My Visit to the Warsaw Ghetto" to be published in the magazine *The American Mercury* as he was correcting the proofs of his book.[78] This was the first time that he allowed his underground name to appear, and it would be his from then on.

In the Warsaw ghetto, Jan Kozielewski became Jan Karski. There, he discovered the annihilation of the Jewish people, the entire Jewish people. The first sign was those who were absent: old people, the first to die of deprivation and disease, the first to be transported to Treblinka to be gassed, had disappeared from the streets. As for the emaciated children, they were "play[ing] before they die[d]." The absent elderly, the children pretending to be children: "A cemetery? No, for these bodies were still moving. . . . They were still living people, if you could call them such. For apart from their skin, eyes and voice, there was nothing human left in these palpitating figures. Everywhere there was hunger, misery, the atrocious stench of decomposing bodies, the pitiful moans of dying children. . . . To pass that wall was to enter into a new world utterly unlike anything that had ever been imagined."[79] Karski described "shadows of what had once been men or women," a world in which the living were the dead, like animals with "their eyes blazing with some insane hunger or greed." Animals could be hunted, and that was the game played by two teenagers in Hitler Youth uniforms, who shot at human targets as if they were competing in a "sporting event."

When he arrived in Washington, DC, in the spring of 1943, Karski, as "Mr. B.,"[80] gave a long interview to the journalist George Creel, who published an extensive version in two articles in *Collier's Weekly* that fall:

> Do you know why we are so desperately resolved to protect and train our youth, putting it against every other underground activity? It is because we see what evil teaching has done to young Nazis. . . . Thousands of German

boys are schooled in Poland, barracked like soldiers. Believe me, sir, when I tell you that they are more cruel, more savage, than their elders. Governor General Frank has granted them the right to carry revolvers and rifles, and after school hours, it is their favorite sport to go into a ghetto and hunt the Jews as though they were rabbits in a warren. With my own eyes I have seen them shoot women down, and with my own ears I have heard them yell, "No, no, Hans, that one is mine. You had the last one."[81]

The "hunting" episode, featured in all of Karski's accounts from 1942 to 1945, was positioned as part of an exaltation of the Polish resistance, which educated its young people to protect them against "debauchery and defilement": "In every possible way, the Nazis try to deprave our youth. . . . A large percentage of the Germans in Poland are homosexuals. . . . In the cities, Black Shirts are under orders to abuse our boys, and the guards in concentration camps and labor camps, recruited from the slums of the Reich, practice perversions in every form on their young prisoners."[82] When, in early 1943, *Les Cahiers du Témoignage chrétien* devoted an issue to detailed descriptions of the tragedies of Catholic Poland, moral perversion was also emphasized: the "satanic depravity" of a population in which "alcohol and pornography flow freely."[83]

Karski expressed himself differently according to his perceived audience. Detailed accounts of cruelties against the Jews had to demonstrate the Nazis' sadism and justify the targeted killings by the Polish resistance—viewed very poorly in the United Kingdom and the United States. Karski glorified the Poles' moral, intellectual, and spiritual resistance with an ecumenism that included Protestants, an infinitesimal minority in Poland but not in the United States: "A whole people—Catholics, Protestants and Jews—have had a deepening of devotion. . . . I say this from my own experience." Naturally, he spoke at greater length about attacks against the Catholic religion. In Wilno archdiocese, hundreds of priests were being "murdered and imprisoned, and at Oswiecim, gray-haired prelates are cleaning latrines with their hands. . . . The revered head of the Polish Protestant Church, eighty-year-old Doctor Julius Bursch, was sent to the hellhole of Dachau, where the Gestapo beat the life out of his frail body." When it came to the Jews, he spoke only of material destruction: "Of all the stately synagogues, none remains for Jewish worship. Such as have not been burned are now stables and storehouses."[84]

Karski did not speculate who in Poland had availed themselves of these new stables for their animals, confining himself to demonstrating that the Nazi "swine" wanted to destroy all Poles: "It is spiritual resistance that calls for all of our courage—the desperate, unending fight to keep from being beaten down to animalism by systematic degradations. It is the soul of Poland that the Nazis mean to destroy [by reducing us to] hewers of wood and drawers of water for the Master Race."[85]

Karski tried to educate his American interlocutors—whom he sometimes viewed as almost childlike—by portraying the resistance "as a ruthlessly efficient organization, a combination of the F.B.I. and the Canadian Mounted." He did not hesitate to vaunt the Polish ingeniousness, comparing Poles to "Himmler and his thugs . . . a very stupid lot. . . . I doubt if your Mr. J. Edgar Hoover would give one of them a job." He further described them as "degenerate gangsters, a pack of wild beasts without even animal cunning."[86] Stupid, perhaps, but well trained for their tasks of torture: "There is nothing amateurish about the Gestapo. Everyone is a specialist in cruelty. When Heinrich Himmler came to Poland, one of his first acts was to set up a school in Poznan where men were trained in the art of torture just as you would train a mechanic. . . . Forcing lighted splinters under fingernails were little more than kindergarten lessons, for they went far beyond your Indians in fiendish ingenuity."[87]

The "Train of Death": Izbica

In late summer 1942, Karski's ghetto guides sent him to what he believed—or, at least, what he said—was Belzec. The first gassings took place there on March 17, 1942, in wooden barracks; production-line efficiency was achieved when six concrete gas chambers were built to exterminate 1,500 people at a time.[88] Between March and December 1942, 434,508 Jews—and more souls, with the Roma and Sinti—were killed there during Operation Reinhard. In reality, Karski had arrived in Izbica. This was where he passed into the world of an annihilated people; his descriptions became more detailed, as if the sensations he had had then were returning to haunt him.

In his early published accounts, Karski tried to distance himself by not giving his own name: "eyewitness" for the BBC; Mr. X, Mr. B, or "a Pole" for *Collier's Weekly*. It was not Jan Karski—even less Jan Kozielewski—who had seen these things but an anonymous person. This was because the prison-guard disguise that he used to enter the area surrounded by barbed wire and wooden palisades—in this case it cannot be called a camp—was a subterfuge that could not have happened had the resistance not paid a huge sum to obtain this favor, equivalent to what the corrupt guards stole from the Jews while claiming to save their lives before demanding even more money—or flesh in the form of rape—before finally leading them to their deaths.

Karski's conversation with a guard offered him a direct perspective on collaboration in the extermination enterprise by Ukrainians, Estonians, Lithuanians, Latvians, Belarusians, and Poles, of German origin or not:[89]

> "If he is willing to fork out plenty of hard cash, in advance, then I do what I can."
>
> "Have you saved many Jews so far?"
>
> "Not as many as I'd like, but a few, anyhow."
>
> "Are there many more good men like you there who are so willing to save the Jews?"
>
> "Save them? Say, who wants to save them? . . . But if they pay that's a different story." . . .
>
> I looked at his heavy, rather good-natured face and wondered how the war had come to develop such cruel habits in him. . . . Under the pressure of the Gestapo and the cajoleries of the Nazis, with everyone about him engaged in a greedy competition that knew no limits, he had been changed into a professional butcher of human beings. He had caught on to his trade and discussed its origins, used its professional jargon as coolly as a carpenter discussing his craft.[90]

Karski, though, was consumed by remorse: "I was in fact one of the enforcers. I believe that my action was justified. I could do nothing to stop what was happening, but by becoming a witness, I could give a firsthand report to the civilized world." The messenger had worn the uniform of barbarism; he did not give his name in order to respect the resistance and to hide what was unnamable in him.

Only the barbarian was named. The process of extermination was described through accusations against Friedrich-Wilhelm Krüger, charged by Odilo Globocnik's headquarters in Lublin with destruction of the Warsaw ghetto and the gassing operations in Belzec. This executioner's name was repeated a number of times by he who had no name: "It was Krueger who raised the number of concentration camps in his district from 22 to 41, and who started the practice of putting barefooted men, women and children into boxcars spread inches thick with wet quicklime. It was Krueger who set fire to synagogues after crowding them with Jews and who first conceived the idea of pumping poison gas into halls where human beings were packed like cattle."[91] A drawing portraying what Karski believed to be one of the highlights of the resistance illustrates the article: a successful attack by Poles disguised as Germans against the Nazi officer's car.[92]

The misnaming of Izbica was not Karski's only error—or omission. He traveled at night and arrived at a place that he was told was Belzec, and why wouldn't he believe it? Yet, he had been there previously, in December 1939, and had witnessed mistreatment of Jews on that visit. Because, at the time, the town of Belzec was on the border between the Soviet and German zones, the Nazis sent prisoners, mainly "Jewish families who illegally wanted to cross over to the Bolsheviks," there to dig antitank ditches on the line of demarcation and to build, first, a labor camp, then the facilities for the killing center. Karski's first report was very precise:

Near Belzec . . . the Germans have created a camp of Jews. . . . An enormous proportion walked and slept under the open sky. Very many people [were] without proper clothing or other covering. While one group slept, the other waited its turn, so that outer garments could be lent one another. Those who waited jumped and ran around so as not to freeze. A few hundred people, among them children, women, and old people, run around for hours or jump in place, for if they stand still, they will freeze. After a few hours [the groups] change places. . . . All are frozen, in despair, unable to think, hungry. [They are] a herd of harassed beasts—not people. I watched this for a whole hour, riveted to my spot, frightened, confused. A nightmare—not real. Blue and red freaks—not people. I shall never forget it. Never in my life have I beheld anything more frightening. . . . The "Master Race" is really a nation of madmen, of brutal haters and heartless beings.[93]

The ice used for slow killing brings to mind a 1941 photograph with the legend "Execution of a Jew in an ice hole in the Belzec concentration camp."[94] The man had been thrown, alive, into a hole carved into the ice and had died of cold; in the picture he seems to be still alive, his bearded head fallen forward as if he was praying; his protruding ribs show his state of malnutrition before the final torture.

Why did Karski persist in saying that he had seen Belzec in 1942, when he had been taken to Izbica, and not talk about his actual visit to Belzec in 1939? Why did he never make the connection between the two times that he said he "would never forget," that would haunt him "as long as he lived": deaths by cold, by fire, and by gas (which he had not seen but reported on in his accounts) and the quicklime in the train, which became, once he arrived in London, his piece of "purple prose"? Indeed, it was because of what he termed "the death train" that Karski was an eyewitness to the German policy of extermination of the Jews.

"The camp is situated fifteen kilometers south of the town of Belzec," Karski wrote. "It is surrounded by a fence that runs along a train track about ten meters away. A narrow passageway, less than one meter wide, leads from the camp entrance to the train tracks. This passage is formed by two wooden fences."[95] Arriving in his guard's uniform, Karski discovered in a fairly small space, similar to a storage locker, a mass of people swept up during the *Aktionen* in the ghettos, left outside for three or four days, stripped of everything, with no food or water, not knowing if their relatives were already dead, gone mad with suffering and pain.[96]

The trains leaving Izbica, the planned gateway toward death, were headed for Belzec and its gas chambers. Karski, however, had seen another method devised to ease the crowding in the gas chambers. The trains were bringing too many bodies to kill, and the death machine was grinding to a halt; the prisoners had to be gotten rid of in another way, while training the guards in sadism. Samuel Golfard, who knew that his sister, taken before his eyes in the Przemyslany ghetto, had probably been killed in Belzec, hypothesized that electrocution was used—something Karski also spoke of: "We have been told that people are being put to death there on a suspension bridge charged with electricity, and then the victims are thrown into the abyss."[97] The unthinkable, even for those who saw it with their own eyes, had to follow a human logic: the trains, the electricity, and the suspension bridge belonged to a known form of industrialization, whereas these gas chambers were invented only to kill human beings.[98] And if it was impossible to imagine how they worked, it was because the technology used exclusively for death was no doubt unspeakable. The Polish underground newspaper *WRN*, translated in New York, stated, "The last Jews in Warsaw were systematically annihilated at Majdanek by suffocating gas cameras operated three times a week. As the crematorium is out of order, the bodies of murdered Jews are burned in huge piles."[99] The cameras took pictures of what could not— or should not—be seen; it was therefore said that they were used directly to kill.

The industrial and technical details of cruelty could not sanitize the suffering undergone by the victims: the smells, the screams. Karski placed himself at the heart of the *Hrbn*—the destruction, as Jews in the east said in their language, Yiddish; he offered his eyes and photographic memory as a means of transmission. For it was in fact in Izbica, through his sensory descriptions, that he most accurately conveyed the extermination of the Jews: "The air was full of stenches, odors, excrement, filth, and putrefaction. . . . We were forced to walk on the piled bodies. . . . Each time I walked on a body I was seized by nausea and stopped short, but my guide pressed me forward." The time came to "load" the boxcars headed for the fake labor camp; most knew that death awaited them. The only question was how:

> Around ten in the morning, a freight train stopped. . . . At the same time, the guards at the other end began to shoot into the air and ordered the Jews to get on the train. This way, they created panic among the prisoners to prevent any hesitation or resistance on their part. The Jews, pushed toward the narrow passageway that I have spoken of, rushed, shoving each other, into the first boxcar stopped at the end of the passageway. It was an ordinary car, the kind that indicate "6 horses or 36 men." . . . Three hundred people were pushed or thrown into this first car; I counted them myself. The doors were then closed and locked. The train pulled ahead a bit. The following car was then in place and the scene was repeated. I counted a total of fifty-one cars, into which were squeezed the six thousand prisoners in the camp. Only some thirty of them fell under the guards' bullets during the stampede into the train. Once the camp was empty and the cars full, the train began to move. I heard the end of the story from one of my so-called comrades, the camp's executioners who had been doing this work for several months, sending one or two trains a week.[100]

The Germans had simply issued orders to the effect that 120 to 130 Jews had to enter each car. . . . Alternately swinging and firing with their rifles, the policemen were forcing still more people into the two cars which were already overfull. . . . These unfortunates, crazed by what they had been through . . . then began to climb on the heads and shoulders of those in the trains. . . . [101] The bones cracked and the screams became insane. . . . It seemed impossible to squeeze more people into the boxcar, and yet at that moment the guards, helped by certain prisoners made half-mad with fear due to the gunfire behind them, began to throw people in. Thirty more were thus heaved onto the heads of those inside. Some women's necks were broken.[102]

From Quicklime to Exhaust Fumes

Karski described the extermination tool:

The floors of the car had been covered with a thick, white powder. It was quicklime. . . . Here, the lime served a double purpose in the Nazi economy of brutality. . . . The occupants of the cars would be literally burned to death before long, the flesh eaten from their bones. . . . In the now quiet camp the only sounds were the inhuman screams. . . . Then these, too, ceased. All that was now left was . . . a queer, sickening, acidulous odor which, I thought, may have come from the quantities of blood that had been left, and with which the ground was stained.[103]

The "death train" seemed to tremble from the effects of the quicklime on the bodies from before it left the camp until it stopped a few kilometers away, at which point everyone was dead. The impression of movement came also from the screams. Karski asked a question about the quicklime that is still being debated today, according to sources: was it used to clean, to kill, or both?[104] In April 1942, the Polish government in exile received details on Belzec in which the expression "death camp" was used for the first time; quicklime was delivered there.[105] In a memorandum submitted to President Roosevelt, on December 8, allusion was also made to murders by quicklime: "Masses of Jews were loaded into freight cars in batches of 150 when there was accommodation for less than one-third of that number. The floors are covered with a thick layer of lime or chlorine, sprinkled with water. The doors are sealed. When the trains reach their destination, half the occupants are dead from suffocation."[106] The long text published by the Polish government in exile on December 10, 1942, gave more or less the same description:

> The Jews were suffering for lack of air. The floors of the trucks were covered with quicklime and chlorine. As far as is known, the trains were despatched to three localities—Tremblinka [*sic*], Belzec and Sobibor, to what the reports describe as "extermination camps." The very method of transport was deliberately calculated to cause the largest possible number of casualties among the condemned Jews. It is reported that on arrival in camp the survivors were stripped naked and killed by various means, including poison gas and electrocution. The dead were interred in mass graves dug by machinery.[107]

All of these similar—almost identical—accounts came from a single source: Jan Karski, debriefed in London between late November and early December. When he met Roosevelt six months later, the president did not know that he already had Karski's reports in hand. But had he read them?

In his account for the BBC, Karski gave more technical details about extermination by gas outside a gas chamber: "The chloride of lime on the floor has the property of developing chlorine gas when coming into contact with humidity. The people jammed into the trucks for many hours are compelled, at some time, to urinate, and this (on the lime), instantaneously produces a chemical reaction. Death must in the end be welcome, for whilst they are dying by the chlorine gas their feet are being burned to the bone by the chemically active chloride."[108]

Other reports on the use of quicklime confirmed Karski's. As in Izbica on the way to Belzec, but much earlier—in October 1941—some of the Jews deported, particularly from Konin, were exterminated at Kazimierz-Biskupi, not far from Chelmno. The murderers, in their search for deadly productivity, tested methods that they hoped would be both more effective and less troublesome for the executioners than mass shootings:

> The Gestapo officers ordered the Jews to undress in front of the two trenches. At the bottom of the larger trench I saw a layer of unslaked lime chunks. They then ordered the naked people to jump into the larger trench. The screams and cries were indescribable. Some Jews jumped in themselves; others were

pushed. Some of the mothers jumped holding their babies; others pushed their children aside, while others still threw their children into the pit and then jumped in themselves. . . . Then a truck carrying four vats arrived in the clearing. The Germans hooked up a motor pump, then a pipe poured water into the trench. The Jews began to boil alive. The screaming was so horrific that those of us who were sitting near the clothing tore off pieces of material and put them in our ears.[109]

And so, trial and error by individuals and small groups paralleled the organization of the industrial complexes. A time when bodies and the soil bled. A time of another world, as epitomized by Auschwitz, where another formidable Polish witness, Witold Pilecki, was voluntarily imprisoned in order to organize the resistance: "In my recollections this was a point that marks the moment when I left behind everything I was familiar with 'on earth' and stepped into something beyond it. . . . All the notions we were accustomed to 'on earth' (the established order of things—the law) took a brutal kicking too."[110]

On August 5, 1942, *The Ghetto Speaks*[111] published a special issue on Chelmno, including the "first authentic report received from Poland on the execution of Jews by gas." They were transported to the changing rooms of fake public baths, where they were "appropriately" asked to undress and leave all their possessions; then, terror. The victims were herded onto trucks that the "SS driver-executioners" drove to trenches that had been dug in advance before activating the gas-feed mechanism. The Jewish gravediggers then did "their job. . . . [When the trucks were opened,] all the victims were . . . smeared with excrement—probably because of the effect of the gas and the horrible fear. . . . Two German civilians would again examine every corpse so as to rob the dead of their last belongings. They would fling off rings from the fingers, and lockets, too. With pliers, they would extract golden teeth from the mouths of the victims, and make certain that there were no hidden articles on the backs of the men, or in the sex organs of the women. The desecrated and robbed bodies would then be placed in rows in the grave under the direction of the SS man. . . . The head of one victim would be laid at the feet of another, and in the spare room which remained, children were placed. . . . In mid-January 1942, a precautionary measure went into effect: the layers were covered with chloride powder, so as to remove the nauseating odor."[112] In this account, like Karski's, there were no euphemisms. Everything that had been seen, felt, and heard was made available to secret services, diplomats, then British and American readers, as well as to Europeans via underground leaflets.

When Karski left the scene of horror and returned to the house where he had prepared himself, he quickly got undressed; he could not bear to wear his executioner's uniform for a single second longer than necessary. He washed himself to the point of splashing water all over the bathroom, but he could not rid his mind of the stenches and screams. The reek of death and of blood, excrement, and vomit, the racket of mad screams and gunshots echoed within him, and he vomited over and over. In the scene shot for the film *Shoah* during which he described Izbica, his mouth was twisted into strange grimaces. He tried to swallow, as if to purge his mouth, his ears, his nose of the horrible words, odors, cries that came out.[113] In 1942, he spoke of his nausea and his nightmares, as if he were possessed by the turmoil of death. Did his body, more than his words, express the ultimate truth? By vomiting, he returned to the state of human being, mingling his stench with those of all the others. At the same time, the reification was complete; he had to forget that he was human to be able to bear witness. He was no longer eyes and mouth, "not so to speak a human being, I was purely a camera, a recording machine."[114] And, he wrote, "I have no other proofs, no photographs. All I can say is that I saw it and that it is the truth."[115]

Can the body's language tell the truth? Karski's body already testified to his courage and heroism: arrested, tortured, he had slit his wrists to kill himself so that he would not talk. Taken to the hospital, liberated by the resistance, he would bear the scars of this incident all his life. During his time in the ghetto and at Izbica, his body was again assaulted—this time as a Jew's body; his soul, however, remained intact. As a fervent Catholic, he insisted on attending mass before leaving for London and on wearing the scapular that had been given to him, "the most beautiful of all gifts." Karski was not a priest, and it was a gift symbolizing the importance vested in him: "'I have been authorized . . . to present you, soldier of Poland, with Christ's Body to carry with you on your journey. . . . It will protect you from all evil and harm."[116]

In the ghetto, Karski had recognized Christ's suffering in certain victims he saw, *ecce homo*, but his guide spoke from the point of view of Jews: "'You other Poles are fortunate,' he began. 'You are suffering, too. Many of you will die, but at least your nation goes on living. . . . From this ocean of tears, pain, rage, and humiliation your country will emerge again but the Polish Jews will no longer exist. We will all be dead. Hitler will lose his war . . . but he will win his war against the Polish Jews. No—it will not be a victory; the Jewish people will be murdered.'"[117] Karski relayed these words in *Story of a Secret State*, but he gradually made them his own. Some of his interlocutors in London, starting with Arthur Koestler, were not fooled.

> "Statistics don't bleed. Do you know what counts?
> The detail. Only the detail counts." (Arthur Koestler)[118]

By 1942, the Hungarian-born author Arthur Koestler had had much experience with wars and totalitarianism. An anti-Fascist in Spain, well informed on the Stalinist Moscow show trials, he was imprisoned as a "foreign enemy" in the Vernet internment camp in Ariège, France, from October 1939 to January 1940, an experience from which he drew material for a remarkable autobiographical essay, *Scum of the Earth*. When he went to England, he was imprisoned once again, as an "enemy alien." After he regained his freedom, as a refugee in London, Koestler collected everything published on the fate of the Jews. He met Karski, of course, and, in an ironic turn of events, he was charged by the MI5 counterespionage service with verifying his reliability. Very impressed by the "modest and aristocratic" Karski, he was then involved in creating the script for *Terror in Europe: The Jewish Mass Execution* for the BBC; in fact, he largely rewrote it, although he was "paralyzed by the feeling that the facts are so horrible that nobody will believe them."[119]

Koestler decided to incorporate Karski's account of Belzec into the novel that he was writing at the time. *Arrival and Departure* tells the story of Peter Slavek, an escapee from a central European country who reaches Portugal to enter service for the British: he arrives—*Arrival*—then hesitates, falls ill (the aftereffects of the trauma suffered in Nazi-occupied Europe?), hesitates a bit more as he has various romantic, medical, and political entanglements (the last with Nazi spies, perhaps), and finally decides to leave as a British agent—*Departure*. For the novel, Koestler borrowed from "details" that Karski provided for the BBC script, as well as other information that was circulating in London at the time. The choice of the word "detail" is not insignificant; in Karski's usage, details are flesh itself: they are destroyed souls. Koestler went even further: let us stop counting the suffering, the deaths, the injuries, let us stop treating this knowledge simply as bookkeeping figures; let us feel the indignation and the suffering. This leads to the hallucinogenic account by Peter—who could be named Jan—that takes up twelve pages of the novel. The fictional Peter, like Karski, provokes knowledge that has been taken for granted and shifts it to another level of awareness. In a section on the "mixed transport" trains, Koestler's blending of what we know today about extermination of the Jews, what was known in 1943, and fiction is truly stunning.

> "Nobody who has not been through it can understand it. Terror, atrocities, oppression—that's all words. Statistics don't bleed. Do you know what counts? The detail. Only the detail counts . . ."
>
> "I know."
>
> "No, you don't. You don't know the details. You haven't travelled in a Mixed Transport. You don't know what it is."
>
> "A mixed transport?"
>
> "Yes, that is a detail. There are trains which are scheduled on no time-table. But they run all over Europe. Ten or twenty closed cattle-trucks, locked from outside. . . . Few people see them because they start and arrive at night. I have travelled in one."[120]

"I," Peter, a political prisoner, discovers that the trains were called "mixed" because of the nature of the Jews being transported, who were placed in two groups:

> Two loads of Useful Jews . . . and five loads of Useless Jews, old and sickly ones, who were being taken to be killed. Then there were . . . two trucks with young women who were being taken to army brothels . . . and six trucks with people who were being taken to work in factories and labour camps. That's why it was called a Mixed Transport. . . . After an hour or so the train stopped at a station and they started shunting. One carriage with Politicals was detached from us and two more carriages with foreign labourers attached. . . . Two new carriages . . . contained the women and their children from a razed village where the men had been shot or taken away. At the next station we left

the Useful Jews behind and got instead two wagon-loads of gipsies who, they said, were being taken to be sterilized.[121]

The narrator offers a summary of Nazi persecutions, all categories of oppression combined: "At each station they started shunting us about again, as if playing general post; it seemed a favourite sport with them, perhaps because they enjoy organizing. They gave us nothing to eat or to drink, except for the women who were being taken to the brothels. . . . We had no ordure-bins in our trucks and were packed so tight that we could only sit, not lie. . . . We were treading all the time in heaps of dung."[122]

Koestler then describes in great detail the fate of the "Useless Jews": trucks arrived and parked near the train and men and women were made to get on them, their names and dates of birth ticked off on lists:

> When both vans were full . . . their doors were shut. . . . Both engines began to roar at full strength, but the vans didn't move. We watched the exhaust pipes and saw the pale blue gas stream out. . . . The engines went on roaring as before and the vans remained rooted to the spot, but the gas-jet from the exhaust pipes had disappeared. . . . Then a comrade in our carriage said he smelt gas and began to vomit. . . . After perhaps twenty minutes . . . the officer . . . peeped through what must have been a spy-hole. . . . The sound of the engines ebbed down to normal and the vans began to move. [They returned after half an hour.] They were empty, and their exhaust-pipes puffed merrily, like those of normal, healthy lorries. [The process began again.] After midnight the five trucks with Useless Jews were all empty.[123]

Koestler was combining what Karski had told him about the "death train" with other information available in London at the same time on the gas trucks in Chelmno. He powerfully evoked the fate of the Jews—the "useful" to forced labor, the "useless" to death—even though certain "details" would not stand up to analysis: for instance, the cars were hermetically sealed but gas could be smelled outside the train. Koestler understood the specificity of the "slaughter" of the Jews. He grasped well that Peter/Jan had shifted from eyewitness to moral witness, one who risked his life to speak out. When information was not disseminated with conviction, it disappeared.

Even though George Orwell felt that the novel was "not a satisfactory book" and was even "very thin"[124]—the political hesitations of the hero did not seem credible to him—he acknowledged that it contained "one of the most shocking descriptions of Nazi terrorism that have ever been written." Orwell placed Koestler in the category of authors who wrote in "the special class of literature that has arisen out of the European political struggle since the rise of Fascism": "They are trying to write contemporary history, but *unofficial* history, the kind that is ignored in textbooks and lied about in the newspapers."[125] Orwell would have appreciated the title of Lemkin's autobiography, *Totally Unofficial*, and probably its content.

In 1944, Orwell returned to both *Darkness at Noon*, which dealt with the Moscow show trials, and *Arrival and Departure*: "English disapproval of the Nazi outrages has also been an unreal thing, turned on and off like a tape according to political expediency. To understand such things one has to be able to imagine oneself as the victim, and for an Englishman to write *Darkness at Noon* would be as unlikely an accident as for a slave-trader to write *Uncle Tom's Cabin*."[126]

Others did take the book seriously—in particular the chapter on extermination, which was also published separately. "We forget if we are not nailed to it," wrote the novelist Phyllis Bottome, "that Europe is a torture chamber a few miles away! . . . I also think it will decrease anti-Semitism except among the few determinedly mad."[127] A jibe by the critic Osbert Sitwell showed that even pessimists such as Koestler were far from the truth: "Is that rigmarole of Koestler's intended as fact or fiction?" Koestler's response, in the name of intellectual morality and ethics, was blistering:

> If I had published an article on Proust and mentioned his homosexuality, you would never have asked such a question, as you would "know," even though the proof of this particular fact is less obvious than that of the massacre of three million human beings. You would blush if you didn't know the name of a second-rate contemporary composer, painter, or author. . . . But you have the audacity to ask me if it is true that you are living in the time of the greatest massacre in history. . . . As long as you do not feel, against and independent of all reason, guilty about living while so many others are being put to death . . . you will remain what you are, guilty by omission.[128]

What was the origin of the denials by those who were "guilty by omission"—not only the British—as well as the denials of anti-Semitism and of the ongoing war with its unremitting cruelty? They were the product of a violent recent past, from World War I to the Spanish Civil War. Indeed, Sitwell added, contemptuously, "In ten years' time such information would be revealed as no more accurate than the lies manufactured to blacken the Germans in the First World War."[129] Sitwell, like so many others, remembered only the propaganda and myths of that conflict and had forgotten the true atrocities of the 1914 invasions, the specific violence against civilians, and the extermination of the Armenians. Koestler and Orwell, like Lemkin and Karski, or Varian Fry and Franz Werfel, were faced with the same barrier to memory. It had been only twenty-three years from 1918 to 1941: too many for complete forgetfulness, enough that the myths were still at work.

3

Flashback

From Violence to Myth;
From One War, Another, 1942, 1914

What is happening in Europe is so horrible that the imagination refuses to picture it. . . . The sufferings of 1914–1918, and of much of the period between the two wars, led to a hardening of the hearts. The drain on sympathy began to be unbearable. We are in danger of becoming morally numb.

—Archbishop of Canterbury, 1942

In London in the fall of 1942, although the Nazi horrors were denounced in public demonstrations, things had not moved beyond the stage of moral indignation. The socially engaged author George Orwell reflected on one of the paradoxes of wars: their cruelties were always denounced as those of the other camp and barely analyzed on their own account—when they were not outright denied, as was the case after the Great War. "The truth, it is felt, becomes untruth when your enemy utters it." But, Orwell grumbled, "the truth about atrocities is far worse than that they are lied about and made into propaganda. The truth is that they happen. . . . These things really happened, that is the thing to keep one's eye on."[1] In the summer of 1940, Marc Bloch, a historian and a veteran of two wars, said just about the same thing, also condemning the media, public opinion, and military and political leaders: "They were thinking behind the times."[2]

Too many wars, too many atrocities—and too many rumors? These contemporaries were, indeed, still heavily steeped in the propaganda lies of World War I, which had ended less than twenty-five years before, not to mention the recent wars in Ethiopia and Spain.[3] Many were certain that German barbarism would last forever, including General de Gaulle:

The war on Germany began in 1914. The Treaty of Versailles in fact ended nothing. There was merely, from 1918 to 1936, a pause in the conflict, in the course of which the enemy rebuilt his forces of aggression. . . . In reality, therefore, the world is fighting a thirty-year war either for or against the universal domination of Germany. . . . As for the future, we will make our response. As long as free peoples, of which France was a leader in 1914, are able to liberate it, we answer that the war effort will not cease to grow until it becomes, no doubt, decisive.[4]

De Gaulle, Churchill, and many of their contemporaries who were veterans saw the horrors of the new war, at least until 1942—and some of them for longer—as a direct extension of those of the previous conflict. General Władysław Sikorski, leader of the Polish government in exile, was just as certain, although he added qualifications: "The Germans have always professed their faith in brute force, and their invasions have been marked by torrents of blood. They will refrain from overturning Hitler's regime, as it is the best fit for their national character, which liberates the dark forces of Germany. The year 1918 will therefore not be repeated this time."[5] In the view of Sikorski, a nationalist who had served in the Austro-Hungarian army from 1916 to 1918 and then distinguished himself in the Polish–Soviet War—the eastward extension of the world war—Germanism was certainly at work in Nazism. And yet Sikorksi, whom Karski idealized and who decorated him in London shortly before dying in a plane accident, also expressed the certainty that Nazism would overtake Germanism. How?

"Nazi War on Jews. The New Barbarism. Response of Civilized World."

On December 4, 1942, the *Times* of London blared, "Nazi war on Jews: Deliberate plan for extermination." The headline proved the acuity of its information; it quoted at length a "memorandum by the Polish resistance that has arrived in London"—Karski's. The article stated with certainty, "All other war aims of Nazism will fail in the end—and the defeat of German Fascism is inevitable—but this particular aim, a complete extermination of Jews, is already being enforced."[6] This was the *Times*, not a leaflet put out by the Bund.

The following day, the *Times* published a letter signed "William Cantuar, Lambeth Palace" and titled, "Nazi War on Jews. The New Barbarism. Response of Civilized World."[7] "Civilized world" against "barbarism"? Was the Archbishop of Canterbury seeing a repetition of 1914? In fact, in October

1914, ninety-three celebrated German intellectuals and artists had signed an "appeal to the civilized world" to defend their country, their *Kultur*, against the accusations of barbarism made during the early weeks of what was not yet being called the Great War. Using the anaphora "It is not true that," the ninety-three denied the German atrocities in Belgium in August and early September 1914. They attributed the invention of such accusations to propaganda and reflected them back on their Russian enemies and on wrongdoing by French and English colonial troops. "It is not true that our warfare pays no respect to international laws. It knows no undisciplined cruelty. But in the east, the earth is saturated with the blood of women and children unmercifully butchered by the wild Russian troops." The signatories rejected the accusations made against Germany and emphasized the British and French alliances with different of categories of patent "barbarians" such as the Russians, Serbians, and Mongols—the true Huns, the real Attilas; moreover, the British and French were bringing their colonial troops into line: "Those who have allied themselves with the Russians and Serbians, and present such a shameful scene to the world as that of inciting the Mongolians and Negroes against the white race, have no right whatever to call themselves upholders of European civilization."[8]

Between 1914 and 1918, racism was common to all of the belligerents. After all, the widespread belief that the Germans cut off the hands of Belgian children was born of a switch of images. In fact, in the Congo—the direct property of the Belgian king Leopold II—Victor-Léon Fiévez, leader of the equatorial district, had introduced the gathering of cut-off hands and excrement of the dead, not the living, even though rare cases of mutilation did exist. But this was in the context of staggeringly despicable forced labor, whence the birth of the myth within circles—still very small—of activists fighting against colonial abuses.[9] In the summer of 1914, Belgians, and then the whole world, *believed* that they had seen white hands, which they *had not wanted* or *been able* to see when the hands were black and in the Congo. These mythified hands took the place, in both cases, of real atrocities committed in the colonies since the nineteenth century and during the Great War and then were used as propaganda.[10]

The reader who wrote to the *Times* of London on December 5, 1942, knew one thing for certain: in 1914, true atrocities (atrocities, plural) had preceded the brainwashing. As for the present reality of World War II, it was revealed through a single "atrocity"—expressed in the singular—the horrifying Nazi extermination. And yet, most people, including the majority of those who debriefed couriers in London and Washington, thought exactly the contrary: all of this could not be true; these facts were, at best, gross exaggerations. They would not be deceived again, as they had been about the German atrocities of 1914. Indeed, how could the British and Americans, who were convinced that they had been tricked during the Great War, be persuaded that this time the events were of a different scope and scale than the "atrocities"— the scare quotes proving that they were largely hypothetical—of World War I? No, they would not be deceived again. Numerous members of the British Parliament, intellectuals such as H. G. Wells, and the most cultivated—and motivated—Americans reacted in this way.

It should have been no surprise. In 1978, when Karski was interviewed by Claude Lanzmann for what would become *Shoah*, he gave a detailed account of his meeting with Lord Selborne, chief of the Special Operation Executive,[11] in London in 1942:

JAN KARSKI: I more or less told him the whole story [including his visits to the Warsaw ghetto and Belzec], and then, at a certain point, I finished. Lord Selborne, with typical English correctness, benevolence, tolerance, rationality, answers: "Mr. Karski, during the First World War we were propagandising that the German soldiers were crushing the heads of Belgian babies against the wall. I think we were doing a good job. We had to weaken German morale, we had to arouse hostility towards Germany. The war was a very bloody war. We knew it was untrue. Speak about your problem, your report. Try to arouse public opinion. I want you to know you do contribute to the Allied cause. We want this kind of report. Your mission is very important." He was clearly telling me, "Mr. Karski, you know and I know it isn't so."
CLAUDE LANZMANN: "It's not true, but it's good for propaganda"?
JK: Yes.
CL: The same problem as in the First World War?
JK: Yes.[12]

Lanzmann's questions and Karski's two affirmative responses prove that most historians until the 1990s also thought that the "German atrocities" of the Great War, such as the children's severed or crushed hands, were inventions or myths; they therefore kept them in scare quotes.[13] And yet, in 1921 Marc Bloch had transformed the "false news" of the war into a historical subject by reflecting on precisely this enigmatic episode:

> From the instant when the error made the blood flow, it was definitively established. . . . Even today, the majority of Germans are probably convinced that their soldiers fell victim to Belgian ambushes in great numbers. . . . It is easy to believe what we need to believe. A legend that has inspired momentous acts, and especially cruel actions, is very close to being indestructible. . . . False news always arises from collective representations that preexisted its birth; it is fortuitous only in appearance. False news is the mirror in which the "collective consciousness" contemplates its own features.[14]

In 1914, the German invaders of Belgium and northern France, under the impression that enemy civilians were snipers, felt that preventive attacks were necessary to protect themselves as the war began. This was the reason for their violent reprisals. Then, these real atrocities—civilians used as human shields, taken hostage and shot, women raped—were transformed with the creation of two myths: that of children's hands being cut off and that of enemies being crucified. These myths became so ingrained in memory that the caricaturist David Low attempted to use them, to doubtful humorous effect, in relation to the claimed mistreatment of German prisoners in 1942 by the British: "Reprisals for British atrocities. The hands of some prisoners were bound." "What, only the hands?"[15] On the severed hands, Bloch was once again very clear:

> The popular imagination always distorts. Whatever "atrocities"—alas, too real—were perpetrated by Germans on French soil, they became mingled with accounts that turned facts into the dregs of legends, such as the legend of the "severed hands." This would be . . . a good subject for study. . . . Would such work not be of use not only for clear history, but also for our propaganda, about which, since peace has come, there is still a useful task to accomplish—in Alsace-Lorraine, in friendly or allied countries, even in Germany? The truth loses its strength when it is mixed with falsehoods.[16]

Bloch was right to advocate research on the true atrocities at the same time as that on the acknowledged outrages that had succeeded each other since 1914. Each camp had used both the enemy's real actions and rumors in its propaganda and in order to prove how much its own society opposed the barbarism of the opposing side. Real atrocities and their mythification went hand in hand on the different invasion fronts and were extended into the territories occupied until 1918, and even until 1923 in the Russian civil war and the war between Greece and Turkey. The extermination of Armenians by the Ottoman empire under cover of war was their most extreme manifestation. Already people were seeing only what they wanted to see, even when it was right in front of their eyes.

"Corpse Factories" during World War I: From *Leim* (Glue) to Quicklime

In the 1920s, one of the great anti-German scandals of World War I re-emerged in Great Britain and the United States: the use of the bodies of soldiers—including their own—for unspeakable purposes in "corpse factories." Although some explained—even in a stormy parliamentary debate in London on April 30, 1917—that only animal carcasses could possibly have been used, others remained convinced that the goal was to use human cadavers to extract fertilizers mixed with pig manure, the Germans being portrayed as lewd, repulsive pigs.[17]

Although in 1917 the "corpse factories" processed only animal fat into candles, glycerin, or glue,[18] words led to confusion, due to inaccurate translations, deliberate or not. The German word for glue is *leim*; its homonym in English is "lime" (in this case, short for quicklime), which was associated—until Karski reported on Izbica in 1942—with disinfection, including of bodies and cemeteries. The connection was quickly made:

> "Germans and their dead. A revolting treatment. Science and the barbarian spirit." . . . The trains arrive full of bare bodies, which are unloaded by the workers who live at the works. . . . They are equipped with long hooked poles, and push the bundle of bodies to an endless chain, which picks them up with big hooks. . . . The bodies are transported on this endless chain into a long, narrow compartment, where they pass through a bath which disinfects them. They then go through a drying chamber, and finally are automatically carried into a digester or great cauldron, in which they are dropped by an apparatus which detaches them from the chain. In the digester they remain from six to

eight hours, and are treated by steam, which breaks them up while they are slowly stirred by machinery.

From this treatment result several products. The fats are broken up into stearine, a form of tallow, and oils, which require to be redistilled before they can be used. The process of distillation is carried out by boiling the oil with carbonate of soda, and some part of the by-products resulting from this is used by German soapmakers. . . .

There is a laboratory, and in charge of the works is a chief chemist with two assistants and 78 men. All the employees are soldiers and are attached to the 8th Army Corps. . . . Under no pretext is a man permitted to leave them. They are guarded as prisoners at their appalling work.[19]

By denouncing the paradox of the Germans' science without a conscience in the industrialization of the process, the author wanted to prove that their technical superiority was leading them to commit even more crimes. The numerous caricatures—such as the one in *Punch* in which the Kaiser shows a terrified young recruit the "body factory" under his window with the caption "Know that I'll find a way to use you, living or dead"— proved that there was general awareness that this was the realm of propaganda. And yet, this idea of the processing of cadavers into soap was found in numerous personal diaries, as rumors were no doubt propagated once more, during the Great War, between battlefields and nearby civilians.[20]

The debate over the German word *Kadaver*—animal carcass or human cadaver?—was not settled then. It returned in 1925 when, during a speech in New York, the Briton Brigadier General John Charteris, former information officer for Major-General Douglas Haig, declared that he had invented the whole thing. He had apparently taken the caption for a photograph of dead horses being sent to the knacker and used it under another photograph showing bodies of soldiers being transported behind the front lines for burial. The world press seized on the photomontage. Ten years after the war, the use of images as propaganda was admitted by one of its protagonists; the British authorities, to their great consternation, were accused of manipulation. Debates in Parliament and a press campaign followed. Pacifists such as Bertrand Russell rejected all "German atrocities" wholesale: if some had been fabricated, why might others be real?[21] Had Charteris lied, or not? In 1917? In 1925? Was he a true forger of the false or a false forger of the true? People continued to believe what they wanted to believe.

Greuelpropaganda: Atrocity Propaganda

Such propaganda and counterpropaganda campaigns extended far and wide after World War I, particularly in Germany. In his *Mein Kampf*, Hitler noted that the British had proved to be far superior in spreading disinformation during the Great War: "The proof of this brilliant knowledge of the primitiveness of feeling of the great masses was to be found in the atrocity propaganda that had been adapted to this, thus ruthlessly and ingeniously securing moral steadfastness at the front, even during the greatest defeats."[22] Not only, said Hitler, had British morale been galvanized by the country's excellent propaganda, but the British had even managed to convince Germans of the truthfulness of their assertions, including those about the corpse factory. Thanks to this *Greuelpropaganda*, or atrocity propaganda, external enemies had enabled their domestic accomplices—socialists and, especially, Jews— to sharpen the daggers with which they would stab Germany in the back. The certainty that external and domestic conspirators had been created thanks to the false atrocities that spread during and after World War I would be found at the core of Nazism in 1933, as Victor Klemperer, an inspired observer of the language of the Third Reich, noted. Klemperer was not surprised that the same words, myths, and debates reappeared:

> Foreign Jews, particularly those from France, England and America, are today frequently referred to as "global Jews (*Weltjuden*)." . . . Does this mean that Jews are to be found everywhere on earth, except, that is, in Germany? And where are they within Germany itself? The global Jews disseminate "atrocity propaganda" and spread "horror stories" and if we report so much as a scrap of what happens here every day then we too are guilty of disseminating atrocity propaganda and are punished accordingly.[23]

In Nazi Germany, the myth of the snipers (*franc-tireurs*) was the first to resurface: it was now taken for granted that Belgian civilians had been involved in the war during the 1914 invasion and that the German army had simply defended itself. The *Manifesto of the Ninety-Three German Intellectuals*, written in 1914, makes this point: "It is not true that our troops treated

Louvain brutally. Furious inhabitants having treacherously fallen upon them in their quarters, our troops with aching hearts were obliged to fire a part of the town, as punishment." Starting in 1940, the Nazis did all they could—with archival research in Belgium, once again occupied—to prove that the Allied campaign on the atrocities of World War I was false, that the Kaiser's troops had only defended themselves against the combined assault of troops and civilians.

But the Third Reich was not a continuation of the Second Reich, particularly in the east, where even in 1940 there was no attempt to "correct" propaganda. At the time of the invasion of Poland, it was claimed that the civilians were barbarians, and Reinhard Heydrich proclaimed that the Jews were snipers and plunderers who had to be dealt with separately.

Among the Allies and resisters in occupied countries, the myths of the Great War were also brought back into service. "*Franc-tireur*" was given a positive gloss; it was—a random irony—the name of the resistance group to which Marc Bloch belonged.

Some of the most hackneyed rumors resurfaced in 1942, even in credible reports of the extermination of Jews. For instance, in the Foreign Office report of September 11, 1942, someone wrote on a typed text, "The facts are quite bad enough without the addition of such an old story such as the use of bodies for the manufacture of soap etc."[24] "Slain Polish Jews Put at a Million. One-third of number in whole country said to have been put to death by Nazis. Abattoir for deportees. Mass electrocutions, killing by injection of air bubbles described in reports."[25] The *New York Times* reported this British information on Belzec (the Karski effect), which had come to it through Rabbi Wise, and specified that human fat was being processed into fertilizer or soap. Those who thought that the victim numbers were greatly exaggerated raised an outcry. The detail—the soap factories—was used to deny the central information, the mass extermination. Similarly, up to 1945, *Christian Century*, a relatively moderate newspaper, returned to both the false figures and the false atrocities: "The use of corpses to produce fat and soap very unpleasantly reminds us of the lie of the 'corpse factory' that was one of the propaganda triumphs of World War I."[26]

And yet, a Canadian war correspondent in Poland in July 1945, Raymond Arthur Davies, reported on his visit to a "human soap factory ... with

corpses from prisoner camps and concentration camps." He included photographs of decapitated heads with his account.[27] Experiments conducted
by Dr. Rudolf Spanner at the Danzig Anatomic Institute, mentioned by the
Soviets at Nuremberg, have been central since 1945 to the belief that the
Nazis produced soap with the bodies of their Polish, Russian, and Jewish
victims. Historians have recently established with certainty that this was
not the case, even though human fat in the process of being saponified was
in fact found in the abandoned laboratory.[28]

Karski kept a copy of Davies's book in his personal library, and even
today many are still convinced that the stories about soap factories are true.
This raises the question: why, during World War II, was there a general refusal to believe in the atrocities of World War I, still so fresh and reflected
in the moment, and then a return to the rumors afterward?

"Our skepticism has been fortified by our experience of 'atrocity stories' during the last war" (Varian Fry, "The Massacre of the Jews," 1942)

The denial of atrocities during the 1914 invasions became a central issue in
1942, at the very time when information on extermination of the Jews was
emerging with clarity. In a pamphlet published during the summer, *Rescue
the Perishing*, an activist member of Parliament, Eleanor Rathbone, pleaded
with Britons to take in more Jewish refugees, especially in Mandatory Palestine. She felt obliged to begin with a meaningful "appeal to the reader":
"These are not 'atrocity stories,' exaggerated for the purposes of propaganda.
They come from too many sources all of which are corroborated."

Whence the poignant appeals from Schmuel Zygielbojm to save the Jews
in Poland who were still alive in 1942 and from Victor Gollancz, another
of Karski's interlocutors in London: "Nothing is baser than 'atrocity mon-
gering' . . . for the sake of stirring up hatred against the enemy." A militant
pacifist, Gollancz was eager to distinguish hate-induced propaganda produced by both sides since the Great War from the reality of December 1942:
"*Unless something effective is done,* within a very few months these six million Jews will all be dead."[29]

Other men, as diverse as Cardinal Hinsley, Archbishop of Westminster,
and the philosopher Jacques Maritain, who had taken refuge at Princeton
University, made the same observation. Maritain wrote, "If we were tempted
to see the accounts that come to us as 'atrocity stories,' reverberating through

the echoes of horror, that would be enough for us to realize their plausibility."[30] And he returned to the facts, as did William Shirer in the *Washington Post*. In an opinion piece, "The Propaganda Front," Shirer reminded his readers that the Nazi authorities had used propaganda about the atrocities of World War I to mock and reject everything that came from England or the United States, as well as the joint Allied declaration on persecution of the Jews dated December 17, 1942; in this foreshadowing of Nuremberg and the United Nations, the British, Americans, Soviets, and governments in exile warned the world of the "bestial policy of cold-blooded extermination" and promised a verdict: "They reaffirm their solemn resolution to ensure that those responsible for these crimes shall not escape retribution, and to press on with the necessary practical measures to this end."[31]

Proclaiming justice, putting off all action until the end the war. To this, Gollancz responded, "Does it benefit the Jew, as he stands at the door of the execution chamber, that, after his body has begun to pass into the dust from which it came, his executioner also will be sent to the grave? . . . No, the proclamation of vengeance will bring back no single Jew from his nameless grave."[32]

The world had to be convinced not only that there was mass murder under way but also of the need to act quickly, not to put off until after the war the eventual punishment of the murderers. But the atrocity propaganda became entangled with this race against death. For instance, Shirer wrote that "the Nazis had always suppressed the slightest reference to the murder of the Jews" but that a certain number of Germans listened to foreign radio stations, which led to their counteroffensive regarding *Greuelpropaganda*: "The Allied governments had resumed their 'atrocity propaganda' against Germany. . . . It was a campaign similar to the last war, when the Allies claimed that Germans chopped off the hands of Belgian children."[33] In another article, "The Propaganda Front: No Atrocity Stories, Facts," Shirer reported on a survey taken in Detroit that revealed that the woman and man in the street did not "believe any of the stories about Nazi atrocities. . . . They were dead sure that the present reports about Nazi atrocities were similar to those we heard about the Germans in the First World War and therefore no more true." He therefore tried to find explanations for his compatriots' general skepticism after more than a year of engagement in the war. "In the two decades that followed the last Armistice, our vast disillusionment over the peace degenerated into a silly sort of super-cynicism and super-skepticism. We would believe nothing. In the weird process, we lost track of the true currents of contemporary history. The result was a terrible and costly confusion." Shirer was even more alarmed because he knew that "the Nazi themselves have admitted atrocities that have no parallel in the First World War. . . . The openly avowed aim of Nazi Germany is to destroy us. There is nothing secret about this aim. There is no earthly reason for us not to believe it."[34]

No reason, and yet every reason. If it was difficult, even in 1942 or 1943, to convince people that Jews specifically were being persecuted and that mass deportations were under way, then very few would be able to believe in the total extermination of the Jewish people. Gerhart Riegner, the secretary of the World Jewish Congress, who, in August 1942, sent the first telegram to the English and American diplomatic corps on the mass extermination, recalled this in his memoir. In a section titled "Why We Failed," he wrote, "The first reason . . . is that . . . there was no precedent for the Shoah." "A second factor, little known but extremely damaging," he went on, "was the precedent of reports on German atrocities during World War I, which after the war proved to be false. This caused us serious problems and we were always being told, 'That's all made up, just like during the First War.' We had to make enormous efforts to convince people of the veracity of our reports on the Shoah."[35] Although in 1998, when he wrote his book, Riegner was still confusing the real atrocities of 1914–18 with the consubstantial propaganda myths, he accurately reconstructed the climate of doubt in Great Britain and the United States, also confirmed by Raymond Aron for free France, where they "did not indulge in *Greuelpropaganda*, the expression the Germans had created in 1914 to denounce Allied propaganda accusing them of atrocities."[36] It was this doubt that Karski, Lemkin, and Varian Fry struggled with.

Fry, an American, had been expelled from Vichy in 1941. The Emergency Rescue Committee, which he had created in Marseille to save Jews who were being hunted, had been closed. In his own country, he was ignored, even spied on; he would never again have responsibilities matching those he had had in Europe. And so, he wrote a masterful article, "The Massacre of the Jews":

We are accustomed to horrors in the historical past, and accept them . . . as phenomena of ages less enlightened than our own. When such things occur in our times, like the Armenian massacres, we put them down to the account of still half-barbarous peoples. But that such things could be done by contemporary western Europeans, heirs of the humanist tradition, seems hardly possible.

Our skepticism has been fortified by our experience with "atrocity stories" during the last war. We were treated, during that war, to many accounts of German atrocities. We were told of the rape of nuns, the forced prostitution of young Belgian girls, of German soldiers spearing infants on their bayonets, or deliberately and wantonly cutting off their hands. Later . . . most of these atrocities were found to have been invented. The natural reaction was to label all atrocity stories "propaganda" and refuse to believe them.[37]

In 1939–40, Fry had been certain that most of the World War I atrocities were the product of rumor and propaganda; more specifically, he confused the myths born of the distortion of true atrocities with the actual atrocities. He admitted his own difficulty with "believing" the early Nazi cruelties perpetrated on the Jews in Germany. But by 1942, he was convinced: even if the Nazis lost the world war, they would have won the war in occupied Europe and murdered the Jews.

Fry then talked about a situation specific to World War I, that of the occupied territories in which harsh conditions and atrocities perpetrated during the 1914 invasion were extended in the form of requisitions, forced labor, and mass deportations and culminated during the 1918 retreat and the evacuation of these territories in the final destruction: "When we remember that, even after the war of 1914–18 was hopelessly lost and the German army was retreating in confusion on the Western Front, it still found time, and the will, wantonly to destroy the factories and flood the mines in the path, we may well believe that this time it will be even more thorough, go even more berserk."[38]

In the summer of 1942, before publishing this article, Fry sent a report to Eleanor Roosevelt; he was attempting through her to reach her husband, who was opposed to "fighting the war of the Jews." She asked Undersecretary of State Sumner Welles if she could mention it in her column as a form of protest.[39] Welles's response is not known, but Fry's exasperation with the procrastination was eloquent: it moved a man whom Fry did not yet know, Raphael Lemkin.

Lemkin, Legal Activist: Jews and Armenians before and after the Great War

Barely had he set foot in the United States, in 1941, when Lemkin was giving well-attended speeches on the sufferings of the Poles, in which he compared the horrors of the two world wars. But when it came to the destruction of entire peoples, he faced the systematic lies about the atrocities of World War I. "I found complete unawareness that the Axis planned destruction of the peoples under their control," he wrote. "Some answered that Washington would not believe it, and many still remembered the 'atrocity stories' told about Germans in the First World War. I thought: genocide is so easy to commit because people don't want to believe it until after it happens."[40]

In fact, in 1942 reports were coming from all over occupied Europe, but many thought they were highly embellished. Moreover, there was total confusion between Nazi atrocities in general and the specificity of the extermination of the Jews—what the historian Raul Hilberg, long after Lemkin, called "functional blindness." Indeed, many Americans—before Karski arrived in the United States, his reports having preceded him as Britons and Americans shared his data—invoked the lack of eyewitnesses and the doubts (many of them legitimate if one thinks of Katyn) about information coming from the Soviet Union.

Lemkin, however, knew that the real violence against civilians in 1914 had been both underestimated and mythologized, especially when one added the atrocities prolonged under different occupations—from Belgium and northern France to Serbia and Lithuania—and the extermination of the Armenians, the true scope of which had not yet been exposed. During his exodus and period of waiting in Sweden, he conducted a study comparing the occupation policies of the Nazis with those during World War I, and he collected the documents with which he would work in the United States to produce his master opus of 1944, *Axis Rule in Occupied Europe*, in which the word "genocide" appeared for the first time.[41]

In early 1942, the newly arrived Lemkin had reason to be bitter: he was simply a stand-in at Duke University despite the kindness of his colleagues. Almost no one understood the importance of his legal work in Poland and his participation in the great project of the League of Nations, the effort to unify criminal law.

Lemkin had realized very early, without expressing it clearly, that extermination wasn't an accidental cruelty but the essence of this type of war against civilians, the goal of which was to homogenize peoples and religions. In fact, this is what had happened during World War I in the processes of internal reconstruction of the Ottoman and Russian empires: population displacements took the form of social or ethnic reorganization, which included the extermination of Armenians and the deportation of "suspect" populations from Russia, starting with the Jews, the vast majority of whom in Europe were living in the residential zone that had been assigned to them in czarist times.

In his later writings, Lemkin placed less stress on his personal experience of pogroms before and after 1914 in his region under Russian rule than on the extermination of Armenians under the Ottoman Empire. As a Jew, he probably wanted to maintain his ideal of universality, so as not to be accused of taking a special interest in his own people. Although he was only six years old at the time of the Bialystok pogrom, in 1906, he would soon read the poems by Hayim Bialik describing the atrocities in Kishinev in 1903, including his elegy to the abominable, "City of the Killings":

Rise and go to the town of the killings and you'll come to the yards
and with your eyes and your own hand feel the fence
and on the trees and on the stones and plaster of the walls
the congealed blood and hardened brains of the dead.
And you'll come from there to the ruins and stop before the rents
and pass by the pierced walls and shattered ovens,
where the axe's head bit deep, to burst and deepen holes,
bearing the black stone and shears of brick all burned
and they'll look like the open mouths of black and mortal wounds
that have no remedy, that have no cure.[42]

As a student, Lemkin had been subjected to insults and beatings by his fellow students, who called him "Beilis," the name of a Jew wrongfully accused of a "ritual" murder of a Christian child killed near Kiev. Menahem Mendel Beilis was ultimately acquitted in 1913, but between the ages of eleven and thirteen Lemkin had lived with this tragedy, discussed every day by his family, and with the fear of an imminent pogrom.

In 1915, his hometown of Volkovysk—then in Russian territory—was caught up in the war. Although the Germans invaded and occupied it, putting its residents into forced labor, the town was at least spared the most brutal Russian decisions. For in the regions that it held, the Russian military conducted full-scale experiments to test its theories about "suspect populations": it imprisoned its nationals situated on the front line or expelled them to the interior, conducting "ethnic cleansing"[43] of Russian citizens of German origin, as well as Jews, on the pretext that their language, Yiddish, enabled them to conspire with the Germans. At least six hundred thousand Jews were deported, subjected to violence and pogroms, put into temporary camps, or forced to move farther east, taking nothing with them. The artist Abel Pann described and drew these war pogroms: civilians were chased into the forests and abandoned there in the snow, starving, or deported in cattle cars, their hands tied through the crooked floorboards; Cossacks on horseback pillaged, raped, and beat women, children, old people.

> In a few hours they were chased from their homes with unimaginable cruelty. The children were in front, it was all the others that were driven out as if they were the worst criminals. . . . They died there like flies; many lost their minds. . . . They opened the stomachs of pregnant women and filled them with feathers from torn pillows. . . . Jewish soldiers, mutilated, decorated for their bravery, returned to their hometowns and found nothing but corpses and destruction.[44]

The historian Simon Dubnow, whom Lemkin met in Riga in 1940, had witnessed these deportations in May 1915:

> An official campaign was openly conducted with the infernal intention of blaming the Jews for the military defeats. . . . I often think, where does such Judeophobia come from at such a time? Psychologically, it can be explained. In his way, the executioner fears his victim. The Judeophobes who have been tyrannizing the Jews for thirty years have their conscience suggest to them that the Jews would have to take revenge on their persecutors, and this likelihood,

in the executioners' minds, is transformed into something real. . . . The nightmare expands. Crazy and criminal things happen. In a single day several tens of thousands of Jews were expelled from Kovno and its province. In the army's chain of command, the talk was of their mass expulsion . . . and deportation. . . . The unfortunate exiles were shut into cattle cars. When they asked, "Where are we being taken," the answer was "Where we have been ordered to send you." . . . What is happening in Lithuania is beyond the imagination. There is talk of tens of thousands of exiles, who, on Shavuot, flowed into Vilna with babies in carriages.[45]

Since 1916, almanacs and war chronicles had been published to celebrate the resiliency of Jews in the east. These *Zalmbikner*—collections of details of daily life and personal diaries—were instrumental to Jews' becoming aware that they formed a people. Under attack specifically during that world war, they recorded the uniqueness of their lay lives, schools, sports clubs, and charity organizations. Facing them, however, was widespread anti-Semitic violence, which, long based on the idea of the idea of the Jew as "traitor," "infidel," "hoarder," and "speculator," was to grow with impunity thanks to the war: it was now permissible to "break the Yids." These were in fact "war crimes" committed by regular units, adding a new kind of mass violence to the old-style pogroms, and this was before 1917, the two revolutions and the civil war, the "turn to extermination."[46]

All memorial books for this region chronicle the extermination of Jews starting in 1941, dating back to the German, and then Russian, abuses of World War I, as the Jews' condition worsened during the Russian civil war.[47] Volkovysk was destroyed during the war between Russia and Poland in 1920, and Lemkin witnessed the anti-Jewish radicalization from 1918 to 1920 in these border regions between the new Poland at war with Russia, Ukraine, Belarus, and the former Austrian Galicia: from quasi-"extermination *Aktionen*" to the future Nazi sense of the word. In fact, those who were fighting against the Red Army took out their rage on the Jews, perceived as Judeo-Bolsheviks and impure organisms that were destroying the healthy (holy) body of Russia. In 1918, military confrontations between Poles and Ukrainians around the city of Lvov (formerly Lemberg, now the Ukrainian city of Lviv), where Lemkin went to university, ended, after the Polish victory, in a three-day pogrom that resulted in seventy dead and at least five hundred wounded. A *New York Times* headline read, "1,100 Jews Murdered in Lemberg Pogroms."[48]

In these regions, where the German, Austro-Hungarian, and Russian empires were disintegrating, the Great War was prolonged: more civilians than soldiers were mistreated, deported, or killed. The modernity of total war swept everything away between 1914 and the 1920s, and in these "lands of blood," Jews had already paid a higher price than the rest of the population: indeed, atavistic anti-Semitism was transformed into self-fulfilling prophecy when a number of Jews, like other minorities, were seduced by Lenin's promises of emancipation. We have seen, through Karski's eyes when he was in Poland in 1939–40, what happened in the zone occupied by the Soviets.

In 1919, other attacks against Jews took place not only in Galicia but across Poland. In article 93 of the Treaty of Versailles, the new country was ordered to protect its religious and linguistic minorities and to give Polish citizenship to everyone who came, in particular, from the Lvov region. After the pogroms, President Wilson established a commission of inquiry on the situation of Jewish Poles; the commission was chaired by Henry Morgenthau, former American ambassador to the Ottoman Empire, who had witnessed the partial extermination of Christian minorities in the crumbling empire, starting with the Armenians.

"When such things happen in our times, like the Armenian massacres, we put them down to the account of still half-barbarous peoples" (Varian Fry, 1942)

The "total extermination" of the Armenians was an attack that was literally inconceivable. The crimes of the Young Turks were well known and transmitted in public opinion in real time. However, these crimes were poorly understood because they were instrumentalized by the propaganda of the Entente: condemnation of them became a new war aim, a way to strike at the Central Powers through their Ottoman allies. As the deportations and massacres of Armenians were occurring, in 1915 and 1916, commissions of inquiry were publishing White Paper after White Paper on the atrocities committed against civilians in Belgium and Serbia in 1914. A 1916 caricature denounced the deportations from Lille during Easter of that year: *Boche* brutes are carrying away women and children as a soldier in a pointed helmet remarks,

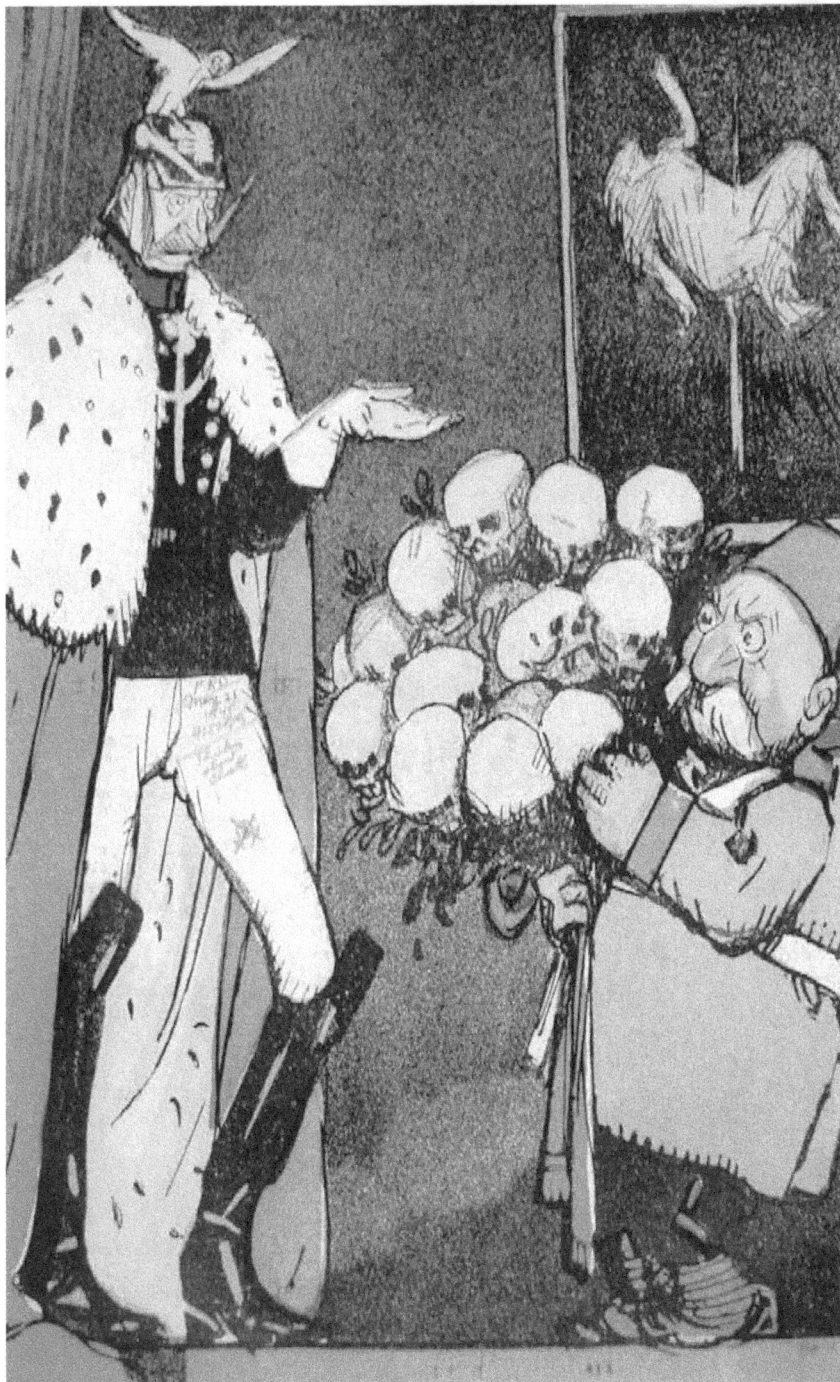

"Accept them in memory of the last massacre of Christians." *L'Asino è il popolo: utile, paziente et bastonato*, Italian magazine published by Podrecca e Galantara, December 5, 1915.

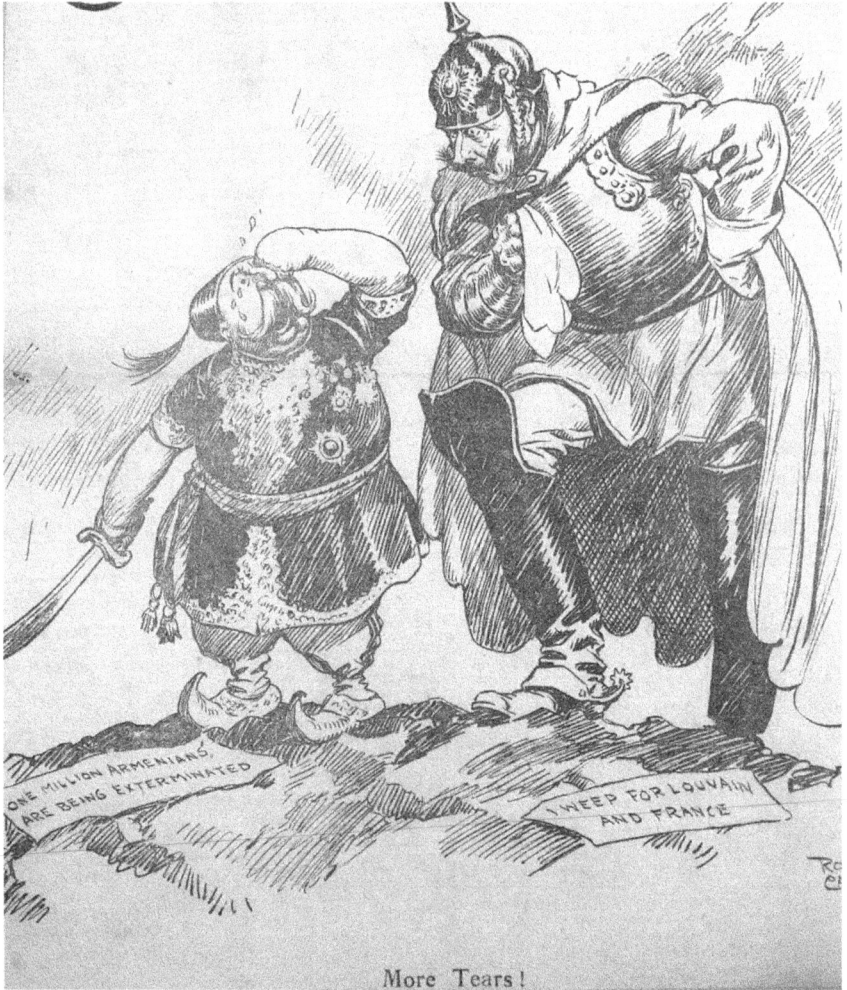

"More tears!" The Sultan and William II cry crocodile tears contemplating their crimes: "One million Armenians are being exterminated." "I weep for Louvain and France." Drawing by Robert Carter, *New York Sun*, 1915.

ironically, "They complain. But what would they say if they were in Armenia?"[49] Although German atrocities in Belgium and northern France continued to be compared to the terror perpetrated against Armenians, some were already aware that something extraordinary was happening in the Ottoman Empire.

Talaat Pasha, a member of the triumvirate leading the Young Turks, described the deportations as the logical retribution for "traitors" bankrolled by the Russians. In the view of the Young Turks, the Armenian—pejoratively singular—was a potential traitor, an "irregular," "unwholesome." The domestic "enemy" was animalized, his ontological humanity denied. What remained was to "sideline" him, a euphemism for killing him.[50] Even in 1918, a French-language Turkish newspaper was denouncing the barbarism—of the Armenians:

One trembles to see the scenes of atrocities that they have committed. . . . They have killed everyone they encounter, they have burned villages, slaughtered animals. . . . The Armenian organizations are systematically applying their plan to wipe out the Turkish race. . . . History will certainly pronounce itself one day on the actions of these civilized criminals. As for today, these madmen must know that their crimes will cost them dearly. It is not up to a handful of Armenians . . . to exterminate the Turkish race, which is so strong that it is guaranteed by nature and God Himself against obliteration. Furthermore, these crimes and atrocities will provoke unforgettable indignation in the world at large, stretching as far as the Chinese border, and as the Armenians are by God Himself condemned to live in the middle of this world, in whichever hands they find themselves, it will become hell for them. This can be the only outcome resulting from so many crimes![51]

In a mirror effect typical of mass murderers, the Turks attributed their own base acts to their victims and claimed to be defending themselves from these "civilized criminals," an oxymoron that defined the Turks themselves perfectly. It was the genocide-denial conviction of executioners who saw themselves as victims and manifested "apocalyptic racism" even as they exterminated Armenians by the thousands.[52] The Ottomans lost the war, but they won their battle: they obliterated the Armenians. Those who were not actually exterminated were destroyed in other ways. Rapes, conversions, forced marriages, and children kidnapped and raised as Muslims eradicated them as a people, as Christians, and their ancient culture was ravaged as churches and libraries were burned. And the seizure of their homes and belongings enabled the Turks to win the economic peace. Without Armenians.

"Crimes against humanity and civilization," "Murder of a nation": How Can the Extermination of the Armenians Be Defined?

In a telegram sent in May 1915, the French, English, and Russians called the "atrocities" committed against the Armenians "crimes against humanity and civilization." It was a vengeful observation, a paradigmatic case of war violence become "crime against humanity" and "genocide" before the legal concepts—and the terms—were invented. And it was difficult to agree on the words: "crimes against Christianity and civilization" or "crimes against humanity and civilization"?

This was a glaring semantic reversal. In the nineteenth century, the concept of "laws of humanity" was used in the positive sense, and actions were sometimes taken in the name of such laws. Now, there were "crimes against humanity." The Russian diplomats deemed the notion of "humanity" too vague and reintroduced "civilization." This represented *the* war aim of the Entente. One of the ironies of the May 1915 telegram is that it constituted verbal belligerence in response to the first Armenian massacres in winter 1915, which resembled the massacres of the past; it was, above all, a way to compensate for the lack of intervention during the massacres of 1894–97 and 1909. Jean Jaurès had thundered in 1896, "In the face of this violation of France's word and of human rights, not a single cry has left your lips, not a word from your consciences, and you have witnessed, mute and therefore complicit, the utter extermination."[53]

In April 1915, several months before the mass deportation of Armenians led to their extermination, the Allied declaration was based mainly on the world war underway, waged this time on Turkish soil. For years, the crimes against the Armenians were used to attack the Germans, the top enemy power and Ottoman ally. "The massacres of Armenia," wrote a historian at the time, "Turkey's work, Germany's method!"[54] But if the Turks were simply the puppets of the Germans, they were exonerated of their crimes.

A number of influential Americans, some of whom would meet twenty-five years later with Karski or Lemkin, took a position. In October 1915, Rabbi Wise denounced "inhumanity whether committed by Germans against Belgians, by Russians against Jews, or by Turks against Armenians."[55] But, in the name of strict neutrality, President Wilson wanted neither to seriously condemn the massacres nor to intervene in Turkey.[56] As for future president Franklin Delano Roosevelt, he had taken an interest in persecuted minorities—such as the Boers—as a student at Harvard and joined an organization called Near East Relief in 1921. Perhaps he had read the report sent from the Caucasus by one of his colleagues that mentioned "heaps of human bones and half-decomposed [Armenian] bodies representing the remains of 500 women and children killed in one spot."[57]

The prolongation of World War I in the modern state of Turkey at war with Greece, and in a Russia in the grip of revolution and then civil war, was to provide a further catalyst for these phenomena. Churchill, for example, wrote to the prime ministers of the Dominions about the "infernal orgy" of the sack of Smyrna by the Turks in September 1922, in which twelve thousand people perished in the flames in the Greek and Armenian parts of the city: "For a deliberately planned and methodically exercised atrocity Smyrna . . . must find few parallels in the history of human crime."[58]

"The bloodiest and most disturbing enigma in history" (Heinrich Vierbücher)

"The liberation and resurrection of Belgium and Serbia have been two of the most splendid outcomes of the World War, as the *debâcle* in Russia and the martyrdom of Armenia have been its greatest tragedies," opined *Punch*, almost tritely, in 1919.[59] Few observers at the time could get past the stage of describing the "tragedies," condemning them, and, above all, putting into words what had happened. Heinrich Vierbücher, a German who had served as translator for General Liman von Sanders in the Dardanelles, took an original view in 1930:

> The fifty long years of terror of the Great War found their climax not on the battlefields of Vaux and Douaumont but in the passes of the Caucasus, a Golgotha for the Armenians that went beyond all imagination of horror, beyond even the visions of Grünewald, Goya, and Bruegel. . . . Might the

greatest tragedy of the ordeal of humanity find one day a creator, an artist, a poet capable of capturing the gaze of men—for centuries to come—upon this time of madness, this evil Sabbath, that the self-satisfied, the cowards, and the idiots call the "world order"?

Not only did Vierbücher understand the extraordinary significance of this extermination but he also situated it within a series of massacres through history, as Lemkin would do later when he was refining the concept of genocide in the international debates of 1945–48:

> During the war, the Turks found the Germans just good enough to hold the curtain behind which they slaughtered more than a million innocents, men, women, and children. . . . The extermination of an entire people with the deliberate execution of women and children—this is a development for which the barbarous past was, no doubt, not "ready." One must think of the misdeeds of a Pizarro in Peru, the war of extermination of the red race by the whites, the manhunts by English "Christians" in Tasmania and New Zealand, the savagery of the Boer War, the extermination by thirst of the Hereros, for a simple glimpse of what happened near Kemah in 1915. Despite all the efforts at explanation and the addition of factors—pleasure of killing, rapacity, religious hate, despotism, stupidity—so many things remain incomprehensible that the tragedy of 1915 seems to us to be the bloodiest and most disturbing enigma of history. There will always remain an aspect that is unjustifiable and inexplicable, beyond all logic, and this vestige is unbearable.[60]

The reactions of witnesses who should have been the best informed, from 1894 to 1915 and from 1915 to 1942, are particularly incomprehensible. For instance, during the session of the House of Lords during which the Allied declaration of December 1942 was read, Viscount Samuel, "member of the Jewish community," took the floor: "The only events even remotely parallel to this were the Armenian massacres of fifty years ago, at the order of the Sultan Abdul Hamid, which were also carried into effect largely under the cloak of deportation. They aroused the outspoken indignation of the whole of civilized mankind, and they were one of the causes of the downfall of the Turkish Empire."[61] Except that the massacres of 1894–96, under the reign of the Bloody Sultan, were in no way comparable to the extermination of 1915 in terms of either how they took place or their scope. How could two episodes of the tragic saga of the Armenians be confused in this way?

"Why is a man punished when he kills another man, yet the killing of a million is a lesser crime than the killing of an individual?" (Raphael Lemkin)

The Lemkin family was affected by another consequence of the Great War: the Spanish flu. The global epidemic, which was responsible for more deaths than the war, claimed Samuel, Elias and Raphael's brother, in 1919. Raphael thus lived in a pivotal time, even though he reconstructed it in part in his successive accounts. When he studied linguistics and then law, he was passionately interested in crimes committed during World War I and the debates at the time. It was not by chance that he had first chosen to study philology. He was convinced that languages were key to understanding nations and their cultures. Influenced by the eighteenth-century philosopher Johann Gottfried Herder, Lemkin saw Herder's *Volksgeist* as a universal notion of national spirit, characterizing each national people. He deleted all references to other works, such as those by the Russian-born jurist André Mandelstam, who, like him, cross-referenced the tragedies suffered by the Jews of Russia and by the Armenians, and Lord Robert Cecil, who, in 1919, attempted to apply an international perspective to the persecution of peoples and religions. This allowed him to claim an immediate understanding of the facts that conferred a teleological slant on his autobiographical writings, even though some information, read in newspapers and discussed with friends or professors at the University of Lvov, had deeply touched him.[62]

And so, when the British government decided in 1921 to free 150 Turks who had been interned in Malta in 1919, Lemkin reacted: "I was shocked. A nation was killed and the guilty persons were set free. Why is a man punished when he kills another man, yet the killing of a million is a lesser crime than the killing of an individual?"[63] Seeking a legal and conceptual response to this quandary, Lemkin decided to change his orientation from philology to criminal law, which alone, he thought at the time, could be used to punish such specific criminals.

Also in 1921, Talaat Pasha, who had been exfiltrated to Berlin in 1919, was killed there by Soghomon Tehlirian. In Paris in 1926, an almost analogous act took place: Shalom Schwartzbard, a veteran serving in the French Foreign

Legion, executed Simon Petlioura, the general considered to be primarily responsible for the pogroms in Ukraine between 1918 and 1920. Lemkin followed both trials closely, noting that an Armenian and a Jew whose families had been victims of collective crime had taken justice into their own hands in the countries where the criminals had taken refuge, Germany and France. The societies in those countries could neither condemn nor acquit them; in both cases, they were held not responsible for their acts. Lemkin knew nothing about the real role of Schwartzbard, a communist and probably a GPU agent, in the "Jews' vengeance" or that of Tehlirian, an Armenian activist, in Operation Nemesis.[64]

What Lemkin wondered was why the Germans, who knew that Talaat was living in Berlin, had not arrested him. The legalistic answer, state sovereignty, disturbed the young legal scholar, even though it was implicated in the birth of the new Poland: "But sovereignty of states implies conducting an independent foreign and internal policy . . . [and] types of activity directed toward the welfare of the people. [Sovereignty] cannot be conceived as the right to kill millions of innocent people."[65] Lemkin took a moral point of view: the "crimes" of 1921 and 1926 bore a share of "goodness" because they had made it possible to expose the true criminals. This was also the position of the author Joseph Kessel, who attended Schwartzbard's trial:

> For me, his act was a sort of personal cause, as it was for all Jews who have blood running in their veins. . . . There's no doubt that I would never have committed his act, but simply because I lack the courage. . . . When it may be only to draw the attention of the civilized world to the awful tradition of the pogroms—and this could be done only in Paris, the most sensitive point of resonance, the most vibrant in the universe in this respect alone— Schwartzbard had to do what he did. . . . And that is why, whatever fate you reserve for him, I will ask him, when the debates are over, to do me the honor of shaking my hand.[66]

After Tehlirian's trial—he was acquitted in part thanks to testimony by Pastor Johannes Lepsius—Lemkin wrote an article in which he deplored the absence of any international law to standardize moral norms related to the destruction of national, racial, and religious groups.[67] In a 1949 interview for television, he returned to the roots of his work:

I became interested in the concept of genocide because it happened to the Armenians; and after[wards] the Armenians got a very rough deal at the Versailles Conference because their criminals were guilty of genocide and were not punished. . . . A man, [Soghomon] Tehlirian, whose mother was killed in the genocide, killed Talaat Pasha. And he told the court that he did it because his mother came in his sleep . . . many times. Here . . . the murder of your mother, you would do something about it! So he committed a crime. So, you see, as a lawyer, I thought that a crime should not be punished by the victims but should be punished by a court, by a national law.[68]

Lemkin turned from the moral and personal point of view—and it was even more poignant in 1949, for he now knew how his own mother had been exterminated—to that of a criminal lawyer. Weren't the laws written to judge individuals alone? It was a vicious circle. People could not take the law into their own hands no matter how just their cause, and so there was a need for an international statute: "In a rare moment of clarity that seething indignation instills, I further understood the concept of the crime that I was trying to establish."[69]

Contrary to what he stated, Lemkin was not the only one interested in the Armenians. The Germans, in particular, had closely followed the different testimonies and trials of the Weimar years.[70] But, starting in 1933, the memory of the extermination returned in force in Germany, both to the executioners—Hitler often used this example to prophesize the fate of the Jews and to jeer at his contemporaries' lack of memory—and to the Jews, who found analogies in the two situations. In 1933, Victor Klemperer, a cultured intellectual, made a play on words on the barbarian Germanic chieftain Arminius, who had defeated the Romans, and Armenia: "Instead of Germany, one should call it Arminia. This sounds more like Armenia."[71]

1933: Lemkin and the Invention of the "Crime of Barbarity" and the "Crime of Vandalism"

At the time of the Schwartzbard trial, Lemkin, an assistant professor in comparative criminal law, had just been appointed assistant public prosecutor for the district court of Warsaw. In fact, the First Conference for Unification of Criminal Law was held in the Polish capital in 1927 to address the question of global jurisdiction with regard to crimes against human rights.

The ambitious young lawyer, who lived in Warsaw, took advantage of this opportunity to become a contributor to these international conferences.

His name appeared on the conference's program for the first time in 1931, when it was held for the fourth time; he was tasked with reporting on "crimes that create a common danger." He was only thirty-one years old, but his work in collaboration with the most eminent Polish experts on the Polish, Russian, and Soviet criminal and tax codes had been noticed. We must not, however, subscribe to the retrospective intellectual logic that Lemkin asserted for understanding the genesis of his body of work, as experienced legal scholars had been working long and hard on "human rights" since the beginning of the century. During the congresses at The Hague in 1899 and 1907, there had been previous attempts to regulate war and invent peace. The Russian jurist Friedrich Martens, president of the Third Commission, on the laws and customs of warfare, became an advocate of the "Laws of Humanity," in a declaration—which became known as the Martens Clause— reproduced in the preamble to the 1899 Convention:

> Until a more complete code of the laws of war has been issued, the High Contracting Parties think it right to declare that, in cases not included in the Regulations adopted by them, populations and belligerents remain under the protection and empire of the principle of international law, as they result from the usages established between civilized peoples, from the laws of humanity, and the requirements of the public conscience.[72]

"Laws of humanity and requirements of the public conscience."[73] All of this had been largely swept away during the Great War, in particular with regard to invasions, occupations, pogroms, and even extermination when it came to the Armenians and Syriac Christians. New deliberations began under the auspices of the League of Nations. A personal report was commissioned from Lemkin for the Fifth Conference for Unification of Criminal Law, which was to be held in Madrid in 1933. Lemkin began to think about the possibility of a legal framing of crimes against the law of nations; his report was to be a decisive turning point, even though neither he nor his colleagues realized it yet. First, he situated himself with regard to previous conferences, in which the term "terrorism" had been used. In his view, "'Terrorism' does not constitute a legal concept; 'terrorism,' 'terrorists,' 'acts of terrorism' are expressions employed in the daily speech and the press to define a special state of mind among the perpetrators. . . . Neither 'public danger,' nor the political goal of the action, nor 'terrorization' of the population could constitute the main and exclusive criterion to formulate this crime as a crime against human rights." He concluded, "In this state of affairs, we are of the opinion that the creation of a new offence against the law of nations called terrorism would be useless and superfluous."[74] What should be done?

Lemkin's report now took an unprecedented direction. In effect, he proposed to turn the question around: because the problem involved the international nature of the crimes, the international aspects had to be dealt with first:

The provocation of disasters in international communications, the vile destruction of works of art and culture, barbarous actions against a defenseless population, envisaged as crimes against human rights.

a) Provocation of catastrophes in international communication

b) Voluntary interruption of the exploitation of the telegraph, the telephone, post office, and T.S.F.[75]

To accommodate the modernity of the crimes, the law had to be modernized in order to resolve a paradox: communications were at the core of international life, and it was extremely easy to interrupt them. Lemkin was struck by train derailings: "What could be easier than placing on the railway, in a deserted place, stones or other obstacles? It is very difficult to apprehend the author and the consequences are expressed in the deaths of hundreds of innocent victims."[76]

"Innocent victims": Lemkin used the pleonasm as a commonplace. It was at this point that the report, intended to name specific crimes against human rights, struck out in an unprecedented direction with two terms: "vandalism" and "barbarity."

c) The vile destruction of arts and cultural works (*vandalism*)

The destruction of art and cultural works must be considered as the violation of international properties. The author of such a crime causes an irreversible damage, not only to the specific owner of the property and to the state where the act is committed but also to the civilized world which is linked through numerous relations, and therefore benefits from the efforts of *all its citizens, the most industrious*, whose works appropriate everyone's culture and valorize it. . . . Such an act demonstrates not only a highly anti-social behavior, but also a specific *savagery* which puts its author outside the entire *civilized world*.[77]

Lemkin moved from crimes committed by individuals to their consequences for all of humanity. Citing the destruction of libraries as impeding all scholarly work, he proposed that "works of art and culture" be protected in wartime at the same level as Red Cross hospitals. The influence on him of the lexicon of World War I was obvious when he created a link between international humanitarian law based on the Geneva Convention and international criminal law, not without recognizing his debt to Nicholas Roerich, who advocated protection of cultural assets.[78] His debt to the Italian lawyer and professor Vespasian Pella was even greater: Pella had introduced, at the Criminal Conference in Palermo in early 1933, the term "crime of barbarity" and had worked to create an international criminal court.[79] This was Lemkin's fourth, and last, point.

d) *Barbarous* actions

Acts perpetrated against a defenseless population. These include *massacres, pogroms*, collective cruelties against women and children, treatment of humans in a way that *violates their dignity and humiliates them*. In the conception of such crimes, the following elements are considered: 1) the use of violence that proves the antisocial motivations and cruelty of its authors; 2) the systematic and organized action; 3) an action directed not against specific people, but rather against the population or a group of citizens, that is, an action not only collective in its nature but also an action directed against a certain collectivity; 4) the attacked collectivity is defenseless or is weak (in a contrary case, we would have equal or nearly equal chances); 5) the goal can be the intimidation of the population. . . . If these attacks and ferocities are executed in particularly cruel fashion and they manifest themselves in ways that can be characterized as savage, these acts evoke therefore a vivid reaction in conscience of the entire civilized world. The opinion of the entire world despises it and worries about the future of world culture. . . . The person who has participated in such barbarous actions in their country cannot be left in peace and go unpunished on the territory of another state; but the person must be pursued and punished wherever they are found.[80]

Lemkin's stroke of genius in 1933 was to link the two crimes, vandalism and barbarity; up to then, different criminal lawyers had been interested in these "evil acts."[81] What is more, when the proceedings were published, the order of the two crimes was inverted: the "acts of barbarity" went first.

The Acts of Barbarity
    ... There are offences which combine these two elements. In particular these are attacks carried out against an individual as a member of a collectivity. The goal of the author [of the crime] is not only to harm an individual but, also to cause damage to the collectivity to which the latter belongs. Offenses of this type bring harm not only to human rights but also and most especially they undermine the fundamental basis of the social order. . . . Let us consider, first and foremost, acts of extermination directed against the ethnic, religious or social collectivities whatever the motive (political, religious, etc.); for example massacres, pogroms, actions undertaken to ruin the economic existence of the members of a collectivity, etc. . . . Taken as a whole, all the acts of this character constitute an offense against the law of nations which we will call by the name "*barbarity*." . . . The impact of acts like these usually exceed relations between individuals. They shake the very basis of harmony in social relations between particular collectivities.[82]

In his definitive publication, Lemkin passed from "acts of barbarity," to "acts of vandalism," and finally to acts of terrorism against international communications. He also added a fifth and final point, "propagation of human, animal or vegetable contagions."

Acts of Vandalism (Destruction of the culture and works of art)
    The art and cultural heritage in which the unique genius and achievement of a collectivity are revealed in fields of science, arts and literature. The contribution of any particular collectivity to world culture as a whole forms the wealth of all humanity, even while exhibiting unique characteristics. . . . It is also all humanity which experiences a loss by this act of vandalism.[83]

The combined emphasis on the religious and the national—aside from the pogroms explicitly mentioned—probably grew out of the episode of the Chaldo-Assyrians, then under threat in Iraq. In August 1933, two months before the Madrid conference, three thousand Chaldo-Assyrians, who had been unable to establish an autonomous territory in Syria under French mandate, were pushed back to the Simele District and massacred by Iraqi troops led by the Kurdish colonel Bakir Sidqi. Even as the Ottoman Empire disintegrated, the killings continued: the Chaldo-Assyrians exterminated in large numbers during World War I—today, it would be called genocide— were unable to find, any more than the Armenians, a state under the aegis of the great powers at the time of the "peace" treaties, or later at the League of Nations. They continued to be killed.

However, Lemkin was unable to go to Madrid to personally defend his arguments before his colleagues. A few months after Hitler came to power, the Polish government, drawing closer to Germany, could not accept arguments considered anti-German, and Polish anti-Semitic newspapers such as *Gazata Warszaka* quickly denounced Lemkin as working solely for his own Jewish interests. As Poland hardened its anti-Semitic laws, Lemkin was forced to resign from his official positions and turn to private law practice; he was also a Zionist activist alongside his brother Elias, who was hoping to move to Palestine (an idea that he later gave up on).

Lemkin was still participating in international criminal-law conferences, where his colleagues knew him as—or maintained that he was—a lawyer, not a Pole, and even less a Jew. Ironically, he was unable to attend the only conference at which his legal gravitas might have counted—the one in Madrid. Another irony: in 1934, Poland denounced the 1919 treaty on the rights of minorities, of which Jan Karski would be among the early historians, as he studied it for his dissertation, defended at Georgetown University— a Jesuit institution in Washington, DC—when he returned to his political science studies, interrupted by the war.[84]

In 1933, Lemkin went as far as he could down the path of a legal formula linking crimes against individuals who belong to certain collectivities and crimes against cultures. "Considering the contagious character of any social psychosis, actions of this kind ... constitute a *general (transnational) danger.*

Similar to epidemics, they can pass from one country to another."[85] The medicalized vocabulary was typical of the 1930s, when the biologization of thought infected everything, even fierce opponents of the "Brown Plague." Like his contemporaries, Lemkin could not avoid these words even when he was trying to prevent attacks on individuals, including for the purpose of physical and cultural "triage." He was searching for the missing legal link that would make it possible to punish acts beyond the work initiated in The Hague at the beginning of the century. In vain.

No one, at the time, thought that this conceptual innovation should be pursued. Even Lemkin, though he was very active at the Copenhagen conference in 1935, fell back into line; there was a return to the expression "terrorism," discussed in the same terms as before. Yet, wounded by the lack of support for him in 1933, he returned to the subject in the 1950s, noting that the Nazi danger had not been comprehensible at the time. He often said that he had been uniquely prescient: "Many thought Hitler was just rhetoric. They tried to discourage me, they asked me not to continue to predict what seemed to be fantastical events and to formulate laws that were unnecessary, as this had almost never happened in history." Lemkin thought, on the contrary—as a Jew and a Pole—that this type of crime recurred "with almost biological regularity. We cannot close our eyes to it and hide our heads in the sand like ostriches."[86]

In 1944, the *Washington Post* was honest enough to credit Lemkin with the progress in Madrid: "If his proposal had been adopted then, Sir Cecil Hurst and his war crimes commission at the United Nations would not have found it so difficult to define the culpability of the Nazi oppressors."[87] Karski had testified in front of the same commission in 1943: "I told them what I had seen in the Warsaw ghetto and the Belzec death camp. My testimony was placed on record and I was told that it will be used as evidence in the United Nations' indictment against Germany."[88] When would Karski's testimony finally be heard, and why would it take so long? Delays, memory lapses, and camouflage obscured what World War I and World War II had in common.

One contradiction persisted: if the mental universe born of World War I had, in most cases, impeded comprehension of the destruction of the Jews in real time, conversely it contributed to the early clarity of certain observers and people smugglers in Great Britain and the United States, members of the British Parliament, Lemkin, Fry, and Werfel, as well as Rabbi Stephen Wise, a personal friend of President Roosevelt's, whom Karski met in Washington in the summer of 1943. In 1917, Wise wrote to his wife just after German bombs fell on London, where he was staying to attend meetings organized to provide assistance to Jews and Armenians, "What a noble deed the Germans yesterday wrought in London! Why are they bent upon plumbing the utter deeps of infamy? For centuries German will be synonymous with Hun, and worst of all the armor of their self-approval is impenetrable. I am yet to hear about the noon-day meeting for Armenia. If anything they are suffering even worse than the Jews. And I rejoice to think that I am helping them a little. But who can undo the evil done to them?"[89] In 1942, Wise wrote to his friend John Haynes Holmes, a Unitarian pastor who was a civil rights activist and a pacifist, about what was causing him great anguish at the time. "In addition to all your suffering over everything connected with the war, I have something more, namely the uniquely tragic fate of my people. You will be tempted at once to ask, why do I think of it as 'uniquely tragic'? Is it any worse than the fate of the Czechs, or Yugoslavs, or Poles?"[90] Wise went on to give a long description of the murderous *Aktionen* in the Warsaw ghetto.

At the same time, people who were trapped in the ghettos of Poland testified to this very culture rooted in the precedent of 1914–18. Calel Perechodnik related, with the vividness of desperation, that the *Greuelpropaganda* of the Great War had now been largely surpassed. The killing was real: his wife and child had really been loaded onto a train headed for Treblinka.[91] Franz Werfel's powerful novel on the extermination of the Armenians, *The Forty Days of Musa Dagh*, was also read in Poland. The historian Emanuel Ringelblum notes this in his description of the intensity of intellectual life in the ghetto and the frantic interest in World War I:

> Serious readers have a great interest in war literature. They read memoirs, such as Lloyd George's, great novels of the 1914–18 war, and so on. They savor pages dealing with 1918 and the German defeat. They seek comparisons with present times, they seek to prove that the defeat of the invincible German army is near. . . . For my part, I recently reread the great novel by Van der Meersch on the German occupation in France and Belgium. On each page, the comparison is obvious with the current epoch, which is even more terrible than that

of the preceding war. One thing is identical: the pillages and the pitiless, cold oppression of civilian populations in the occupied countries. The population was enslaved and subjected to forced labor, just as it is today. After reading this book, one must ask the question: What was done to forestall a new Hun power in Europe?[92]

The question posed by Ringelblum in the Warsaw ghetto in 1942 was raised again more than two years later in Washington: an important meeting was held at the White House to "discuss the problem of rescuing the Jews still living in Europe" just after the creation of the War Refugee Board, for which Henry Morgenthau Jr., secretary of the Treasury and increasingly critical of the State Department's inaction, had been an advocate. In fact, Morgenthau raised the first point, as he was "convinced that successful action could be taken, referring to the results of his father, Henry Morgenthau Sr., who, as ambassador to Turkey, had successfully gotten Armenians out of Turkey to save them."[93] A few days later, Randolph Paul, who had worked with Morgenthau to establish the Board, recalled that Morgenthau Sr. "had undertaken a similar operation when he was American ambassador to Turkey and had saved numerous Armenians."[94] Indeed, Morgenthau Sr. had done all he could on the ground in 1915–16 and, after he returned to the United States, from 1917 to 1919 to warn his compatriots about the massacres of Christians, Armenians, Greeks, and Syriac Christians. In June 1917, Felix Frankfurter had accompanied him on a US War Department secret mission to persuade the Ottomans to break away from the Central Powers. The mission also had another goal: to find ways to improve the lot of the Jewish community in Palestine, which was in the process of dying of hunger.[95]

We know how things went for the Armenians: there was more talk than action.

The Jews in Europe also had to wait. In March 1944, two months after the meeting in Washington, Ringelblum, who had found refuge in the Christian district of Warsaw, was shot by the Nazis, along with his family and the Poles who had taken them in.

4

∞∞∞

Naming a Nameless Crime

Lemkin and Karski in the
United States, 1943–45

Germany will go down to utter defeat. But the Jews of Europe . . . have no
assurance at present that a United Nations victory will come in time to save
them from complete annihilation.

—Memorandum submitted to the President of the United States by a
delegation of representatives of Jewish organizations, December 8, 1942

A "Conspiracy of Silence"

Jan Karski arrived in the United States on June 16, 1943. With Polish ambassador Jan Ciechanowski as his guide, he was caught up in the political discord
between those who, like him, supported the Polish government in exile and
those who were already envisaging a "free," Sovietized Poland. In 1943, the
Nazi occupiers made public that the Soviets had murdered Polish officers
imprisoned in Katyn in 1940; yet, most of the Allies continued to claim that
the massacre had been perpetrated by the Nazis. The Poles, however—and
first among them Officer Karski, who had been taken prisoner by the Soviets
and managed to escape to enter the resistance—had known the truth for a
long time.

Karski could not get out of his mind what he had seen in the Warsaw
ghetto and Izbica in the summer of 1942: although the Poles were enduring a
horrible occupation, their suffering was not comparable to that of the Jews.
The information in his possession had been sent to the United States by Great
Britain. In June 1943, what revelations could he bring to a country where not
only the leaders of Jewish organizations but the entire government, including

President Roosevelt, had been alerted to the situation in the spring of 1942? Stephen Wise, president of the American Jewish Congress, had been among the recipients of the Riegner telegram sent in August. On November 25, the *New York Times* summarized the report of the Polish government in exile on Belzec, Sobibor, and Treblinka under the headline "Himmler program kills Jewish Poles." On December 7, an encoded telegram labeled "This is of particular secrecy and should be received by the authorized recipient and not passed on" was sent by the British War Cabinet to the American State Department: "Massacres of Jews in Europe: While it is impossible to obtain confirmation of particular incidents or of allegations regarding the existence of a detailed plan for extermination of Jews, we have little doubt that a policy of gradual extermination of all Jews, except highly qualified workers, is being carried out by the German authorities."[1] And yet, the fate of the Jews did not move the Foreign Office except to the extent that "there is considerable public interest here and early action is advisable." No detail on the form of the killings was given.

In early December 1942, President Roosevelt received a long memorandum: twenty pages of details from every European country on the verified extermination of two million Jews by "caravans of Death, deportation . . . mass murder, organized famine, forced labor in disease-infested ghettos, slave-labor reservations . . . mass shootings in orgies of murder, deportation and extermination centers. . . . Germany will be defeated. But the Jews of Europe, whom Hitler has marked out to suffer utter extinction, have no assurance at present that a United Nations victory will come in time to save them from complete annihilation."[2]

And then Chaim Weizmann, president of the World Zionist Organization, declared bitterly in March 1943, "When a future historian assembles the sad history of our time, he will find two incredible things: first, the crime itself; second, the world's reaction to that crime. . . . He will be stunned at the apathy of the civilized world regarding this enormous and systematic massacre of human beings. . . . He will not understand why the world's conscience had to be stirred. Above all, he will not be able to understand why free nations, facing renewed and organized barbarism, had to be begged to grant asylum to the first and main victim of this barbarism. Two million Jews have already been exterminated. The world can no longer claim that these horrible facts are unknown or unconfirmed. . . . We are being destroyed by a conspiracy of silence."[3]

Did Karski, who had arrived in Washington three days before, accompany Ambassador Ciechanowski to a rally in New York on June 19, 1943, "in memory of the 35,000 Jews murdered in the Warsaw ghetto"? There, Shmuel Zygielbojm, the Bund representative for a free Poland based in London, explained that the past offered numerous examples of "black records of violence and persecution" but that "never in the whole history of mankind have its chronicles registered so continuous, so methodical, so iniquitous, so barbarous, so inhuman a system of cruelty and mass extermination."[4] Adolph Held, president of the Jewish Labor Committee, denounced the tragedies and lauded the sacrifices, including Zygielbojm's. The telegram that Zygielbojm had sent to Churchill in December 1942 was poignant but futile. "I address to you and to your government this last appeal of despair. . . . As [a] man who directly represents the unfortunate Jewish population of Poland I convey to you . . . this last appeal for help."[5] A few months later, he committed suicide, as did so many Jewish leaders in Europe. He sent his last will and testament to General Sikorski:

> The latest news that has reached us from Poland makes it clear beyond any doubt that the Germans are now murdering the last remnants of the Jews in Poland with unbridled cruelty. . . . I cannot continue to live and to be silent. . . . My comrades in the Warsaw ghetto fell with arms in their hands in the last heroic battle. I was not permitted to fall like them, together with them, but I belong with them, to their mass grave.
>
> By my death, I wish to give expression to my most profound protest against the inaction in which the world watches and permits the destruction of the Jewish people.
>
> I know that there is no great value to the life of a man, especially today. But since I did not succeed in achieving it in my lifetime, perhaps I shall be able by my death to contribute to the arousing from lethargy of those who could and must act in order that even now, perhaps at the last moment, the handful of Polish Jews who are still alive can still be saved from certain destruction.
>
> My life belongs to the Jewish people of Poland, and therefore I hand it over to them now.[6]

He who had been treated with contempt during his lifetime and considered, including by the Bund, a poor choice for a representative became one of the heroes of the Jewish uprising, celebrated alongside the ghetto fighters. From Poland to London, and in Washington, DC, those who were collecting archives and telling the story were fighting the same battle. The heroic Jewish discourse that would become that of the first remembrance of extermination emerged in real time: "The Jews who died in Warsaw fought the same cause as allied soldiers in Africa and that their feat would 'be resurrected on the pages of future civilized historians.'"[7]

Jan Karski in Washington: Bearing Witness
Deep in the "most powerful nation in the world"

Karski was seen as a "civilized" witness. He "looked as if he had gone through great suffering and hunger and his burning eyes reflect[ed] keen intelligence coupled with childish candor," a "tall, dark young man, of striking appearance,"[8] and he spared no effort to continue what he had started in London. He gave interviews to the press—he was Mr. B in *Collier's*—and met with everyone deemed influential in Washington. Although he knew that he had nothing new to reveal in June, July, and August 1943, he willingly engaged in a new round of meetings. But did seeing, hearing, or reading him mean understanding him? As he had in London, Karski spoke mostly about the resistance and his mission. Yet, his words were not heard except to the extent that they served the purpose of his interlocutors.

For instance, on July 10, 1943, Assistant Secretary of State Breckinridge Long returned from a requiem mass for General Sikorski, who was revered by Karski and who had made sure that he was sent to the United States—and who had just died in a plane crash (an assassination?). Sikorski had been the guest of the Americans; his farewell speech in New York in early 1943 showed that he was hoping—or was it wishful thinking?—for an American-Soviet victory that would not damage democratic Poland, which he envisaged as a member of a "Central European Federation." Sikorski referred once more to 1914–19: "After the victory, we will be faced with the problem of organizing a just, democratic peace, a peace more durable than that of 1919. . . . Under the guidance of President Roosevelt and Prime Minister Churchill the American and British peoples have realized the meaning of these last two world wars. The first one which started in Belgrade in 1914, and the present one launched by an attack of German bombers on Warsaw in 1939. These two world conflicts have proved that it is no such thing as isolation from common dangers and suffering and that real peace is indivisible and touches the world over."[9]

After Sikorski's death, the Americans became increasingly concerned about the abominable relations between the Poles and the Russians, which were the subject of Long's memorandum: "Sikorski's death settles nothing. He was the only one who could heal the rifts among Poles and keep them together as a nation. No one can replace him. The elites are dying by the hundreds in the German concentration camps. Unfortunately, we have obvious proof: the account by resister Jan Karski that the ambassador told us about yesterday evening leaves no doubt of this."[10] Long, notoriously indifferent to the fate of the Jews, was struck only by the fate of the Polish elites.

On July 28, Lieutenant Karski and Polish ambassador Ciechanowski met with the president of the United States in his office. "This was the very citadel of power. I was to meet the most powerful man in the most powerful nation of the world." All this "power" accounted for twenty-one lines in his memoir and fifteen words about the Jews: "He asked me to verify the stories told about the German practices against the Jews."[11] As a refugee in the United States, Karski was cautious. Ciechanowski, however, reported the interview in 1947, when all was lost for the free Poland that they had envisaged. He had resigned so as not to represent a government in communist hands, whence the title of his book, *Defeat in Victory*, in which he made Karski one of his spokespeople in the cold war that was underway. Eleven pages were devoted to the meeting with Roosevelt, which dealt mainly with the organization of the Polish resistance, the future free Poland without a Danzig Corridor, and the negotiations with Stalin on territorial compensation for eastern Prussia. In the rushes for *Shoah*, Karski recounts that the ambassador had given him detailed instructions: "'Now you be careful. You are going to see the most powerful man on this globe. This man evidently is busy. He thinks in terms of the war, of humanity. . . . He thinks after this war the human race will be organised in such a way: no more wars, and he will play a key role in this arrangement. So, again, be brief, be concise.'"[12]

Karski was clear: the Jewish question was only a secondary problem for the president of the United States. Karski saw things the same way at the time, even though he felt some guilt later, especially when Claude Lanzmann pressed him on the extermination of the Jews: "You realize that throughout my entire mission, for me the Jewish problem was not the only problem. For me the key problem was Poland, the Curzon Line, Soviet demands, Communists in the underground movement, fear of the Polish nation. What is going to happen to Poland? This was the emphasis."[13]

Roosevelt, who had read so many reports, wanted to hear a single voice. Karski talked—but less than Roosevelt, who asked questions about the Polish economy and assured him that a solution would be found for eastern Prussia. Karski did not manage to say one word about the Jews; finally, just before the interview ended, he raised the issue. Roosevelt simply made a gesture. "What was the significance of this gesture? Was it a gesture, or was it an expression of good will of the centre of power, who does not deal with particular problems? I still don't know until today."[14]

Roosevelt knew. He didn't need Karski's information. He also knew that he had a war to wage, advisers and ministers with strongly opposed opinions, and Jewish friends, including Supreme Court justice Felix Frankfurter, who were recalcitrant regarding any specific policy for their people. On the other hand, he had a list prepared for Karski of important Jewish figures to meet, including the justice. Neither in Frankfurter's published memoir nor in his handwritten notes is there any mention of his meeting with Karski.[15] Frankfurter was very well informed; he read the same reports as did the president, as well as the news reports, and he was a long-standing friend of Rabbi Stephen Wise, who had informed him of the gassings in September 1942.

Even in 1978 Karski had not forgotten the stereotypes of his childhood when he described Frankfurter: "A little man. He did emanate brilliance. Very alert, his eyes. Unimpressive physically, a little man, Jewish-looking. Very friendly, smiling, towards me all the time friendly."[16]

"No! No!" Frankfurter, who knew, could not "believe" what Karski had seen and was telling him.

AMBASSADOR CZIKANOWSKI: Felix! . . . [Karski's account] was checked and rechecked ten times . . . He is not lying.

FRANKFURTER: I did not say that he is lying. I said that I don't believe him. These are different things. My mind, my heart, they are made in such a way that I cannot accept it. No! No![17]

Karski was not discouraged. On August 9, 1943, he addressed the representatives of Polish Jews in the offices of the World Jewish Congress. These men had been fighting the State Department for months—as their British counterparts had been fighting the Foreign Office—for action, finally, to save European Jews. Two avenues were proposed: to attempt actions in Nazi-occupied Europe and to authorize refugees to move to temporary refugee camps in southern Italy or liberated North Africa.

Karski presented himself as an apostle of truth, an "envoy" in an almost-religious sense of the term:

> I have been asked by the leaders of Polish Jewry to tell you of Jewish sufferings and to inform public opinion of the plight of the Jews in Poland—so that at some later date no one may arise and claim that the world was not aware of the tragedy of the Polish Jewry. I can give you my personal guarantee that everything I report to you now is authentic and true. I speak from personal knowledge as well as from well-authenticated reports given to me. I am ready to testify to the veracity of everything I say under oath.[18]

The messenger repeated the accounts he had given in London: "I have given a report of the Jewish situation in Poland to leaders of the British government as well as to the British Labor movement. . . . They can make no pretense of ignorance of the true state of affairs." He dissected the system of "terror, starvation, ghettos, deportation, extermination," the reports by executioners, victims, and neighbors, and the information that had reached the British and Americans. He went into more personal detail, recounting how he had saved an old friend, a Jewish officer in the Polish army, from the Otwock ghetto; asserting that the Polish were active on the black market; and defending Jewish councils in the ghettos against accusations that they had sent their own people to their death by saying that it was impossible for them to do otherwise. He recalled that many of them—including Zygielbojm[19]— had committed suicide in response to the tragedy.

As a Polish resister, Karski also wanted to preserve the honor of his homeland. Too much so? "Poland has no traitors. We have no Quislings. The Poles know that their country lives and will live on and that only the Polish Government is qualified as the mouthpiece of the Polish People."[20]

One of his interlocutors in London, Ignacy Schwarzbart, would say in 1945 that he had lost all trust in the resistance couriers, "for in none of them, even in Karski, did I feel a heart for the Jews."[21] Yet, Karski remained very clear on the mediocre assistance provided by the Poles to the Jews. If the resistance conducted reprisals against informers, that was because there were in fact informers. "I do not mean to say by this that all Poles have changed their attitude against the Jews, but I can testify that all are opposed to the tortures they are enduring."[22]

Karski noted that Poles who helped Jews risked the death penalty. But he went further than this constantly repeated argument. Yes, Poles were put into forced labor, undernourished, subjected to terror and cruelty, but "they are not murdered outright by the Nazis as are the Jews. . . . At the time when I left Poland, the German terror was still raging. The Jews feel that the situation will become even worse. The Poles are now afraid that Hitler will turn against them and will murder them as he did the Jews. But the Nazis were determined to wipe out the Jews, as a people and as individuals. It was their intention to exterminate them as a race, systematically, without exception. The massacres of Jews that were committed were therefore without historical precedent. It was mass murder, pure and simple."[23]

"It was the murder of the truth: suppression of the notice of murder" (Raphael Lemkin, 1943)

And yet. In Washington in 1943 the same phenomenon occurred as had occurred in London a year earlier. The British, starting with the Foreign Secretary, Anthony Eden, had questioned Karski in order to corroborate their information on the Polish resistance. On both sides of the Atlantic, some thought that all this, which would lead to rescuing the Jews—even if they truly realized that the Jews were the Nazis' main, if not only, target—might compromise the main war effort. It took almost the entire duration of the conflict for this wait-and-see attitude, or even denial, to end—two more long years, during which almost all the Jews in Europe would perish.

Although Karski had accomplished his mission, he had the impression that words remained just words, that neither the Americans nor the British were taking—or wanted to take—the true measure of the crimes. It was for this reason that he decided to write his memoir, *Story of a Secret State*, the main subject of which was his Poland and its resistance. But it was when he was describing the fate of the Jews that he used the words "annihilate," "wipe out," "exterminate," "massacre," and "mass murder."

In his personal archives are pamphlets that he referred to while writing his memoir, all of which speak first of the fate of Catholic Poles. One is *Oswiecim Camp of Death*, published in Polish in 1942 and translated into English in February 1944. After forty pages devoted to the fate of the Poles in the main concentration camp, Oswiecim, an appendix gives a mapped typology of the hundred concentration camps scattered around Poland; it shows "camp districts," "temporary concentration camps," and "general concentration camps," including the largest one, Oswiecim, "recently greatly expanded by . . . [a] *'camp of death'*" (emphasis added; though not named, this was Birkenau), as well as camps situated in Germany (Dachau, Mathausen, Ravensbrück, and others) in which Poles were imprisoned. Also listed were "forced labor camps," "concentration camps for clergy," "camps for 'improvement of the race,'" "camps for 'correction of youth,'" and "concentration camp for children, so-called 'educational institutes.'" Between the camps for clergy and those for "improvement of the race" appears the category "Concentration Camps for Jews":

> These camps have been established in conjunction with the Nazi campaign to liquidate the European Jews. Some of them are simply places of execution where Jews from Poland and the rest of Europe are asphyxiated, electrocuted, and machine-gunned. The most notorious of these are:
>   Belzec
>   Sobibor, near Wlodawa
>   Tremblinka [*sic*] III
>   Six other camps for Jews are located in:
>   Starogard II
>   Potulice III
>   Kosow Podlaski
>   Trawniki
>   Pomiechowek II
>   Between Chelm and Wlodava (the name could not be ascertained)
>   In these camps, too, the Jews are murdered, but mostly by starvation, disease, torture, and forced labor.[24]

The information was detailed, and the distinctions were well described. But there was a concept missing, a word that did not yet exist, a word that Raphael Lemkin was looking for at exactly the same moment.

In fall 1943, Karski was cited by leaders in the Treasury Department who were in favor of taking action against the "timorousness"—an understatement— of the State Department. Indeed, the small group working around Treasury Secretary Henry Morgenthau Jr. to establish the War Refugee Board was devastated: "Mr. Cox: . . . In the first place this is a problem which we have gotten facts on. It covers all of occupied Europe. . . . German policy has been clearly one of extermination of the Jews, complete and final, and we have talked to people from the Polish underground, who also, incidentally, have talked to the president about that firsthand observation. . . . Unless you get effective action . . . many of these people are turned back. . . . It means certain death as far as the Germans are concerned. . . . Now, the President has heard that fellow, Karski, who came out of the Polish underground. He knows what is happening there."[25] This verbatim account underlines that President Roosevelt was affected by what Karski had had to say, even though he did not decide to renounce his wait-and-see approach.

The British, who did not want to put undue stress on their strategy in Mandatory Palestine, blocked Jewish emigration as of 1939. Morgenthau and his advisers could not have criticized this move more harshly—to the point that they were comparing the British policy to that of the Nazis.

> Mr. Paul: I said that there isn't any difference between the British position, as you have described it there, and the German position. If anything, the Germans are somewhat more merciful. They proceed much more rapidly. How can we ever accuse the Germans of cruelty to these Jews in Europe when we decree the same sort of death, or a more lingering death for them?
>
> Mr. Dubois: . . . There is a group of Jews the Germans are not killing, and that is the group who have visas for Palestine. They are specifically setting them aside in camps so after the war, they can say that the United Nations were just as much to blame as Germany: "Here is a group of Jews who had visas for Palestine whom we were willing to let out, and they would not let them come out."[26]

A plan formulated by the World Jewish Congress was considered: find the financial means to help neutral countries that would take in exfiltrated Jews by making payments to the Nazis. "Extraordinary measures to take to save the Jews of Hungary," deported in 1944, were now sought. Karski's testimony was evoked once again:

> He expressed his conviction that it would be possible to gain agreement from the German government to release a considerable number of Jews:
>
>   a) If a certain number of countries declared themselves prepared to receive them;
>
>   b) If a large ransom were paid to the German authorities. The catastrophe that is befalling the Hungarian Jews pushes us to resort to methods as extraordinary as those suggested by Mr. Karski and the Jewish leaders in Slovakia.[27]

Karski was well aware of the appalling corruption of the Nazis and their henchmen in Poland. But the State Department was not planning to offer extra visas or to become involved in the corruption of rescue for ransom. Giving money to the enemy seemed neither politically nor morally acceptable.

Could large-scale immigration to Turkey or Iran be organized, with the Jews returning when "Europe was purged of Hitler"?[28] But how, after the war, would survivors be able to return to their countries purged of Jews? Or should transit camps be opened in zones where the Americans had landed: North Africa—which the French and de Gaulle were blocking—Sicily, southern Italy, Sardinia? All these proposed solutions came to naught.

It was then that two of the most senior executives at the US Treasury Department, Randolph Paul and John Pehle, seriously challenged the State Department and Assistant Secretary Breckinridge Long. In their *Report to the Secretary on the Acquiescence of this Government in the Murder of the Jews*, they wrote, "Since the time when this Government knew that the [European] Jews were being murdered [summer 1942], our State Department has failed to take any positive steps reasonably calculated to save any of these people."[29]

The Treasury Department moved from observation to attack: those who did not act were guilty of complicity in murder. The executives at the State Department had, in effect, falsified the statistics on immigration to the

United States: "The most glaring example of the use of the machinery of this Government to *actually prevent the rescue of Jews* is the administrative restrictions which have been placed upon the granting of visas to the United States."[30] The tenacious Long had continually lied about the number of Jewish refugees accepted into the country in order to make the president believe that the country was concerned with their fate.[31]

The highly detailed report of errors since 1942 was unusually forceful: "If men of the temperament and philosophy of Long continue in control of immigration administration, we may as well take down that plaque from the Statue of Liberty and black out the 'lamp beside the golden door.'"[32] The Secretary of the Treasury, Henry Morgenthau, sent another secret report. The pressure became too great: on January 22, 1944, the War Refugee Board was created. The very name is striking: even though it was known that Jews were the refugees involved, it was only war refugees in general that were mentioned.

More than a year after Karski's visit to the White House and six months after the creation of the War Refugee Board, President Roosevelt reaffirmed the principles proclaimed by the Allies since the signature of the Atlantic Charter: win the war, punish its instigators: "Please express to those gathered at the meeting to protest the *deportations and cruelties* visited upon the *remaining Jewish community* of Europe my feelings of abhorrence of these desperate acts of the enemy. I repeat to all concerned my earlier warning that those who participate in *these acts of savagery* shall not go unpunished."[33] This message proves once more the president's cynicism—or realism?—with regard to the specificity of the war being waged against the Jews. He knew; he knew everything: "the remaining Jewish community of Europe," "deportations and cruelties," "acts of savagery." But he did not say the word "extermination." At what point did silence, restraint, and prudence become complicity? This was what Lemkin was wondering, too.[34]

Lemkin Confronting Denial: Finding the Words

"Data compiled by Dr. Raphael Lemkin when he was on the faculty in Stockholm, Sweden and at Duke University, North Carolina, then as consultant for the Board of Economic Warfare."[35] When Lemkin arrived in Washington, his experience of occupied Europe was validated, but his 1933 conceptualization, "crimes of barbarity and vandalism," was not. He felt totally abandoned: not only were the Jewish people in the process of "disappearing from Earth," as Hitler had prophesized, but the Allies were participating indirectly in the crime by their procrastination.

Lemkin was absolutely determined to meet with President Roosevelt, who he felt was lacking information. To his dismay, he was allowed only a brief memorandum: "How could I compress the pain of millions, the fear of nations, the hope for salvation from death onto one page?"[36] Then, it was weeks before advisers responded that he had to be patient. Mortified that neither President Roosevelt nor Vice President Wallace, for whom he was working directly, had perceived the urgency of the situation, his sense of foreboding grew: "'Patience' is a good word for when one expects an appointment, a budgetary allocation, or the building of a road. But when the rope is already around the neck of the victim and strangulation is imminent, isn't the word 'patience' an insult to reason and nature?"[37] He was shattered to discover that "this was a conflict not between the Jewish people and the German, but between the world and itself":

> The impression of a tremendous conspiracy of silence poisoned the air. There was no escape from this feeling. . . . A double murder was taking place. One committed by the Nazis and the other by the Allies. Were the Allies refusing to make it known that the execution of nations and races had already begun? . . . The silence of murder started the day the first reports of mass executions reached London from Warsaw late in 1942. It lasted until December 1944, almost two years. No acknowledgment was made of the death of a nation that had given the world the belief in one God, whose Bible was still read every day in the Allies' churches. It was the murder of the truth: suppression of the notice of murder.[38]

"A dog run over by a car upsets our emotional balance and digestion; three million Jews killed in Poland cause but a moderate uneasiness. Statistics don't bleed; it is the detail which counts." (Arthur Koestler)

Lemkin and Karski were not the only ones to express the idea that the complicity of silence also meant complicity in murder. For instance, Samuel Golfard said, shortly before he was murdered in a Polish ghetto, "The Germans are not alone guilty of our tragic fate. The English and the Americans who tolerated the acts of the German nation are also guilty. They fattened Hitler and nurtured the present regime in Germany."[39] Once the war was over, in 1948, Isaac Schneersohn—the French Emanuel Ringelblum, founder in April 1943 of the Centre de documentation juive contemporaine, secret at the time, in Grenoble—expressed the same despair in his recollections:

> The nations that were to defeat Germany did nothing to top its barbaric madness against the Jews. They allowed it; they stayed quiet. They did not use reprisals. They later feigned that they had been unaware of the excesses of these crimes. An unacceptable excuse when one thinks of the sources of information of all sorts that the wartime secret services were providing to them. . . . The Allies opposed nothing. When the political assault against Europe became an assault against the essential principles of modern humanity, they undertook no counterattack. They never thought to make good use of their advantages, as their victory advanced and the Germans began to weaken, to break the only front on which the latter continued to win and to persevere even more desperately: the Jewish front.[40]

On February 7, 1943, an article of rare invective appeared in the *New York Times*, written by an author who had been living in the United States for a long time, Sholem Asch. If the unusual length of the article did not catch the reader's eye, the drawing of a swastika crushing a landscape empty of people but populated by scavenging crows in flight certainly would.

"In the Valley of Death. That valley is the scene of Hitler's mass murder." Asch described Polish ghettos and extermination camps, "dumping ground and a clearing house"; the Jews of Europe were transported there in "sealed, unventilated, lime freight cars which are death traps" (Asch had read Karski). "Those that survive become as human waste to be thrown into mass-slaughter houses which the Nazis had created for all Jews. These houses of death consist of gas chambers and blood-poisoning stations. . . . Regardless of origin, age, or sex, all are being killed." Following were accounts of the extermination of children and adults in three health-care and charitable institutions that Asch had visited before the war in Warsaw, including Dr. Korczak's orphanage. Asch not only described the killing of all the Jews by the Nazis; he also searched for their friends and excluded no member of the human community:

When I think of the state to which Hitler has brought humanity, I am disturbed by one thought: after all, Hitler belongs to the human race and so do the other Nazis. They were accepted as a part of us, I daresay a part of the system in which we are living. They are not a cause, they are the results of our behavior, of our psychology. . . . Never would Hitler have dared to select a people for annihilation had not the way been prepared for him by all kinds and degrees of anti-Semites. A person's constitutional rights are secure only when his social standing in a community is secure. If a people is singled out for hatred, as a group, if the fact of just belonging to this group is considered enough to count as a crime, that people loses, in the eyes of its persecutor, the dignity and mysticism in the eyes of a human being. . . . All who have prepared this ground of hatred toward the Jews and other races are exactly as responsible for the bestial slaughter of the Jews in Poland and others as Hitler and his clique. . . . Hitler only gathers the fruits of their well-planted seeds.[41]

In January 1944, Arthur Koestler, also infuriated, published an article in the English and American press, illustrated in the *New York Times* with a drawing of Hitler and Himmler calmly conversing in front of a scene of hanged people and piles of cadavers: "It is the greatest mass-killing in recorded history; and it goes on daily, hourly, as regularly as the ticking of your watch." Increasingly desperate, Koestler returned to what he had said in 1942. He set the number of deaths at three million—and yet he was far from the actual count—as he contemplated a double-sided nightmare: on the one side the reality of the atrocities and on the other side the refusal of the English and the Americans to see it. Koestler placed himself among the "screamers," those who yelled as they unveiled photographs, films, books, witnesses—nothing was missing, and yet nothing changed, despite the insane risks taken by the "resisters who came from Poland." Then, "Nine out of ten average American citizens, when asked whether they believed that the Nazis commit atrocities, answered that it was all propaganda lies, and that they didn't believe a word of it! . . . [It is the same in England.] They don't believe in concentration camps. They don't believe in the starved children of Greece, in the shot hostages of France, in the mass graves of Poland; they have never heard of Lidice, Treblinka, or Belzec." Were the screamer-messengers as certain that they would lose the game as the "prophets of the Old Testament" or "Cassandra"?[42]

Koestler offered an explanation: "In reality both 'knowing' and 'believing' have varying degrees of intensity." It is easier to believe what is close in time and space and what one is capable of integrating.[43] Faced with the absoluteness of Nazi crimes, people remained speechless. "A dog run over by a car upsets our emotional balance and digestion; three million Jews killed in Poland cause but a moderate uneasiness. Statistics don't bleed; it is the detail which counts. [This sentence was taken from the mouth of his protagonist, fashioned after Karski, in his 1943 novel *Arrival and Departure*.] We are unable to embrace the total process with our awareness; we can only focus only on little lumps of reality. . . . When we approach the sphere of the Absolute, our reaction ceases to be a matter of degrees."[44] What to do? Think specifically about the murders. Koestler took the example of a British lecturer—the publisher Victor Gollancz, who had been so upset by his meeting with Karski in 1942—who imagined what the victims had suffered: "One day he tried to feel what it was like to be suffocated by chloride gas in a death-train; another day he had to dig his grave with two hundred others and then face a machine gun."[45] Koestler recommended that newspaper readers undertake such an exercise for two minutes every morning to break through their oblivious normalcy.

As some accurately described the mass murder of European Jews by the Nazis and accused the Allies of inaction and public opinion of being complicit in the silence, others sought the underlying causes, starting with anti-Semitism. Raphael Lemkin chose to take both paths to try to tear the Jews away from their executioners. He directly addressed the American people—and, beyond them, the world—to break the "conspiracy of silence" in a book, *Axis Rule in Occupied Europe: Laws of Occupation, Analysis of Government, Proposals for Redress*. He reported on the sacking of all of Europe and the exterminatory exactions, proposed concepts to explain them, and expressed his wish for a quick turn to action. Lemkin sought words, the word, to describe this form of violence that was both "ancient" and so contemporary.

"How strange that I was among both the mourners and the dead" (Raphael Lemkin, 1943): Toward the "Genocide Pact"

Since the 1920s, and especially since the advent of the paired "crime of barbarity"/"crime of vandalism" in 1933, Lemkin had become an activist—

a soldier for his cause—in the debate that had raged since the invention of his concept: what is a genocide? Or, rather, what are genocides? For the plural was obvious to him, but because the word was coined by a Polish Jew in 1943, it was quickly assimilated with the Genocide (with a capital G) of the Jews. This is a mistake, if one analyzes his writings. Lemkin blurred comprehension of his work by predating his invention, referring only to the legal concept even as he made himself the historian of his own life. He was Jewish, a member of a national minority that the League of Nations, for which he had worked so hard to standardize international criminal law, had not been able to protect. He had become a victim of the concept that he had theorized. Although he probably created the word "genocide" in the name of dead Jews—his own—he was convinced that he could mourn as an individual only on behalf of all humanity. And so, he reconstructed his final days in Poland with his family and other inhabitants of the shtetls, which he described in his autobiography: "It was like going to their funeral while they were still alive. The best of me was dying with the full cruelty of consciousness."[46]

> During the war, forty-nine members of my family perished from genocide, including my parents. . . . Suddenly I felt that the earth is receding under from under my feet and the sense of living is disappearing. I transformed my personal disaster into a powerful moral force. . . . Was it not the best form of gratitude for my mother, who had awakened me to the idea of these persecutions, to engrave "genocide pact" as an epitaph on her symbolic gravestone to ensure that she and millions of others had not died in vain? I decided to make this law my strength, and to make my work a respite from my sorrow.[47]

Horrified by his own apocalyptic visions, Lemkin told many morbid stories in which he depicted himself, traumatized, in the place of all victims: "I myself am living in a procession of the afflicted, following the bodies of dead nations. Strange that I was among both the mourners and the dead. Strange to feel my living body as my soul was taking to its grave. . . . All over Europe the Nazis were writing the book of death with the blood of my brethren."[48] In his papers was a profession of faith, *This I Believe*, in which he proclaimed his faith in a law opposing inhumanity in almost mystical terms. Although he used the word "genocide" in this essay, indicating that it was written after 1943, he dated this description of his flight across Poland to 1939–40:

In the forest, I pronounced to the dead and to the living that if I survive I will devote the rest of my life exclusively to outlawing genocide. I reviewed my history through memories of my eyes. I believe that memory stimulates conscience. Looking at the stars, I asked myself . . . The same sun shone . . . over the [illegible] of the Huguenots before the night of St. Bartholomew's, shone on the Catholics in Japan in the seventeenth century, and shone over Warsaw, where neighbors from the frontier came to kill my people. Sameness, oneness, but yet no recognition of the place of the component parts in mankind. . . . The words of love must be spoken, although it fills the heart with serene silence. . . . [Doing] constructive work while bombs [are] destroying the forests fully and dying trees crying over groaning of man. Two beliefs from forest: 1) Realization of parts to be allotted by law so they may not be destroyed. 2) Belief in ultimate victory of constructiveness over the destructiveness. The lesson of the arts.⁴⁹

Lemkin, the intellectual, kept his impulses to himself, even though he knew how to transition in his public writings from the personal to the universal, in both present and past: "History provides us with other examples of destruction of national, ethnic, and religious groups. The destruction of Carthage; those of religious groups during Islamic wars and during the Crusades; the massacres of the Albigensians and the Waldensians."⁵⁰ But, he also affirmed, genocide is "a modern crime," and he reduced his field of application to the twentieth century and the two genocides that had taken place during his lifetime: those of the Armenians and the Jews, to whom he added the Gypsies. For the rest of his life, he would be faced with this quandary: whether to make genocide a spatially and temporally universal concept or to limit it to the contemporary. If the latter, the "crime of crimes" would be punished in the present in the name of the recent past and prevented in the future thanks to the "law of laws," in parallel with the humanitarian and legislative progress of the nineteenth and twentieth centuries.

The concept gestated over an extensive time and space, the 1920s and 1930s in Europe, but was invented specifically in the United States in 1943, when Lemkin wrote chapter 9 of his *Axis Rule*, titled "Genocide." Once the book was published, in 1944, the concept passed into the public domain: it was commented on, critiqued, and escaped its inventor, who undertook an international lobbying effort for its recognition at the Nuremberg court—in vain—then for its legitimization by the United Nations: committees, com-missions, amendments, votes, rejection. Although both the concept and its inventor were growing in influence, Lemkin was also dispossessed of his initial project. It was therefore difficult to establish who thought what about genocide, including Lemkin himself.

For Lemkin was acting with a tenacity approaching obsession, capitalizing on his credentials as a legal scholar and his participation in the prewar ses-sions on the standardization of international criminal law. To better attract and convince his interlocutors, he presented himself as Polish, Jewish, a Polish Jew, an American, an immigrant, or a friend of Armenians and thus of Christians. At the very time when he was inventing his concept, his beloved mother was murdered. "Genocide hit his family home."[51] His accounts always began with his mother, who made him read Henryk Sienkiewicz's *Quo Vadis* when he was very young.[52] That book would serve the cause that Lemkin opportunistically reconstructed in the 1950s: his extremely precocious inven-tion of the concept leading to the word "genocide." Sienkiewicz was Polish, and he described the fate of Christians "collectively sentenced to death for no reason except that they believed in Christ. And no one could help them."[53] He received the international recognition of the Nobel Prize for Literature in 1905, and the blockbuster movie adaptation premiered around the world in 1951.

The Creation of a Barbarism: Genocide

Lemkin built the argument of *Axis Rule* around an analysis of "German techniques of occupation," culminating with the chapter "Genocide." His compilation of European laws under Nazi domination was particularly remarkable given that he was working in Sweden until 1941 and then in the United States. This did not keep him from reading everything about what was happening, as the war never cut off the flow of information, notably via the neutral powers.

If the table of contents, from chapter 1, "Administration," to chapter 7, "Labor," seemed banal for the study of the occupation, chapter 8, "The Legal Status of the Jews," singled out in four pages their fate deriving from the statute adopted in Nuremberg in 1935: "The treatment of the Jews in the occupied countries is one of the most flagrant violations of international law, not only of specific articles of the Hague Regulations, but also of the principles of the law of nations as they emerged from usage among civilized nations, from the laws of humanity, and from the dictates of the public conscience."[54] The last sentence of chapter 8, introducing chapter 9, noted, "The Jews being one of the main objects of German genocide policy, their particular situation in occupied Europe has been additionally treated in the chapter on genocide."[55]

At the moment when the word "genocide" was offered to the world for the first time, there was no ambiguity: it referred to Jews. Or, more exactly, to Jews as a group. Lemkin brought together the different forms of belonging to Judaism—paradoxically, in the way envisaged both by the Nazis, to better hunt down and exterminate them, and by Jews themselves, particularly Zionists, for whom this group constituted a people. Yet, after singling out Jews as specific victims of the Germans, Lemkin combined them with other European peoples under Nazi tyranny, group by group.

> *New conceptions* require new terms. By "genocide" we mean the *destruction of a nation or of an ethnic group*. . . . Generally speaking, genocide does not mean the immediate destruction of a nation, except when accomplished by *mass killings* of all members of a nation. It is intended rather to signify a *coordinated plan* of different actions aiming at the destruction of essential foundations of the life of national groups, with the aim of annihilating the groups themselves. The objectives of such a plan would be *disintegration of the political and social institutions, of culture, language, national feelings, religion, and the economic existence of national groups, and the destruction of personal security, liberty, health, dignity, and even the lives* of persons belonging to such groups.[56]

Lemkin reflected on the targeted groups and the individuals who composed them, and on those who targeted them; such a plan could be "coordinated" only at the national level. This violence, flowing from a deliberate policy, presumed intention and preparation and was identified with different acts of persecution and destruction that ultimately formed a whole: genocide. The word was composed of two parts: the people or ethnic community targeted, *genos*, and that which kills, *occidere*. By combining a Greek and a Latin root, Lemkin, an excellent linguist, deliberately built a semantic monster, a barbarism, to express the barbarity of barbarities, the "crime of crimes." In fact, it was no longer possible for him to use the German term *Völkermord*, as he had for the extermination of the Hereros and Armenians, for German was the language of the annihilators of his parents, their culture, and their language, Yiddish. However, the adoption of his invention in Polish, *ludobojtwo* (murder of a people), in a note by the government in exile, must have gone straight to the patriot's heart.

Some of the documentation presented in *Axis Rule* in 1944 was dated, however, as Lemkin had begun to think about the texts he had gathered before he left Sweden in 1941. He said so clearly when he sent his work to the War Refugee Board on April 14: progress on the book was already quite advanced, and he thought that it would be useful to the committee created several months before. However, it was his 1942 compilation of laws that he sent,[57] not his list for the book, although the two had some texts in common, and so the word "genocide" did not appear in it. Were these documents from 1941 and 1942 useful to the War Refugee Board in its frantic struggle to avoid the massive deportation of Hungarian Jews in 1944?

Lemkin also collected laws and declarations on the separation and "legal" persecution of Jews, published in the form of posters or leaflets aimed at occupied populations. Nothing that was secret—the trial and error and experiments with extermination—appeared in his compilation, because this was in fact not a legal matter.[58]

Here is an example of the laws collected by Lemkin for the case of Yugoslavia:

Anti-Jewish Legislation
    AN ORDER concerning Sheltering of Jews, of December 24, 1941. (Verordnungsblatt des Militärbefehlshabers in Serbien, No. 27, 1941, p. 196.) . . .
    Section 1—Any person who
    a) shelters or hides Jews
    b) accepts (from Jews) for safekeeping objects of value of any description, furniture, and money, or acquires them by way of purchase, barter, or any other transaction shall be punished by death.[59]

If Lemkin was working in this way, through accumulation, it was because he wanted to start on the basis of occupation laws and thus on what still formed, in appearance at least, the undergirding of a "law of war": the Hague Conventions, the idea of law of nations, the Geneva Convention for International Humanitarian Law. But the Nazi war aimed to transform European demography as a whole—to Germanize it—while destroying or enslaving other peoples. What was acquired through prolonged occupation would be perpetuated whatever the outcome of the war: "Their general plan consisted of *winning the peace*, even if the war was lost, and this goal could be obtained by permanently reversing the European political and demographic balance in favor of Germany. . . . They were very close to achieving their goal in terms of extermination of Jews and Gypsies in Europe."[60]

"Winning the peace": that is what the Young Turks had done by wiping out the Armenians in their Anatolian homeland and replacing them with Turks. The Nazis, for their part, exterminated the Polish Jews and their world, the *Yiddishkeit*. Lemkin's "winning the peace" dovetailed with two categories established by today's genocide researchers: that of the "frenzy of the victors" in 1941–42 during the murders by gunfire in the Soviet Union and that of the "triumph of the defeated" when, as the war was about to be lost, the Nazis made the killing system even more efficient—for instance, exterminating four hundred thousand Hungarian Jews at Birkenau in summer 1944—even as the older methods continued to be used until May 1945.[61]

But—and this was behind the ambiguities of the concept—Lemkin did not reserve the term specifically for Jews. The Poles, the national and religious majority, were also described as victims of genocide. Lemkin contradicted himself twice: he based his concept on all the crimes of mass murder in history even as he said it was a "modern" crime, and he universalized it even as he dwelled upon the primary victims, the Jews.

Lemkin's Campaign: From 1944–45 to 1914–18

"Dr. Raphael Lemkin, distinguished Polish jurist, economist, authority on international law, author and traveler, will tell of his experiences of World War I and II tonight at the Woman's National Democratic Club."[62]

In the United States, Lemkin explained the coherence of the "thirty-year war": in his country-by-country analysis of the occupation of Europe, he took his readers to the occupied territories of World War I—the deportations, the forced labor, particularly in Belgium. Indeed, he had been informed of the situation of civilians in these countries by his Belgian friends and colleagues encountered during international conferences. In 1939, he had thought of moving there; by 1940, this had become impossible.

The Nazi desire in 1940 to repair the consequences of World War I provided Lemkin with a link between the occupation policies instituted during the two conflicts. The 1914–18 precedent was central to his demonstration—particularly the case of Belgium, where an order was issued for the "restitution of the rights of persons persecuted . . . because of their collaboration with the German Army of Occupation during the war of 1914–18."[63] In effect, the Nazis wanted to wipe clean the legal slate of those who had collaborated between 1914 and 1918 and were sentenced in the 1920s. Whence the annulment—in the name of German honor—of legal decisions made by the Belgian state to punish acts of collaboration—deemed uncivil—after 1918. The Nazis ruled that "Wrong demands restitution. In the war of 1914–1918, inhabitants of this country tried to adopt a loyal attitude toward the German Army of Occupation and to obey its rules. For this they were persecuted by the state and certain sections of the population. They suffered penalties of death, hard labor, and imprisonment. . . . At that time, as today, these regulations had to be enforced just as did the Belgian laws. And so the persecuted people were acting in a way that was by no means unlawful."[64] As the new rulers of Belgium, Lemkin opined, they wanted to go even further, "[trying] to disintegrate Belgium by creating and exaggerating differences between the Belgians and the Flemings [*sic*], and the latter collaborating with Germany were given special privileges."[65]

Lemkin had access to the works of American legal scholars such as James Garner, who concluded from the Belgian archives that in 1917 the United States had joined the "good camp," that of the law, in this war of laws. Conversely, in 1914 the Germans had begun a war of atrocities, counter to the values of humanity and international law; the deportations of civilians from the occupied country proved it:

> By tearing away from nearly every humble home in the land a husband and a father or a son and brother, they have lighted a fire of hatred that will never go out. . . . [It] will impress its horror indelibly on the memory of three generations, a realization of what German methods mean, not, as with the early atrocities, in the heat of passion and the first lust of war, but by one of those deeds that make one despair of the future of the human race, a deed coldly

planned, studiously matured, and deliberately and systematically executed, a deed so cruel that German soldiers are said to have wept in its execution, and so monstrous that even German officers are now said to be ashamed.[66]

The forced labor imposed twice on the occupied populations of Belgium and northern France were of particular interest to Lemkin. In chapter 7 of *Axis Rule*, titled "Labor," he quoted General Erich Ludendorff in 1917 to explain the Nazis' choices in 1942:

"The existence of a large mass of unemployed labor is a danger to public safety. With a view to averting that danger, men may be sent compulsorily to any place where they are needed; whether at home or abroad is immaterial."[67] . . . By deporting millions of able-bodied men and women from the occupied countries, Germany moreover hopes to disrupt centers of political resistance . . . and . . . by separating families and keeping the men far away from their homes, a policy of depopulation is being pursued.[68]

The 1914–18 period was used as an argument. At that time, the laws of war and occupation were violated—the Germans were not the only ones to do so—and, especially, the innovation of which World War II was the extreme consequence was introduced. The battle was waged not only on men wearing uniforms who might be protected by international humanitarian law when they were out of combat, wounded, or taken prisoner. Civilians were at the center of the conflict, physically, in reality, and in propaganda. And yet, international humanitarian law did not cover them. Not yet. Lemkin differentiated between groups "selected" for who they were and "collateral victims," who found themselves in the wrong place at the wrong time:

When, in 1918, a German shell fell on Église Saint-Gervais in Paris, a large number of people belonging to a specific religious group were destroyed. Yet although this was a war crime (because civilians were killed), it did not constitute an act of genocide, as it did not involve the destruction of a specific category of civilians; there was no selection of the victims.[69]

Departing in an original way from his contemporaries, Lemkin wanted both to invalidate the propaganda and rumors of the Great War and to observe the new forms of violence. Although numerous doubts subsisted regarding the "German atrocities," the occupations and forced labor in Belgium and northern France, the pogroms against the Jews in Russia and Poland, and the extermination of the Armenians had actually taken place, even in the opinion of the most skeptical.

Yet, paradoxically, Lemkin put aside the extreme violence against civilians that he knew the best, that against the Jews of Eastern Europe and the Armenians of the Ottoman Empire, at the very moment when he launched his campaign for recognition of the word "genocide," between 1944 and 1946. He retained only the military and occupation violence of 1914–18, returning in a classic way to the Great War.

In 1945, Lemkin wrote to Robert Jackson, who had just been appointed prosecutor of the Nuremberg Trials, to offer his services to the Americans in two ways: participating in the prosecution and judgment of Nazi criminals and making his new concept central to the court. He was in fact engaged as an expert by the American team, but he went to Nuremberg only occasionally, as he was confined to Washington, DC, most of the time to prepare documentation for the Office of Strategic Services (the forerunner of the CIA) and its War Crimes Office. Although he knew a number of influential figures, few of them considered him, whether for good reasons—he was very individualistic, sharing little with the team—or, above all, for bad ones: the highest-profile lawyers at the time were thinking mainly in terms of war crimes until Hersch Lauterpacht's "crimes against humanity" concept was adopted, and not in terms of genocide. Yet, Lemkin was strongly committed to his concept. He wrote to Jackson, "I am taking the liberty of sending you my article 'Genocide.' This article contains a statement by the recently captured Marshal von Rundstedt . . . that points to the particular responsibility of this man as a major war criminal."[70]

Why was Lemkin so interested in von Rundstedt? Because at the time he was charged only with "criminality of groups and criminal organizations." Lemkin wanted to see him charged differently, for the archives left no doubt about his participation in the "crime of genocide." Indeed, he had "approved and transmitted to his troops" a document by Walter von Reichenau, on October 10, 1941: "The most essential aim of war against the Jewish bolshevistic system is a complete destruction of their means of power and the elimination of Asian influence from the European culture. . . . The soldier in the eastern territories is not merely a fighter according to the rules of war but also a bearer of ruthless national ideology. . . . Therefore the soldier must have full understanding for the necessity of a severe but just revenge on subhuman Jewry."[71]

Lemkin returned yet again to World War I in his description of von Rundstedt "aping the Fuhrer": "'One of the great mistakes of 1918 was to spare the civil life of the enemy countries, for it is necessary for us Germans to always be at least double the numbers of the peoples of the contiguous countries. We are therefore obliged to destroy at least a third of their inhabitants. The only means is organized underfeeding, which in this case is better than machine guns.'"[72]

Lemkin presented the Nazis as capable of conceptualizing depopulation through the indirect extermination brought about by hunger or murder because of their experience in World War I, their heritage, their mental universe. "Hitler was right. The crime of the Reich in wantonly and deliberately wiping out whole peoples is not utterly new in the world. It is new only in the civilized world as we have come to think of it. It is so new in the traditions of civilized man that he has no name for it. It is for this reason that I took the liberty of inventing the word 'genocide.'"[73]

Lemkin had an encyclopedic knowledge of Nazi Germany that was very valuable to the prosecutors. This was why, in 1942, he was hired by the Board of Economic Warfare, an extension of the War Trade Board formed during World War I. Vice President Wallace, who led the board, was also convinced that the new world after 1918 had not been well understood, and he might have supported Lemkin. But he came into permanent conflict with the State Department, and Lemkin may have been the victim of this conflict. When Lemkin asked Wallace to promote his book, Wallace answered coldly, in keeping with his political calculations: "Thanks so much for delivering a copy of your book. It seems to me to be an extraordinarily competent job in a very complicated field. . . . PS: I am returning the literature that you were kind enough to leave with my Secretary."[74]

Lemkin "alerts the world to genocide"[75]

Wallace had Lemkin pegged: "extraordinarily competent job in a very complicated field." In contrast to the image of the solitary researcher that he—or certain of his later sycophants—cultivated, Lemkin was now well established in Washington and knew how to slip in everywhere, from newspaper pages to commissions of experts, from London to continental Europe. He published his book, to favorable criticism, and wrote short articles that he had translated into various languages. The "genocide" chapter had been written between 1943 and early 1944, and the book came out in November. On December 3, 1944, the *Washington Post* published the first article with the word in the title, directly inspired—even dictated—by Lemkin, who knew the newspaper's editor well. Reprinted widely in the American and British press and then in all other countries with a free press, the editorial informed hundreds of thousands of readers about the contents of the enormous tome that they would never read, with its precise facts and obscure definitions.

The editorial was introduced by the War Refugee Board's report of the preceding week: to the "shock" and "shame" of having to write about such "atrocities" one could contrast the response of the new concept:

In Birkenau, between April 1942 and April 1944, approximately 1,765,000 Jews were put to death in ingeniously constructed chambers; their bodies were then burned in specially designed furnaces; their ashes were distributed as fertilizer. . . . It is a mistake, perhaps, to call these killings "atrocities." An atrocity is a wanton brutality. There were unspeakable atrocities at Auschwitz and Birkenau. But the point about these killings is that they were systematic and purposeful. The gas chambers and furnaces were not improvisations; they were scientifically designed instruments for the extermination of an entire ethnic group. On the scale practiced by the Germans, this is something new. And it is this purpose that human beings find it difficult to believe or understand. Yet it is a purpose that Hitler has openly avowed.

We have never even had a word for it until now. But one has been recently coined by a noted Polish scholar and attorney. Professor Raphael Lemkin . . . has devised the term "genocide."

The author emphasized the unique extermination of the Jews, yet closely associated them with other Europeans:

Thus Jews were gassed at Birkenau and Aryan Poles and Russians and Slovenes were otherwise butchered, not for any crime or any resistance to Axis authority but because the Nazis wished to terminate the ethnic groups to which they belonged. . . . The Germans have committed genocide in virtually all the countries of Europe that they occupied. They have struck deliberately at the culture, language, religion, political institutions, and economic existence of the peoples they conquered—all with a view to undermining their national identity and weakening them, physically and morally, so that they would become subservient to German rule.[76]

The concept was broadened to include all national groups that had been victims of Nazism; it also explained the hundreds of pages of *Axis Rule* devoted to exactions, including forced labor. This does not seem to have caused many problems, and would not do so for some time, as could be seen in the Jewish press itself. For instance, the *Palestine Post* printed the following: "The nature of this crime, which was practiced against the Poles as well as against the Jews, is a systematic attack on the different aspects of life of captive people."[77] Then, *The Polish Review* devoted an article to Lemkin and Karski: the thinker and the soldier did not know each other, but they were brought together in the Polish patriots' newspaper.

It is easy to see Lemkin's hand behind the *Washington Post* article, which referred to his 1933 proposals in Madrid for "crime of barbarity and of vandalism," predating the term in a rather dishonest way: "As long ago as 1933, Professor Lemkin proposed the recognition of genocide as a crime under international law."

So that American readers in 1944 would come to the desired conclusion, they had to be convinced that an international law was essential to the indictment, judging, and sentencing of those who were found guilty of crimes throughout the conflict, and particularly the crime of genocide. This way, the sovereignty of nations and morals would be respected. But the contradictions led to criticisms. To a *Post* correspondent who asserted that the Hague Conventions would suffice for the War Crimes Commission to act, Lemkin pointed out the shortcomings of the 1907 convention, according to which decisions reached under its provisions would apply only to the treatment of populations under military occupation; in fact, in Madrid he had proposed that war criminals be arrested and tried in the countries that may have given them asylum. He had in mind the Turkish killers exfiltrated to Germany in 1919.

In 1944, Lemkin's response was based on the idea of the general guilt of those whom he would soon call "genocidists." To judge them, a new international law was needed here and now:

> If we treat the mass murders of Birkenau and Oswiecim as simple murders, only the comparatively few who were directly involved could be prosecuted. For the murder of several million people, only some hundreds of officials and subordinates could be directly accused. As I have defined genocide for the purpose of an international treaty, all persons who incited the population to committing and approving this crime and who provided the legal bases and machinery for its commission should be considered accessories to the crime. Thus, Goebbels and his many associates would be equally responsible for Birkenau, although they may not have given the direct orders to kill. . . . We should not fail to create a more readily enforceable machinery . . . for the fight against the onslaught of barbarism.[78]

Lemkin's definition of genocide remained vague at this stage: this was why he cited both Birkenau, referring to the gassing of Jews, and Oswiecim, the Polish name of which pointed to the martyrdom of Poland as a whole.

Nazi Guilt, German Guilt?

In late December 1944, the literary critic for the *Washington Post*, in his turn, urged "all intelligent Americans" to read Lemkin "on trial and punishment for international gangsters. . . . Unfortunately, millions of Americans do not believe that the Germans have systematically practiced 'genocide,' the calculated extermination of national and racial groups." The writer scathingly derided the "smug individuals . . . the party of those who know nothing," who he felt represented the majority of his compatriots, those who "want a soft peace." He counted upon the lawyers to inflict a "hard peace," one that was definitive, on their enemies; otherwise, the war would return to haunt their own grandchildren. Like Lemkin, he established a continuity among all Germans: "No mercy should be shown a nation that has made national heroes of aggressive tyrants, that has fed its youth upon Clausewitz, von Treitschke, Nietzsche, Bernhardi, and the paranoic vapors of Adolf Hitler."[79]

The *New York Times*, for its part, assigned its senior critic to open the book section with a review of *Axis Rule*, a rare honor. But beyond the praise for the intellectual performance that exposed the skeleton of the "twentieth-century Moloch," Nazism, the critic wondered whether the accusation made against all Germans as a perverted race was not counterproductive; he even posited that Lemkin, as a Pole, "would not want to be held personally responsible for all the acts of the Pilsudski regime."[80]

A *Washington Post* reader also noted that genocide, founded on a biological argument, was "dangerously close to Nazi theories. One only has to translate genocide as '*Völkermord*' and one finds oneself with a classic Nazi slogan: it's even incredible that the Nazis haven't thought of this themselves." These critics did not understand not only that Nazism was a crime against humanity—I use this nonlegal wording here deliberately to expose the various hesitations—but that genocide also defined something else, despite its gaps and ambiguities: "Nazism is a crime against the spirit and not against a biological notion, and if we need a new international crime, why not call it simply Nazism, instead of trying to incorporate by a Greco-Latin word what we have been fighting against during the last few years. If we don't find the spirit of man worthy of protection, the biological notion of nation does certainly not seem to be worthy of protection either."[81] Another stated with dark irony that the Czech government in exile, which was preparing to require a million Sudeten Germans to adopt the Czech language and culture, would be guilty of a "perfect genocide."[82]

"A cry of horror from the abyss"[83]

Lemkin had written a relentless book, but so full of statistics, texts of statutes, decrees, and contradictions that it is difficult to follow. Meanwhile, Jan Kozielewski set out to write his memoir while working at the Polish embassy under his resister's name, which was now his. His clandestine identity had been discovered by the Nazis, who accused him on the airwaves of "spreading lies about the Third Reich." The war had turned him into a different man, with a different name, Jan Karski. Published in fall 1944, *Story of a Secret State* became a Book of the Month Club selection the following December and January. The publisher advertised heavily in most American newspapers, including in Chicago, the city with the largest Polish immigrant population in the United States. The intense campaign bore some resemblance to that which had preceded the publication of Erich Maria Remarque's *All Quiet on the Western Front* in 1928. Remarque, who had barely seen the front, had nevertheless written a novel that was taken as the reality of the Great War. Karski's autobiography was presented, conversely, as a thriller, a spy novel: "Jan Karski has emerged from the Polish underground to reveal how his countrymen built a whole secret government under the Nazis' noses";[84] "Spine-Curling Saga of the Polish Underground."[85] The book garnered numerous reviews, promoting both Karski's incredible courage and the various miracles by which he had escaped the "Nazi Gehenna." "Here is the Jeremiad of western civilization, realistic, appalling."[86]

The handsome young Pole had to get Americans to understand what was playing out in Europe. During this time, when newsreels and news photographs were essential, many organizations put together exhibitions and conferences on propaganda. Karski went to the exhibition in New York glorifying Polish heroism, inaugurated in September 1944 by his host, Ambassador Jan Ciechanowski: "If ever a nation has won its right to freedom, then surely Poland's record in this total world war has won her that right. . . . Her people have uninterruptedly fought and suffered. . . . They have been ruthlessly decimated by methodical extermination, and yet they have never faltered."[87] Playing on his charming modesty despite his heroic aura, Karski posed across the country in front of posters for the exhibition *The Secret Polish State* taken from pages of his book. The images vaunted the entire Polish nation, standing up against the Nazi evil, denouncing forced labor and the enslavement of an entire people. Everywhere, children exalted the renaissance. In Los Angeles, they waved Polish and American flags in front of a poster: "Poland: First to Fight." Front and center were the soul of the Poles and the attacks against their culture, such as the destruction of sculptures of Chopin: "The conquerors were not able to break the Polish spirit of resistance, so now they want to erase their culture."[88] At the New York Public Library, an exhibition of old Polish books pointed out how important the collection could be in helping with the cultural reconstruction of the devastated country. The final display was organized around Karski's book; in just a few weeks he had become the paradigmatic Pole—he who had suffered, resisted, and who would make it possible for his country to be revived, as it had been in 1918. A photograph often reproduced shows an inscription of the resistance in Warsaw: "*Deutschland Kaputt, 1918–1943.*"[89]

"Jan Karski bridges the all but unbridgeable gap between American civilians who have suffered virtually nothing in this war and the harassed, starving, mortally wounded masses of conquered Poland. If anyone can pierce the elephantine skin of the callow noncombatant, Karski can."[90] A gentle caricature by a compatriot portrays him in front of his book, his finger pointed as if on a military propaganda poster, issuing an invitation to astounded American visitors: "Poland's Heroic Spirit."[91]

And the Polish Jews? Although they weren't forgotten, they were simply an adjunct to their nation's suffering. The major exhibition held at Freedom House in New York, inaugurated by such eminent American and Allied figures as Eleanor Roosevelt and the Czech diplomat Jan Masaryk, drew a parallel between the resistance in Warsaw in 1944 and that in the ghetto in 1943. The Jews were not hidden away, but their specific fate was marginalized: given the terrible suffering of the Polish people in general, how could extermination be classified? The article that announced the Book of the Month award for Karski was, however, divided into two equal parts, one on the fate of Poland in general and one on the two chapters describing the Warsaw ghetto and "Belzec"; the author of the review slip, Clifton Fadiman, considered these chapters the most important and quoted Karski: "I know history. I have learned a great deal about the evolution of nations, political systems, social doctrines, methods of conquest, persecution, and extermination, and I know, too, that never in the history of mankind, never anywhere in the realm of human relations did anything occur to compare with what was inflicted on the Jewish population of Poland."[92] Fadiman wrote that Karski "record[ed] the kind of facts about the Germans which, for some mysterious reason, the American people all through this war have not been particularly encouraged to learn. The basic truth about this particular aspect of the conduct of the German people is that, as Karski *proves*, 1,800,000 Jews have been murdered. Not killed in battle. Not even executed for 'crimes.' But murdered, sometimes quickly, sometimes slowly, but murdered. Murdered by Germans, tens of thousands of Germans (many of them not 'nazis'), and murdered with every appearance of alacrity, not to say profound pleasure."[93]

These sentences were published in December 1944. Majdanek had been "opened"[94] by the Soviets in July; the abandonment of Auschwitz-Birkenau was underway, and its survivors were being forced into wintertime death marches.[95]

"The nightmare that is a reality"[96]

Yet, as the American and British troops discovered for themselves the horrors of the camps (although never specifying exactly which "camps"), the debate over belief and nonbelief resumed. It was the Soviets who discovered the extermination sites such as Treblinka, and in 1943 they established their commissions of inquiry; on January 27, 1945, they entered Auschwitz-Birkenau.[97] The Americans and British, in the west, liberated concentration camps—including Dachau and Buchenwald—where survivors of the death marches, deported from Birkenau, were imprisoned.[98] This furthered the incomprehension, the difficulty with creating a hierarchy of horrors: it was hard to know which was which. For instance, how could people interpret the photograph, taken on April 16, 1945, by soldier H. Miller, in which skeletal people, their bulging eyes overwhelming their entire faces, are squeezed four by four onto cots? The *New York Times* published the picture on May 6, 1945, with the caption "Crowded Bunks in the Prison Camp at Buchenwald." Today, we recognize long-term deportees at Buchenwald, as well as the young Elie Wiesel and other Jews from Hungary who had survived the death marches and had recently arrived from Auschwitz-Birkenau.[99]

The United States was much quicker—due to anti-Japanese racism and national pride following the Pearl Harbor attack[100]—to denounce the atrocities by the Japanese than those by the Nazis, as Paul Winkler noted: "The cruelties committed by the Germans are at least as great as those of the Japanese. Members of the various European undergrounds go to great risks to smuggle out reports on these matters, but they get pitifully little hearing in the United States."[101]

Once more, it was the cartoonists, with their talent for immediacy, who brought to light the confusion that arose from the geographic and mental distance between the American people at war and devastated Europe. A young mother proudly shows her toddler in a playpen surrounded by barbed wire to her friend who has come for tea: "We want him to be better prepared to meet the facts of life than we were," she says.[102] A reader returns two books to the library, saying, "I don't think I can stand another concentration camp." Or "I thought the whole thing was terribly dated. Nobody ever murders with prussic acid any more."[103] And a reader besotted with Karski tells him that the passage in his book where the Gestapo begins to torture him is so beautiful.

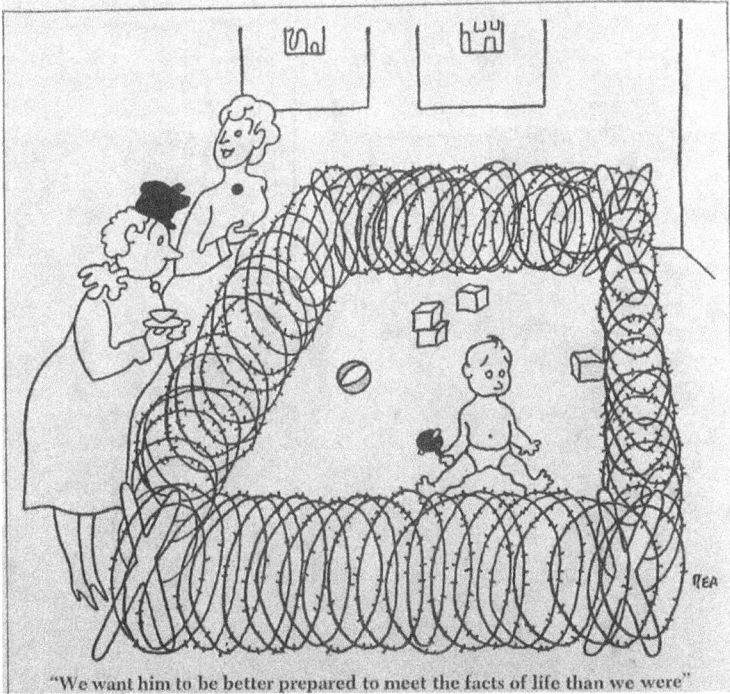

"We want him to be better prepared to meet the facts of life than we were"

Cartoon by Garner Rea published in *Colliers*, February 19, 1944.

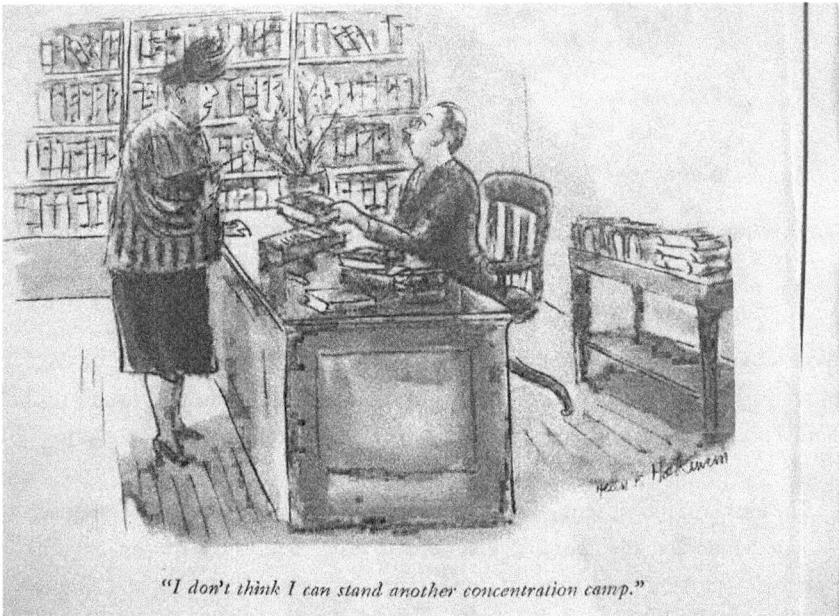

"I don't think I can stand another concentration camp."

Cartoon by Helen Hokinson published in *The New Yorker*, May 20, 1944.

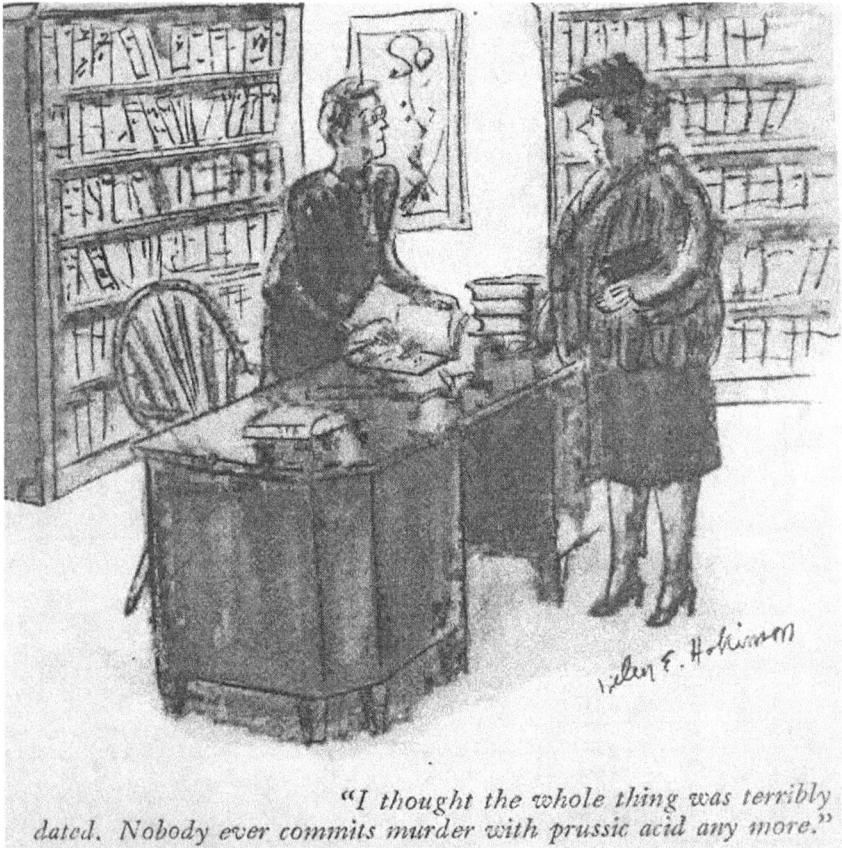

"*I thought the whole thing was terribly dated. Nobody ever commits murder with prussic acid any more.*"

Cartoon by Helen Hokinson published in *The New Yorker*, May 13, 1944.

The critic at *The New Yorker* tried to figure out why the eyewitness accounts were so limited: the Pole, Karski, had written the "best book" on the resistance in Europe, and yet it was not possible for him, who had fought, who had seen, "by writing books, to catch up with the terrible reality." Why?

The events of the present war . . . have burst the barometer of human response. The demands made upon our emotions so exceed our ordinary capacity for either sympathy or excitement that we almost cease to feel at all and simply begin to things for granted. The feverish exploitation of glory by the jingo, still so much in evidence for the last war, has become almost as impossible as the indignant humanitarianism of the liberal and the socialist. . . . Books and articles . . . all alike seem fatally inadequate to make us realize either the dimensions or the profound effects of what is going on.[104]

Inadequate—truly fatally inadequate? And all of this because it was impossible to believe in old rumors, traces of World War I? Late in 1944, however, the Gallup polling firm, surveying Americans again on the "atrocity stories," reported that 76 percent of them believed that the Germans had murdered "many people" in the concentration camps, 12 percent weren't sure, and 12 percent did not believe it at all. But among those who said "many people," all underestimated the number, and only 12 percent thought that the reports had assessed it at more than two million. The *Washington Post* headline emphasized this underestimation, as the report by the War Refugee Board, which situated the number of dead at 1,765,000 for the Auschwitz camp alone, had just been published, but the author acknowledged, "Regardless of the numbers involved, the American people are fully prepared to believe atrocities have taken place."[105]

This poll was published in the *Washington Post* on the same day as the editorial titled "Genocide," the first time that the word appeared in the press. Readers did not necessarily make the connection between the two, and they continued to mix all the atrocities together, from one war to the other. How could it be otherwise?

When the American soldiers arrived, in their turn, in the concentration camps, they finally became aware, at least, of the reality of the exactions. For instance, when Ohrdruf was opened, "The *Post* correspondent, who had been a skeptic ever since the last war when men argued about Edith Cavell and the Belgian babies who were supposed to have had their hands cut off, drove all the way to Ohrdruf to join in the grim procession. The thing we had heard about was right before our eyes in the yard of the concentration camp. . . . A soldier of one of Patton's Infantry divisions . . . murmured, 'Good Lord' [then] 'This is hard to believe when you read about it . . . but there it is.'"[106]

"The casting into doubt of atrocity stories after World War I is probably partly responsible for the current rejection of the World War II stories. But this time, the skepticism is not justified," stated Shirer.[107] Again on May 6, 1945, a *Washington Post* reader recalled "Lord Bryce's committee on the supposed German atrocities in 1915 and the prison camp in Wittenberg. Today, our forces occupy Wittenberg. During World War I it was as terrible as Buchenwald today. . . . We have forgotten Wittenberg. For how long will we remember Buchenwald and Dachau?"[108]

By invoking the burden of the rejection of World War I atrocities, Lemkin had perceived very early what many discovered in 1945, including *The Christian Century*, which finally made an honorable amend: "We have found it hard to believe that the reports from the nazi concentration camps could be true. . . . Or perhaps they were just more atrocity-mongering, like the cadaver factory story of the last war."[109]

Concentration camps, extermination sites—the confusion was at its height, including among those ready to accept the word "genocide." It was still very far from Marcel Cohen's clear response: "I knew, very young, the unfathomable distance between slavery and mass slaughter, between what one could still attempt to express and the silence of the factories. One of my aunts was selected for labor. . . . Speaking of the laborers, she said 'us.' About those, in another line, on the ramp at Birkenau, who were going to their death, she bowed her head and was silent."[110]

5

The War Is Over

Weep for the Dead, Find the Living, Judge the Criminals

Throughout the ages, the victims of genocide have filled history with their
pain to the point that humanity can no longer avoid identification of the
consequences and its own moral responsibility.[1]

—Lemkin

"All wiped out. No more family."

Devastated, in shock, Raphael Lemkin gradually learned about the abominable conditions under which the Volkovysk ghetto was destroyed and his
parents were murdered. Might he really have thought that the sufferings
of Jews were intermingled with those of others in the disaster of Europe, or
had he wept for them in private, even as he was pushing forward his universal conception of genocide?

In 1946, the "crime of genocide" began to be integrated into certain proc-
lamations, as it was into the UN resolution of December 11 of that year:
"Genocide is a denial of the right of existence of entire human groups, as
homicide is the denial of the right to live of individual human beings."[2] But
1946 was also the year of the Kielce pogrom, on July 4: forty dead, more
than eighty wounded. Everywhere in Poland, Jews who had survived ghettos, labor camps, and concentration camps or who had returned from the
Soviet Union were either killed or so worried that they preferred to flee again.
Their former neighbors had taken their belongings or, finally freed of their
"Jewish problem," were not keen to see them come back, even though barely
three hundred thousand out of the three million had survived.[3]

As Lemkin was visiting displaced persons camps, he was unaware that his older brother, Elias, with his wife and two children, was at Neu-Freimann in Bavaria, not far from Nuremberg. The two brothers were among the *lebensgeblibenen*, Yiddish for "Jews who stayed alive." Raphael was more of a *survivant*—he had escaped in time—whereas Elias was more of a *rescapé*.[4] But these considerable semantic differences in French do not exist in the English language, which uses a single word, *survivor*.

In 1944, the Allied General Staff created the status of "displaced persons," a provisional and imprecise term. Among the eleven million people moving through the Western zone, at least eight million transited through Germany. It was a paradoxical situation: although the country responsible for the tragedy was in utter ruins and occupied, it was where displaced persons found a temporary safe harbor—including 250,000 Jews, most of them from Poland.[5]

At first, the Allies didn't separate the Jews from the other refugees; the idea was to create a contrast with Nazi ideology. However, they ran into specific difficulties, as reported disapprovingly by Earl Harrison, President Truman's envoy to these camps: "The Jewish refugees . . . are in need of attention and help. Up to this point they have been 'liberated' more in a military sense than actually. . . . They feel that they, who were in so many ways the first and worst victims of Nazism, are being neglected by their liberators."[6] Indeed, certain Baltic, Polish, and Ukrainian refugees repeatedly harassed Jews gathered in the same locations. Harrison also deplored the fact that some former concentration camps, such as Dachau, were serving as displaced persons "camps." Finally, he was surprised that the desire of most Jews to immigrate to Palestine was not being taken into account. His report ultimately had a broader scope, as it made it possible to identify Jews as a people and thus, indirectly, to better apprehend Zionism.

And so, separate camps for Jews were organized and managed by the American Joint Distribution Committee. The Joint, as it was known, had been created in November 1914 to assist Jewish populations in Central and Eastern Europe and in the Middle East, notably those in Palestine under Ottoman domination, who were suffering from a terrible famine. Henry Morgenthau Sr., American ambassador to the Ottoman Empire and father of Treasury Secretary Henry Morgenthau, had been active in the Joint. In yet another way, one world war was extended into the next.

An amateur film shot in fall 1946 shows General Dwight Eisenhower visiting the Neu-Freimann camp. School, synagogue, warehouse: the common buildings were labeled in English and Yiddish. Crowds—Elias Lemkin's family among them, perhaps—pressed forward to welcome a relaxed Eisenhower.[7] The conquering general, who, staggered, had declared at the Ohrdruf camp in 1945 that now American soldiers knew why they were fighting, could never comprehend the unprecedented tragedies that these people had just gone through. For instance, in the extended Lemkin family, the survivors wept for some fifty dead.

The files of the Red Cross are overflowing with both details and poignant gaps: "Elias born in 1895, his wife, Lea Winograzka, in 1899, their two sons Sholom and Samuel in 1928 and 1935. Jews from Wolkowysk, Poland." Elias was a "farmer" and "office employee" until 1941; the family were then "*Statenlos*" [*sic*], stateless, and wished to immigrate to Canada or the United States, because they thought they had relatives there. In 1945, Elias tried to reach his brother, Raphael, through an American journalist he met in Moscow, as he thought he recognized him in a photograph taken in Nuremberg: "Your brother, his wife, and their two sons are looking for you, they have a decision to make that will affect their entire life. . . . Your parents and the rest of the family stayed in Volkovysk and we have never heard anything about them. The only thing they know is that all the Jews were deported by the Germans and no doubt perished with the millions of other victims of the Nazis."[8]

Elias did in fact still have a brother, but Raphael never received the letter. A sister also reached Palestine, but in those years, when millions of refugees were on the move, it was impossible to find her. Also, to the question "Do you want to return to your home country?" Elias answered "*Nein.*" If no, why not? "*Alles vernichtet. Keine Verwandete.*"[9]

The forms left little room to describe how the Lemkin, Pomeranz, and Winograzky families had been "wiped out" or how some had survived. It was mentioned that Elias, his wife, and their two sons lived in Volkovysk, near Bialystok, from 1936 to 1939; then, starting in 1941, they were "wearing the Jewish star" and "living illegally"; they were "liberated by the Russians in 1944." They did not figure on the "legal" (in the Nazi sense) lists of deportations and camps. They hid—they therefore encountered saviors during their ordeal—then reached the Soviet Union.

The salvation of the Polish and Baltic Jews who fled east is sometimes minimized, even though we must not forget those who were deported, transported, or killed. In fact, without intending it, the Stalinist USSR saved hundreds of thousands of Jews. Soviet citizens of Jewish origin who were deported (most of whom survived the conditions of forced labor and transportation) or evacuated and those who fled were the only ones to escape the Nazi genocide in Eastern Europe. About 10 percent of the five hundred thousand deported from the "new territories" (including eastern Poland) after 1939–40 were Jewish, as were 40 percent of the seventeen million evacuees. Of course, many thousands of them would not live to see the end of the conflict: the mortality rate in the nonoccupied USSR during the war, and especially in the camps, exile zones, and refugee zones, was two to three times higher than the average during peacetime. Nevertheless, a huge number of "evacuees" and "forced settlers" escaped the certain death reserved for them by the Nazis.[10] Late in 1943, several American senior government officials summed things up: "The Soviets did more for the Jewish refugees than any other state in the world."[11] They remembered that in 1942, when they had tried, from Washington, to set up refugee camps in North Africa or liberated southern Italy, their own hierarchy and their allies—from the British to the free French—had barred them from doing so.[12] After the war, however, these Jews did not want to stay in the Soviet Union, which is why they traveled west, among them Elias's branch of the Lemkin family.

Elias's family managed to obtain Canadian identification papers. They tried to get their hands on some reparation compensation and persisted in the search for the rest of their family. "All wiped out. No more family"; at each stage of their journey, the same words were repeated. They kept quiet about their hunt, however, and about the places where they had hidden throughout Poland after 1941, their arrival in Moscow, their survival thanks to the Anti-Fascist Committee, their return via Bialystok, the desolate void of a Volkovysk in which not a single Jew still lived, their departure for Berlin, and finally their transit through the displaced persons camp at Neu-Freimann before reaching Canada.

One of their cousins, Daniel, born in 1919, the son of Raphael and Elias's uncle, Benjamin Lemkin, reached the Bamberg displaced persons camp in Bavaria. He lived there until late 1950 and then left for the United States via Bremen after an incredible voyage that is recounted in his papers. On the

Red Cross forms, the list of the main camps was printed in advance; the camp or—more often—camps that had been "visited" could be simply ticked off: "1.8.41–15.8.43, forced laborer Bialystok; 18.8.43 KZ Maidanek; 28.12.43, KZ Blizics; 15.10.44 KZ Auschwitz ZaL Kirchhof; 18.11.44–11.4.45, KZ Buchenwald, liberated."[13] After his liberation in 1945 and before his arrival in Bamberg, in 1947, Daniel returned to Volkovysk. Did he meet his cousins there; did they discover together their town empty of Jews? He then wandered for two years before reaching a camp of another type, free but having become destitute. Almost three more years of steps followed before he could emigrate. Between the beginning of the war in 1939 and his arrival in the United States in late 1950, Daniel, a typographer and bookbinder, suffered eleven years of the worst mistreatment in forced labor camps and in extermination camps where all of his relatives died and then wandered through a totally destroyed Poland and Germany, where he was classified as a "stateless Jew." Surviving. But living?

Could even a man such as Raphael Lemkin feel what his family members had experienced, displaced in the Soviet Union or confronted with mistreatment and death? He had experienced the beginning of the war, the difficulties of immigrating to the United States, the long voyage across the USSR, Japan, and the Pacific Ocean. But that was nothing in comparison with what they had gone through. By escaping, he was able to bring the world a new concept: genocide.

A Mitigated Victory: The Term "Genocide," 1945 to 1948

Two days before May 8, 1945, under the title "Retribution," the *Washington Post* ran an anonymous article explaining Germany's defeat as due to its immorality and its total lack of honor and humanity. Its punishment had to be proportionate to the catastrophe it had wreaked upon the world: "Death, sorrow, degradation, hunger prowl through Germany . . . because the world did not allow the completion of the pitiless plan for the entire destruction of other peoples that was to satisfy Nazi ambitions. . . . Their weakness was not military. It was their total absence of morality and respect for human rights."[14]

In fact, Lemkin had written the article. He was aware of the difficulty of importing the new concept into the great trial that was being prepared, because laws could not be applied retroactively. The Nazis had practiced "genocide" before the concept was invented and defined by international bodies. Therefore, he stressed, Hitler and the Nazis were common-law criminals. He raised the problem both of the German population and of collaborators in Poland, France, Norway, and other countries. "When one man is murdered, it is murder. We cannot accept the proposition that organizing the murder of millions is less than murder."[15] This was exactly what he had said about the Turks between 1919 and 1933. In 1944–45, however, Lemkin put his research on the Armenians aside. It was not until 1946 that his lobbying in favor of calling a vote on a convention against the crime of genocide caused him to return to the Armenians and then to what he called victims of all genocides through history.

The small American legal team led by General Taylor was far from operational when it was formed in May 1945 to prepare for the Nuremberg trials: "The first question a prosecuting attorney asks in such a situation is 'Where's the evidence?' The blunt fact was that, despite what 'everybody knew' about the Nazi leaders, virtually no judicially admissible evidence was at hand. . . . In fact, the OSS [Office of Strategic Services] included a number of able and learned experts on the Third Reich [Franz Neumann[16] and Raphael Lemkin were specifically mentioned in a footnote here]."[17] Although Neumann (the main representative of the Frankfurt school in New York) and Lemkin offered avenues "valuable as background information," this was "neither documentary nor testimonial evidence suitable for court use."[18] Taylor's team used the word "genocide" in relation to "the extermination of racial and national groups . . . particularly Jews and Poles and gypsies and others,"[19] but without a legal definition genocide simply did not exist, even if Sir Maxwell Fyfe, the British prosecutor, included it in some of his cross-examinations; it was therefore just a descriptive term.

Hersch Lauterpacht, a British lawyer who also worked on preparations for the Nuremberg trials, recommended that the extermination of the Jews be called a "crime against humanity." In an extraordinary coincidence, Lauterpacht was born in Lvov, where he studied law, like Lemkin; he then went on to Cambridge, where he became a professor in the late 1920s. Simultaneously promoting the introduction into the international legal arsenal of the concepts of crime against humanity and genocide were two Jews who had studied in Lvov. The city has been known, successively, by four names—

Lwow, Lemberg, Lvov, and Lviv (the Polish, German [Austrian], Ukrainian, and Russian versions)—symbolizing the upheavals in European boundaries.

Lemkin, not taken seriously, having heart problems, often hospitalized, tried—not without difficulty—to carve out a place for himself at Nuremberg, where he believed he could make his concept known to the entire world. But Lauterpacht was ahead of him. Celebrated in Great Britain, he had given lectures in the United States and knew Robert Jackson, the American prosecutor.[20] However, Lauterpacht disapproved of the concept of genocide and was fiercely opposed to the book by Lemkin, whom he called a "pale lawyer." In his view, both criminals and victims were individuals: justice was rendered against the former; for the latter, there was no group that applied—neither Nazis, nor Germans, nor Jews, nor Poles.

Lemkin thought exactly the contrary: in his view, groups and their members, not individuals, were the targets: "Genocide is the crime of destruction of human groups, just as homicide is the crime of destruction of individuals."[21] But he convinced no one. He and his concept were relegated to the sidelines when it came to settlement of the conflict. Some of his self-important colleagues on the United Nations War Crimes Commission went so far as to question his skill as a linguist because he had mixed Greek and Latin in his neologism. *Le Monde* did the same in its editorial of December 11, 1945, in which the term "genocide" was used in French for the first time one year before the UN declaration was issued:

Now we have been enriched by a monster. Of course, the man who, according to Professor Lemkin's definition, committed the "genocide" is himself a monstrous person. But was it necessary to coin, to designate his crime, one of those barbarous words made of the coupling of a Greek and a Latin root? The Latin *gens* would have done just as well as the Greek word *genos* to say what he wanted to say, and the analogy with homicide, fratricide, regicide, etc., for example, would have been complete. But we wager that, in a time when words get used up so fast, this one will cause an uproar for one or two seasons: by synecdoche—or else by catachresis—it will be used in disputes to express the highest degree of contempt.[22]

At the same moment, Dr. Leo Alexander, a physician and an expert witness at Nuremberg who described the Nazi doctors' "quest for the ecstatic pleasure of death," was searching for a term including *thanatos* (death) as the medical equivalent of "genocide." He questioned Lemkin, who confirmed that the Nazis' medical "experiments" had been conducted for a single purpose, to develop the "science of murder,"[23] and proposed two variants for the "techniques" of murder and of sterilizations or castrations: *ktenotechnics* (from *ktenos*, "murder') and *sterotechnics* (from *steirosis*, "infertility"). Alexander approved, and he coined "ktenology as a scientific technique of genocide." The term was not widely adopted, but the episode proved Lemkin's mastery of Greek, as he had deliberately opted for a loaded linguistic barbarism to define the barbarity of barbarities.[24]

At the War Crimes Commission, Lemkin compiled thick bibliographies on the three indictments finally chosen for prosecution at Nuremberg: crimes against peace, war crimes, crimes against humanity. Did he know the role played by Lauterpacht in the attempt to unite Americans, British, French, and Soviets around "his" crime against humanity? Lemkin, who never gave up trying to convince, added paragraphs to his previous texts, including chapter 9 of *Axis Rule*:

> The concept of genocide gives a formula for covering not only the destruction of the Jews but also of other peoples, like the Russians, Czechs, Poles, Yugoslavs, Frenchmen. If one should stress only the Jewish aspect of the crime of destroying peoples and races, it would invite further attempts on the side of the defendants and their supporters to use the court for antisemitic propaganda. However, if the broader concept of genocide would be used more prominently the defendants would have to declare themselves as enemies of all other nations to justify their actions. Therefore, the use of the term genocide in any further proceedings is also important from the point of view of trial strategy.[25]

Lemkin was never short of ideas. When the films of Nazi atrocities were screened—for the first time ever—at the international court, he came up with the idea of the International Film for Discovery of War Criminals: to use films not only as clues to crimes but also to hunt down perpetrators. He proposed that the defendants be filmed and that the films be shown to survivors in displaced person camps, as well as "in countries where a number of victims may be found, such as New York, Palestine, Sweden, Portugal, and

Shanghai."[26] To modern criminality, a modern response; to global crimes, a global response. Once more, Lemkin was innovating. Later, he made a film strip from still images called *Le Génocide, le plus grand des crimes* (Genocide: The Greatest of Crimes): "The first part presented an imaginary group, the Extabians, who were persecuted by their government, not allowed to marry; sent to a labor camp, and eventually died there."[27]

"The guilty should be punished like common criminals and the world protected from the Crime of Genocide"

At Nuremberg, the word "genocide" was used more often than Lemkin acknowledged; he was annoyed that it wasn't mentioned in the indictment or the conviction statement. The day the trial opened, French lawyer Pierre Mounier spoke the word for the first time in a court of law, under the heading of "war crimes." He was followed by the Soviet lawyer, who situated it within "crimes against humanity," also a first in a courtroom, after attempts to invent the term during World War I in relation to the extermination of the Armenians. As we recall, at that time, it was a term of revenge against the enemies of the Turks, not a legal charge. Lemkin, left behind in Washington, was disappointed: the trial continued, day after day, without his concept being cited again, but only "crimes against humanity." Why had this term, which hadn't existed in international law before Nuremberg any more than "genocide" had, received the court's favor when it was just as retrospective?

Bitter, Lemkin insisted, "The inclusion of the word genocide in the verdict would help to create an atmosphere likely to prevent the repetition of such acts of barbarism." The "crime of barbarity" dated from 1933; it had now become "genocide." Thirty years of intellectual battles, a second world war, and yet a legal void persisted that the concept of genocide alone would be able to fill, whether it was physical, biological, or cultural: "We cannot continue to speak to the world in interminable sentences: 'Do not assassinate members of national, racial, or religious groups; do not sterilize them; do not steal their children.'"[28]

Lemkin was convinced that the Allies were being too timid because the Nuremberg trials were military tribunals, and war crimes or crimes against humanity were linked to combatants. The crime of genocide, however, concerned civilians, whose fate the military forces were incapable of envisaging.

But he was wrong; although crimes against humanity were not yet totally detached from the notion of "armed conflict," their defenders were using the term to account for the fact that civilian populations had suffered more from the war than had soldiers.

During this period of intellectual gestation, "crimes against humanity" referred to the question of protection of civilians and genocide to the protection of minorities. This was in fact how Sir Hartley Shawcross, prosecutor for the United Kingdom, understood it when he included the word "genocide" in his closing argument devoted to "crimes against peace." Benjamin Ferencz, the young American prosecutor at Nuremberg who tried the "subsequent" cases in the American occupation zone, was the first to truly distinguish "war crimes" from "crimes against humanity" in his indictment opening the trial against the Einsatzgruppen in 1947. He was thus the first to slip genocide into the category of crimes against humanity, whereas at Nuremberg it had remained an act underlying war crimes. Yet, he could not have spoken more harshly of Lemkin in 1945: the team around Jackson had no time to waste with his "'obsession' with genocide."[29]

Indeed, Lemkin's colleagues continued to lash out at his work for legal, political, or personal reasons. Some lamented that he had not analyzed the real content of the laws described, as if compiling them was enough for an understanding of how Nazism worked in Europe or to judge those responsible. In a review of *Axis Rule*, Melchior Palyi, an economics professor at the University of Chicago, was venomous:

> This case is typical of the conflict between the impassionate pursuit of a political goal and the purposeful political approach. It is the case of the ethically indignant prosecutor who unconsciously assumes the role of the judge—so common among students of law doubling as "social scientists." The field of international law, in its vague incompleteness and its lack of positive authority, is especially fit for the confusion of ultimate standards. Dr. Lemkin's case is a tragic one, too. His highly refined legal apparatus which is to serve against the Nazis could be turned on the Allies as well. Almost every one of the . . . international crimes he charges to the Nazis has been duplicated . . . by Allied occupational authorities.[30]

Palyi seized on the lack of precision in the definition of genocide, which made it an easily manipulated concept: "Allied practices include, in effect, even the worst of Nazi excesses—'genocide,' the mass extinction of civilians, as the fate of millions of Germans driven, under inhuman conditions, from their homes in east-central Europe. Of course, there is this substantial difference: that the Nazis shamelessly displayed their intentionally planned misdeeds, while the western Allies stumble into illegal practices and cover them with humanitarian or other formulas."[31] He was alluding—rightly—to the Soviets' lies at Nuremberg, starting with their transfer of responsibility for the murders in Katyn to the Nazis.

The French jurist Eugène Aroneanu, who had performed the enormous task of compiling Nazi crimes for Nuremberg and done pioneering work on witnesses (even though he mixed up "ordinary" concentration camps and extermination sites), would deliver the mortal blow against the term "genocide":

> Too narrow to embrace all crimes against humanity . . . but motivated by true legal imperialism, this vaunted "genocide" adapts to every reality to accomplish its conquests. For instance, it is proposed that we allow "biological genocide," "cultural genocide," etc., which, in my opinion, is a real monstrosity. . . . Only the introduction of crimes against humanity will impede a policy of the crime in the future, as it has already triumphed, in the past, over Nazi officials. To rechristen the "crime against humanity" . . . is to try to destroy a living reality through a quarrel over words. I am pointing out the double danger that there would be in replacing the law itself by a convention and the institution of the crime against humanity by an ersatz.[32]

Genocide of the Jews: A Singular Event?

"Ersatz," "monstrosity": the concept of genocide seemed to be destined for stillbirth and Lemkin for a return to oblivion. He did find allies, however. At Nuremberg, due to differences of interpretation among the four Allies, including on the notion of the "Jewish people"—some felt that Jews had nothing in common but religion—and on crimes against humanity, the coherence and centrality of the crimes against Jews could not be recognized as "as a unit in fact and in law."[33]

Lemkin then crossed paths with the lawyer Jacob Robinson, a Lithuanian Jew who had created the Institute of Jewish Affairs in New York, where he had arrived as a refugee in 1940. Robinson, like Lemkin, thought that during the early discriminatory measures and violence the Jews had served as "lab rats" for Hitler's war in a "cold pogrom," starting in 1933.[34] The failure of the future Allies to agree on the refugees, for instance at the Évian conference in 1938, had armed Hitler with a detestable argument, which was reiterated in following years. The entire world claimed not to understand the specificity of the Jews' fate, even after 1941 and 1942, when it involved physical, biological, and cultural extermination—what Lemkin was now calling "genocide."

Robinson and Lemkin agreed on the factual aspects of the extermination and on the comparisons with the massacres of Armenians in the preceding war, as well as on the impossibility of a legal sanction for the Turks' crimes. Where they diverged was in Robinson's single-minded interest in the Jews. Lemkin, due to his obsession with bringing the word "genocide" to global awareness and into the international legal vocabulary, "de-Judaized" it in order to universalize it. It became necessary to relativize the burden of the Jewish catastrophe, even though it weighed so heavily upon him. Breaking away from the time span of the war and proving that acts of genocide had been committed starting in 1933, he wanted to apply the crime during peacetime. Robinson wanted above all to establish a "conspiracy against the Jewish people": the Nazis had intentionally thought out a grand plan of destruction of the Jews "directed not only against the Jews under their control but also against those beyond their reach."[35]

Jewish survivors closely followed the Nuremberg trials. Although some found them balanced, others felt that the main victims of the Nazis were not made central to the deliberations, as there was more talk of the executioners than of them. And yet, the accumulation of testimony on the Einsatzgruppen, Treblinka, Birkenau, the Warsaw ghetto, and other locations had given a real Jewish flavor to the tribunals. Moyshe Feigenbaum, who participated in the historic commissions on the displaced persons camps, felt that it was also up to Jews to make up for the deficiencies in the verdicts with their personal, private experiences. There would have to be a transition from the "final solution"—the expression of the executioners—to *Hrbn* ("destruction" in Yiddish) or "catastrophe," the victims' expression:

[The documents in the trial] show only how the murderers behaved toward us, how they treated us and what they did with us. Do our lives in those nightmarish days consist only of such fragments? On what basis will the historian be able to create an image of what happened in the ghettos? . . . Therefore each testimony of a saved Jew, every song from the Nazi era, every proverb, every anecdote and joke, every photograph is for us of tremendous value.[36]

Toward the Convention on the Prevention and Punishment of the Crime of Genocide, Paris, 1948

It is always an arduous task to have a new concept admitted into international law. It was even more difficult at the beginning of the Cold War: how could pro-Americans and pro-Soviets be brought together to reflect, at a time when negotiations on the creation of the state of Israel were concluding, by a Polish Jewish refugee in the United States? No nation wanted to be looked into in peacetime—the Soviets no more than the Americans. And yet, Lemkin succeeded. The editor of the *Washington Post* wrote a portrait of him that became a portrait of the concept itself: "'The crime of genocide.' The word invented by a refugee will become a treaty. There is not a bomb, bullet, or torpedo in Raphael Lemkin's story. Yet this is one of the more fantastic stories of World War II. It is the story of an idea and a word."[37]

Lemkin was particularly satisfied by the UN declaration on December 11, 1946, on the "crime of genocide": it both laid the groundwork for a convention and finally distinguished genocide from crimes against humanity, to which it had been confined in Nuremberg the previous year. The Convention on the Prevention and Punishment of the Crime of Genocide was adopted on December 9, 1948, by the UN General Assembly in Paris.

For Lemkin, what was now essential was the prevention of genocide. He emphasized this in an interview in the French newspaper *Le Monde*: "never again" could not serve simply as a mantra; it was necessary to take action for peace through international law. His determination was never as strong as during these years. He was convinced that Hitler had intended to exterminate the Jews; in fact, "he had begun to exterminate German Jews" in 1933. Although criminals were punished in Nuremberg—not fully, because the crime of genocide had not been recognized—now, no criminal in power could become a Hitler. Under the convention, "a new Hitler could be arrested as an international criminal long before he had crossed any border with his armies." And in the *Washington Post* Lemkin ironically recalled the words of his detractors in Madrid in 1933: "But there is no such thing as exterminating whole groups of people."[38]

Lemkin doggedly returned to his compilation work. For example, he annotated a report on Czechoslovakia: "Horrible crimes done by Germans about looting and kidnapping of children from all nationalities in the occupied countries have been uncovered. Special orders have been issued concerning the germanisation of Polish and Czech children and families." He made a list of the names of children from the Czech villages of Lidice and Lezaky kidnapped after their parents were killed and placed with German families and of fifty-seven Germans, from nursery-school employees to directors of *Lebensborn*, from the director of the Lodz ghetto prison to members of the Gestapo to simple truck drivers.[39] The fate of the children would be central to the definition of genocide in the UN convention, which the Economic and Social Council was charged with writing.

During the preparatory sessions, Lemkin stood toe to toe with his opponents, both lawyers and politicians. In the more than two thousand pages of reports and debates, the Cold War and the year 1948 figured more prominently than the first half of the twentieth century: there was no allusion to the Armenians and few to World War II and the extermination of the Jews, even though the Soviet delegate remarked that his own country knew the most about genocide: "We know all about Maidanek and Babiy Yar. We waged this struggle in actual fact. . . . We shall carry on with the struggle."[40]

Lemkin, meanwhile, was using the word "civilization" to add universal scope: "I realized that the real issue at stake in the war was civilization not as a propaganda slogan but as a palpable reality."[41] Civilization stripped of propaganda: here again, World War I, when barbarity was the essence of the German Other, surfaced, and in World War II the reality of the Nazi crimes enabled the Soviets to camouflage their own crimes. Lemkin wanted to give real meaning to the overly manipulated terms "humanity," "civilization," and "culture"; in his drafts he constantly scribbled "cultural genocide."

In his essays on cultural genocide, he took Jewish culture as a first example, with the Bible as the founding document:

In 1939 the Germans burned the great library of the Jewish Theological Seminary at Lublin, Poland. This was reported by the Germans as follows: "For us it was a matter of special pride to destroy the Talmudic Academy. . . . We threw out of the building the great Talmudic library. . . . We set fire to the books. . . . The Jews of Lublin were assembled around and cried bitterly. . . . We summoned the military band and the joyful shouts of the soldiers silenced the sound of the Jewish cries."[42]

Then, he exalted European culture:

How impoverished our culture would have been if the people condemned by Germany, like the Jews, had not been capable of creating the Bible or bringing into the world an Einstein, a Spinoza; if the Poles had been unable to offer the world a Copernicus, a Chopin, a Curie; the Czechs . . . Huss, Dvorak; the Greeks . . . Plato, Socrates; the Russians . . . Tolstoy, Rimsky-Korsakov; the French . . . Voltaire, Montesquieu, Pasteur; the Dutch, Erasmus, Grotius, Rembrandt; the Belgians, Rubens, Maeterlinck; the Norwegians, Grieg; the Yugoslavs, Negosti; the Danes, Kierkegaard.[43]

No example was given from outside Europe; although the peoples of Africa and Asia were still largely under colonization, Latin America had been of great assistance to the UN. The first signatory state of the convention, in December 1948, was the Dominican Republic.

"Camouflaged genocide"?

Lemkin made a living teaching at various universities, but he was only a guest lecturer for limited terms, looked down on by his colleagues. He tried to find a position via the Emergency Committee in Aid of Displaced Foreign Scholars, which had assisted him so generously in 1941. He put forth his main specialty, financial law and international payments, convinced of its importance in settling the war.[44] He lashed out at legal scholars who disdained him and clung to the Nuremberg categories—not including genocide—in order to "reap jobs, honors, and Mandarin ceremonies." As for his political and diplomatic opponents—particularly the British and the Soviets—they joined forces to bury the convention project "in perfumed coffin committees."[45]

The reporter for *The New Yorker* in Paris for the 1948 UN session sketched Lemkin aptly: "Lemkin is a sad, witty, man born in eastern Poland. . . . He became a lawyer, which he now regrets, because he feels that lawyers are against progress. In the course of studying genocide, he has, he says, discovered that when authorities burn books, they are likely to start burning people next, and he wants a law against both."[46] Burning books, burning human beings: Lemkin, shameless, did not credit the German poet Heinrich Heine, but he plainly showed his disappointment. At first, he had divided evil, crime, into seven "fields of genocide techniques"—political, social, economic, biological, physical, religious, and moral—which he subsequently reduced to three: physical, biological, and cultural genocide, "a violation of the integrity of the group and selected members of this group. . . . If one kills a man without regard to the fact that he is Polish, Armenian, Huguenot, or Muslim, this is a simple murder, but if one kills a man because he is Polish, Armenian, Huguenot, or Muslim, it is a case of genocide."[47]

To emphasize intentionality, the delegate from the Netherlands invented the incisive formula of "camouflaged genocide": "It will have to be established beyond doubt, however, that so-called camouflaged genocide will equally be punishable; this covers cases in which the defendant might plead that the incriminated action, although it did in fact lead to the destruction or frustration of a group, was not aimed against that group."[48]

But, by the time it was being adopted, the convention no longer really corresponded to what Lemkin was arguing for. When he began his work, he took the example of other peoples to prove the universality of genocide and had his articles translated into many languages. In an interview during the UN session in December 1948, he talked about the consequences of the "crime of crimes" in relation to the forced departure of victims (a subject as current in 2018 as in 1948): "The victims of genocide do not simply wait patiently for death to arrive. They flee to other countries that are not always prepared to accept them. The problem of displaced persons and children in distress is only one direct result of genocide. Certain countries are called upon to pay the costs of crimes committed elsewhere. This crime is thus international because of its ramifications for international life."[49]

ς

Lemkin was plagued by bad luck: on the eve of the vote on the convention, the Universal Declaration of Human Rights was itself voted on. After suffering the blows of Lauterpacht and Jackson, he had to face competition from René Cassin and Eleanor Roosevelt.[50] Indeed, many thought that the first fight of the twentieth century, the protection of minorities under the law, should now give way to protection of individual rights—a feeling shared also among Lemkin's supporters, although he was convinced of the contrary:

> The Declaration of Human Rights is only an enunciation of general principles. It has no binding force as international law. ... The Genocide Convention is an international treaty. It can be enforced both as an international law and as a domestic law. Dealing with international crime, it carries with itself penalties and the highest degree of legal and moral condemnation. The Genocide Convention is a definite and precise commitment before the world not to murder peoples and races.... The Declaration of Human Rights is only an engagement; the Genocide Convention is a marriage.[51]

This was quite ironic, coming from a man who had never married. Perhaps he had never even had a love affair, except with his concept.

"There are some jurists who are still hesitating . . . but there are fewer of them than of those who are horrified by genocide and want to stop it. The convention must become a living force in the global community."[52]

After the vote in December 1948, the fight for ratification began, as the signatures of twenty nations were necessary for the convention to become law. Given the combination of the word "genocide" and its new legal definition, the reticence of legal scholars, and the reality of planned extermination, the "founder of the movement to outlaw genocide" looked in every direction. He dared to lie outright to Eleanor Roosevelt, telling her that in 1943 his memorandum had convinced her husband of the relevance of the concept; as we recall, he was furious when he learned that Roosevelt likely hadn't read it! One of his colleagues, Betty Hight, reported to him, though, that "the President expressed his great interest . . . and that he believed in this cause; that such a treaty would not apply to past genocides cases but would be very beneficial for the future."[53]

Persuaded that his argument was legitimate, and sometimes not without bad faith, he wrote relentlessly. For instance, to Léon Blum: "You know
about this tragic problem, alas, better than any statesman in the world. Your
entire life you have fought for the principles that are the essence of this convention. . . . If France ratifies it, quickly, I am convinced that all other members will follow its example."[54] France was indeed an example, but of what
all nations were thinking: the crime of genocide was always for others. As
a French member of the human rights mission to the UN wrote at the time
of ratification in 1950, "Genocide, which is the systematic destruction of a
human group, is a crime that France will never commit and that it will never
approve nor excuse. There is no reason for France to defer its ratification."[55]

Even though twenty nations ratified the convention in 1951, it was quickly
weakened by the lack of an international tribunal, notably, and by the prolonged refusal of major states, including the United States, to ratify it. Up
to the present, United Nations bodies have made scant use of the concept,
in inverse proportion to its common and often inappropriate use by the
public.

Lemkin remained the target of attacks. Some felt that the notion of genocide
contributed nothing tangible. Others, conversely, felt that he was minimizing their own persecution by not characterizing it as genocide. These debates
have continued for seventy years. For instance, at a time when segregation
had just been abolished in the US army but remained legal throughout
the country, certain African Americans wanted to appropriate the concept:
"Yet this powerful weapon [racist hysteria] is responsible for the extermination of three million European Jews, what a prominent jurist, Dr. Raphael
Lemkin, calls 'genocide.' Warsaw and Brooklyn may not be the same, but it
can happen here and with the most appalling consequences for the Negro
people."[56] In 1951, William Patterson, secretary of a civil rights association,
went even further, presenting the UN with a petition accusing the United
States of genocide on behalf of "fifteen million black Americans, the vast
majority of whose lives are deliberately warped and distorted by the willful
creation of conditions making for premature death, poverty, and disease."[57]

Again in 1953, after Lemkin had once again maladroitly evoked discrimination against blacks in the South in an article on the "nature of genocide,"
Oakley Johnson asked him to reexamine his definition of the term in a

country involved in "terrorizing colored people, that is terrorizing a whole race of people who are colored. . . . They terrorize all Negroes, regularly, systematically, all the time. . . . We have here discrimination as a factor in genocide, just as the yellow badge of racial inferiority was forced on Jews by the Nazis." And Johnson added, "In view of the importance of this subject in the United States and its international importance too (South Africa; the whole colonial set-up) . . . you and other authorities should clear up the meaning and application of the term 'genocide.'"[58] This gave rise to a current of thought that has come to prominence in the early twenty-first century, a current that aims to define the slave trade and racialized enslavement not only as crimes against humanity but also as genocides.[59] Even though Lemkin rarely addressed racism, colonialization, and colonialism, his term has been seized upon—proof of recognition of its effectiveness. The concept has become more political than legal, which explains why some social sciences researchers hesitate to use it, even today.

Tirelessly, until the end of his life, Lemkin justified his body of work. For he had only one goal: to have the convention ratified.

Like any new concept, genocide was amalgamated with others. Some confuse genocide and discrimination. That is false:

a) Genocide implies destruction, death, annihilation, whereas discrimination is a *regrettable*[60] denial of certain life possibilities. Being treated unequally is not the same thing as being dead.

b) Genocide is an international crime whereas discrimination is comparatively minor; it is not a criminal phenomenon.[61]

Lemkin was not without political cunning. His correspondence gives multiple examples of his about-faces. For instance, he wrote to Andrey Vyshinsky, the Soviet representative at the UN and a prosecutor at the trials in Moscow. Not hesitating to use medical metaphors, as was the style of the day, he tried to cajole the mass criminal by explaining that not all progress meant a plot against the USSR: would Vyshinsky vote against penicillin?[62]

Yet, he supported peoples—such as the Greeks and the Baltic peoples—who were accusing the Soviets or their satellites of crimes of genocide. In a text sent to the International Labour Conference in London, he protested against communist "genocidal ideology": "Although human rights violations

exist in democracies in different forms of discrimination, genocide is practiced only in Russia."[63] And when African Americans returned to the fray,
he explained to them that they were directing blame against the United
States, when the real tragedy was happening to peoples dominated by the
Soviets.[64] "From the present communist campaign it becomes clear that
action is directed against the Jews in the entire area under communist control. Although Genocide affects now parts of the Jewish people, there is a
danger that under the influence of Soviet propaganda, which assumed the
dimensions and techniques applied by Streicher and Goebbels, the action
will spread rapidly so as to cause the destruction of the entire Jewry."[65] Lemkin did not deny the local anti-Semitism in different Soviet and Sovietized
territories; on the contrary, he rightly emphasized in his writings of the
time that both ancestral and recent lands were susceptible to this new campaign: "The communist campaign is facilitated by the pogrom traditions
in the areas involved which have developed and matured through centuries.
The Russian soil is saturated with the blood of hundreds of thousands of
Jews, and the local population can be easily aroused to participate now in a
large scale genocide action."[66]

Therefore, when the USSR ratified the convention, in 1954 (one year after
Stalin's death), Lemkin could not rejoice fully, as he realized that this signature invalidated his work. But the attacks against Jews by the Soviets
and their satellites (Lemkin cited the Czechs, the Poles, the Hungarians, the
Romanians, and the Bulgarians) were not the only reason for his uneasiness, and his argument was far from being only about the Cold War. In 1951,
he pointed out the major error by the United States, which stubbornly refused to sign the 1948 Convention. He concurred with Adolph Berle, former
assistant secretary of state and now chair of the International Law Committee of the New York City Bar Association: "Failure to ratify the convention
deprives us of a powerful weapon against communism. . . . The Communists unquestionably would use our reluctance to accept the convention in
an attempt to undermine our moral leadership. . . . There is evidence that
the Soviet Union was engaged in genocidal acts against the population of the
Baltic Republics—Lithuania, Estonia and Latvia. Thousands upon thousands
of their male citizens were being deported to Siberia, and their women to
Turkestan. . . . Lemkin warned against the delusion that the crime of mass
extermination had died with the Hitler Regime."[67] Berle, an eminent figure,

was briefed by Lemkin, who was still obsessed with "his" genocide, and he pointed out two fundamental aspects: the convention had a moral, ethical aspect, and American democracy had to recognize it to prove its superiority over Soviet communism. In addition, the Soviet Union was continuing to practice genocide against its own peoples, in particular in reprisal for their "collaboration" with the Nazis during World War II. Lemkin spoke out publicly about the Baltic states, but he also mentioned the Crimea-Tartars, the Caucasian people, and the Volga Germans.

This was when Lemkin turned to examine the Soviet past, and it led to his decision to campaign to have the Great Famine in Ukraine in 1933 declared a genocide. He gave a well-documented speech for the anniversary of the Great Famine in Ukraine on September 20, 1953, six months after Stalin's death: "It is the classic example of Soviet Genocide, its longest and broadest experiment in Russification—the destruction of the Ukrainian Nation." He described the genocide of the Ukrainians in three parts, starting with the destruction of its

> religious, intellectual, political [elites]. . . . The first blow is aimed at the intelligentsia, the national brain, so as to paralyze the rest of the body. In 1920, 1926, and again in 1933, teachers, writers, artists, thinkers, political leaders were liquidated, imprisoned or deported. . . . Second an offensive against the churches, priests, and hierarchy, the "soul" of Ukraine. . . . The third prong of the Soviet plan was aimed at the farmers, the large mass of independent peasants who are the repository of the tradition, folklore and music, the national language and literature, the national spirit of Ukraine. The weapon used is perhaps the most terrible of all—starvation. Between 1932 and 1933, 5,000,000 Ukrainians starved to death.[68]

Lemkin's vision was true: the famine sponsored by Stalin—the Holodomor, as the Ukrainians called it—was a "classic" genocide, with no doubt as to its intention. Prominent historians are unanimous on this fact today, even as the debate over the legal qualification of the crime of genocide continues.[69] For although Lemkin did indeed include political and cultural motivations in his personal definition of genocide, it must be said that the historically recognized definition was not that used by the legal scholars in 1948—whence the debates continuing to the present day, and not just on Ukraine.

The Ukrainian Parliament voted to recognize the Holodomor "as a deliberate act of genocide" in 2006, and many monuments memorializing the famine, the most imposing of which is the Museum-Memorial of Kiev, bear lines from Lemkin's "Soviet Genocide in Ukraine." Nevertheless, some Ukrainians see the events in Babi Yar, in Kiev—site of the largest open-air massacre of Jews—and of the extermination of Jews by Nazis in general—in which many Ukrainians participated—as unfair competition for victimization: had the Ukrainians not suffered enough? These Ukrainians don't like to remember that Lemkin, whom they are happy to canonize as inventor of the term "genocide," was Jewish and Polish and that he had studied in Lvov, now Lviv.

The Armenians Appropriate the Word "Genocide"

How happy Lemkin would have been had he known that Chavarche Missakian, who had been tortured and had survived the first deportations from Constantinople on April 24, 1915, and who had become editor of the Armenian daily in Paris, *Haratch*, had titled his editorial of December 9, 1945, "Genocide":

> A new word . . . coined by an American professor, Lemkin, who explains its meaning in a recently published book. . . . We follow the Nuremberg trials and our mind draws us to a distant world, where "war crimes" were similarly committed according to a plan designed and premeditated yesterday—actually, thirty years ago—to annihilate a people abandoned and left defenseless during the Great War. . . . At that time, where were the lawyers and judges of today? Had they not discovered the word, or was the bloodthirsty monster so powerful and beyond apprehension that they could not grasp it? . . . Has the world improved, from Istanbul and Malta to Nuremberg, Berlin, or Auschwitz? . . . These hyenas of genocide should be summarily judged and sentenced! But where was the first "exemplary" lesson of the present-day genocide inaugurated?[70]

Missakian wrote "war crimes" in scare quotes and adopted the word "genocide"—the neologism *Tséghasbanoutyoun* in Armenian—the word that he would have so wished for in 1915.

Disaster? Massacre? That was yesterday! A genius would have to be born to conceive of this form of extermination and transmit it to barbarians. Another genius was now necessary to find the word describing the fait accompli. No modern language had this word. . . . Today's words seem risible to character-ize this catastrophe. "Massacre," "slaughter," and "war" are all innocent words.[71]

To make his case for the urgent need for the Convention on Genocide, Lemkin, the "genius," now oriented his campaign to Christian institutions. In a letter to the Council of Methodist Women, he linked the catastrophes affecting Christians in the two world wars:

This convention is a matter of our conscience and is a test of our relationship to evil. I know it is very hot in July for work. . . . Let us not forget that the heat of this month is less unbearable to us than the heat in the ovens of Auschwitz and Dachau and more lenient than the murderous heat in the desert of Aleppo that burned to death the bodies of hundreds of thousands of Christian Arme-nians victims of genocide in 1915.[72]

Lemkin was well known at the time, as he had given an interview broad-cast on the CBS television network. After summarizing the principles of the convention, he gave a long description of the Armenian genocide. In the background were images of Ottoman soldiers hunting down Armenian children and adults, over which the moderator, Quincy Howe, commented, "These folks . . . are running for their lives. . . . Men on horseback . . . let's say they are modern cavalry out on orders of their commanders. They are huntsmen out on the chase. Only the prey doesn't happen to be a fox. The prey is people. These [Armenians] were the victims. . . . Why? Well, the rea-son given was that they were friendly to the enemy of their rulers; that they were a fifth column; that they were spies. Every one of the 2 million of them—women, men, and children." Then, Lemkin explained that the annihilation of the Armenians and the impossibility of indicting the criminals had led to his interest in genocide. He recalled Soghmon Tehlirian, the murderer of Talaat Pasha in 1921, with whom he identified directly; both had lost their mother and their native tongue and culture. "[His] mother was killed in the genocide. . . . And he told the court that he did it because his mother came in his sleep . . . many times. . . . The murder of your mother, you would do something about it! So he committed a crime. So, you see, as a lawyer, I thought that a crime should not be punished by the victims, but should be punished by a court."[73]

Lemkin sought in history the intellectual arguments needed for ratification of the convention, even though he knew that it was a political act—whence his complementary readings, in particular on the Armenians. By allying with the Christians, he was pursuing the universalization of his concept, and in looking back at 1915 he was defining his mission to span the entire century. It was in these years that the Armenian genocide returned to being the matrix of his intellectual scaffolding, as it had been in the 1920s and 1930s. Thus, he wrote, in reference to cultural genocide, "The Armenians tried to assemble the names from all their communities who were victims of the genocide. Libraries around the world are collecting all these facts. It would be morally wrong to think that they are being collected for purely scientific and historical reasons. Each Armenian finds himself in each of the documents of the time."[74]

In Lemkin's papers is a book by James J. Mandolian, *What Do the Armenians Want?* (1946), in which Lemkin would have read, "The Armenian case is an old case and a forgotten case which is being revived."[75] He was still emphasizing his affinity with the Armenians in his last published work, a book review that can be read as a testament:

> Father Naslian expresses a judgment that is particularly close to the author's heart. It is that the victims of genocide through the ages have filled history with their pain to the point that humanity can no longer evade either identification of the consequences or its moral responsibility. . . . The sufferings of Armenian men, women, and children thrown into the Euphrates or massacred on the road from Deir Ez-Zor prepared the way for adoption of the Convention on Genocide by the United Nations and morally forced Turkey to ratify it. . . . A million Armenians died, but a law against the murder of peoples has been written with the ink of their blood and in the spirit of their ordeal.[76]

Satisfied that fifty countries had ratified the convention by 1959, Lemkin forgot that it might be absolutely counterproductive. Indeed, the Turks had signed in July 1950, but with the certainty that the Armenians had not suffered a genocide, as Lemkin had made sure not to speak to them about it.[77] Up to the present day, the Turkish state has maintained its position of genocide denial.

"Mr. Lemkin of the Genocide" (Mgr. Roncalli)

Lemkin twice met with Monsignor Roncalli, the future Pope John XXIII, who offered him a beautiful title of nobility, "Mr. Lemkin of the Genocide."[78] Convinced more than ever that the "genocide catastrophe"—the constantly recurring killing of "other" people—formed the nucleus of world history, Lemkin launched himself into writing, publishing numerous articles and planning two books, an autobiography and a history of the concept of genocide, designed as a kind of encyclopedia, in which he intended to describe every destruction of peoples from antiquity to contemporary times.[79] For the latter book, he created or adopted a number of concepts in order to clarify his thought on genocide, revealing himself to be an original cultural researcher. His transdisciplinary vision brought together history, demography, international relations, anthropology, art history, geography, law, sociology, and political science, and his subjects ranged from the Assyrians to the Tasmanians, in alphabetical order. Unfortunately, only a few fragments and a detailed table of contents remain from the original work.

As he was particularly interested in psychology, Lemkin sought to define the interrelationships among three groups: "victims," "genocidists," and the "outside world." There is little chance that Raul Hilberg had read his manuscript when he created his three categories for destruction of the European Jews: "victims," "perpetrators," and "bystanders." Hilberg's "bystanders," analogous to Lemkin's "outside world," reflected more accurately the ambivalent reality than did the concept of the French word *témoin* (witness), as it encompassed seeing, not seeing, participating in the crime, resisting.[80] At the same time as he was theorizing genocides for the final time, Lemkin was also writing his autobiography: in the Belarusian, then Polish, village of his youth, he had been able to observe his disreputable neighbors (or bystanders).[81]

Like the psychiatrist William Niederland, Lemkin described "survivor syndrome," from which he was trying to recover.[82] He knew from experience that the extreme situations with which combatants were confronted had little in common with those facing victims of genocide. After a war, the number of survivors—male, uniformed veterans—is always higher than the number of dead. Coming home from the military front, they return to domestic life and their families. As Lucien Febvre wrote in 1946, "I, a survivor, confronted with cemeteries where the dead of two generations, mown down in their prime, rest uneasily."[83] Conversely, there are very few survivors of a genocide, and they are without family, without support, often forced to go into exile, without a home, without photographs, without personal effects.[84] This explains why so many of them have problems that Lemkin called the "psychological responses of fear; defeatism; loss of self-respect; resistance; and revenge."[85] True to his method, he took specific examples from his readings, encounters, the Nuremberg trial records. It was a prodigious work, in which everything led to genocide. He also alluded to the sense of guilt for having survived, explored in depth in the 1960s by authors from Niederland to Primo Levi. The catastrophe—*Shoah* in Hebrew—was irreparable, it was still spreading, and again, one did not live (*vit*), one survived (*sur-vit*), a semantic nuance that Soazig Aaron reinvented as "subviving" (*sous-vivant*).[86] *Introduction to the History of Genocides* was to be the masterpiece that Lemkin, who had crossed the Atlantic in time, would offer to victims of the crime of crimes: "The very fact of having survived thanks to geography leads to the perpetuation of painful memories." At the time of the Eichmann trial, in 1961, there were some who missed him: "Lemkin, the man who could have abolished future Eichmanns; the man who fought, the fight of a single man, for a single science. A modern Don Quixote who charged the windmills of the world and offered a major contribution to save humanity."[87]

But Lemkin died in 1959. Although the last people to visit him claimed that descriptions of his misery and solitude were being exaggerated—he had even been nominated for the Nobel Peace Prize—his strong feeling of exclusion was like a metaphor for the general indifference to the word "genocide" for many years, inversely proportional to its excessive use today.

> "I was alone, with no money, in a foreign country.
> I had to start my life over." (Jan Karski)

While Lemkin was fighting to save his conception of genocide, Karski was losing his Poland. In May 1944, as he was feverishly writing his memoir, he sent a telegram to London suggesting that "his impressions of England and the United States be publicized in Poland, including the political problems with postwar aid to Poland in world opinion."[88] His book *Story of a Secret State*, a call for mobilization in his country, an implicit order, was intended to be used to prove the rights of the democratic Poland arising from the government in exile. "Poland grew no Quislings, but under the Nazi terror there has grown a secret democratic state. This book is the story of a people who for four years have lived and worked under an invisible government."[89]

But the Soviets who let the Nazis crush the resistance would soon occupy Poland, bringing it under their domination. After Yalta, Karski, the militant patriot, was quoted as saying, "Another Munich for Poland."[90]

For American communists guided by remote control from Moscow, the Warsaw insurrection was a trap, and the resisters who had worked for the government in exile in London were traitors to the true nation and true Poles. Karski was a perfect example. His book was the subject of a critical review in *Soviet Russia Today*, "Not the Whole Story," the author of which paid scant tribute to the courier's courage, presenting him as a naive puppet in the hands of the government in exile. The offspring of a "rather well-to-do family," he was incapable of understanding anything about the struggle of the Polish people and the grandeur of the Soviet sacrifice in 1940.

"In spite of excellent treatment when he was sent to a [prisoners'] camp by the Russians, Karski decides to go back to German-occupied Poland. . . . There he encounters Nazi terror and brutality." While recognizing the importance of his testimony, notably in the two chapters concerning the Warsaw ghetto and Belzec, the critic evoked Karski's treachery: he left Poland in 1943 (in reality in 1942, which would have further reinforced the magazine's point of view) and thus knew nothing further about his country; he was able to survive "easily" thanks to his networks, whereas true Poles were "collectively held responsible for acts of resistance" and massacred. Finally, Karski was working under the auspices of the National Democratic Party: "Every Pole knows that the foundations of this party were laid on anti-Semitism and political and economic struggle against the Jews." Why so much hate, even though the anti-Semitism of certain Polish political parties, before and after the war, cannot be denied? Because Karski was advocating for an Inter-Allied Committee that would administer Polish affairs until free elections were held, which, he hoped, would give birth to a democratic Poland.

For the proponents of a Sovietized Poland, therefore, he lost all the value that he had acquired as a resister. He was no longer anything but "an instrument for the propaganda apparatus of the London Government-in-Exile."[91]

Serving the CIA

So, it is not surprising that Karski agreed to work for former president Herbert Hoover. Hoover, whose political career had been ended by his inability to grapple with the 1929 crisis, in 1945 regained all the energy of his remarkable organization that had supplied occupied Belgium and northern France during the Great War. The neutral powers had sent humanitarian aid to populations threatened with famine and had sold their agricultural production, while accomplishing the feat of having most of the receipts go to the French and Belgian governments. Hoover had also largely saved the Russians from famine in 1921, following the civil war.[92]

Now, in 1945, the important thing was to rescue archives. The documents of former governments in exile, starting with those that the couriers, the agents, often risking their lives, had transported, were in danger of disappearing. Karski accepted this repatriation mission and was to leave for Europe in early summer 1945. On July 5, however, the United States recognized the new Sovietized Poland; the country for which he had fought no longer existed. His mentor, Jan Ciechanowski, handed in the keys to the embassy in Washington. Karski, like most of the staff, did not want to pledge allegiance to the new regime. From refugee, he became stateless.

It was in the service of the United States, of which he became a citizen in 1954—and where his pseudonym "Karski" definitively replaced the name Kozielewski, because that was how he had entered the country—that he went to Europe with the hope, an insane hope for many years (until 1989), of finding a Poland that he knew.

In this context, the search for archives that he conducted from July to December 1945 resembled Dubnow's or Ringelblum's. When all was lost, the traces of the glorious past struggle against the Nazis—and the communists—remained proof of life, of struggle, of hope.[93]

In London, Paris, and Rome, Karski collected hundreds of leaflets during this final trip as a courier. The main thrust of these documents, of course, was anti-Soviet more than anti-Nazi. In *Poland Accuses: An Indictment of the Major German War Criminals*, Poles, who had been absent from Nuremberg in accordance with the wishes of the Soviets, insisted on looking back at 1939 and the German-Soviet agreement on the dismantling of Poland.[94] The time of the Nazis seemed to have been only a short parenthesis in the larger struggle of Polish patriots against the Russians and then the Soviets.

However, Karski continued to carry within himself the great massacre of the Jews. With them he shared an early memory, from immediately after the catastrophe, a private memory recorded in accounts hastily written in 1945–46 and marked by numerous commemorations, especially in Yiddish, in the different countries—France, Belgium, the United States, Australia, Argentina, the Yishuv and then Israel—in which several tens of thousands of survivors found themselves.[95]

Professor Karski

Karski had dreamed of becoming a Polish diplomat, but this was now impossible. So, he returned to studying political science under the aegis of the regent of Georgetown University in Washington, the Jesuit priest Edmund Walsh, whom he had met in 1943. He used his personal documents for his dissertation, "The Great Powers and Poland, 1919–1945," a typewritten copy of which was presented in 1953 at Georgetown University and numerous editions of which formed the basis of his teaching throughout his academic career.

His work as a student and then as a professor was in line with his citizen engagement since 1939: to show the calamities faced by independent Poland, from its resurrection in 1919 to its obliteration by the Soviets in 1945. In chapter 28 of his dissertation, "British and American Attitudes toward Poland, 1941–1943," he explained how Roosevelt's and Churchill's "pragmatism" in winning the war led them to prefer an alliance with the Soviets, who were indispensable to defeating the Nazis, over their commitments to Poland: "Polish interests, whenever in conflict with Russia's demands, rarely seemed important enough to risk antagonizing the Soviet dictator. Stalin realized his worth, and whenever it came to Polish matters, he took full advantage of his position."[96] Military strategy dominated, and, if Poland had to be sacrificed, Poland would be sacrificed. Karski quoted himself:

In August 1943, a courier from the Polish Underground, Jan Karski, was dispatched to Washington with a mission to report on the situation in Poland

and on the Nazi extermination of the Jews. Roosevelt received him with both interest and sympathy. True, he pointed out, Poland would have to concede some territory to Russia, but he was sure that Stalin would demand no more than what was necessary "to save face." . . . "Tell the leaders of the resistance," the president concluded, "that their indomitable attitude has been duly appreciated. Tell them that they will never have cause to regret their brave decision to reject any collaboration with the enemy and that Poland will live to reap the reward of its heroism and sacrifice.[97]

It was 1953, the year of Stalin's death, but the Cold War continued. The fate of the Polish Jews was now secondary. And yet, when, twice in his imposing volume, Karski spoke of the Holocaust, it was as an eyewitness: "In enslaved Poland people lived in abjection, humiliation, lawlessness, and terror. Concentration camps grew larger and more numerous every month. Nazi atrocities were unspeakable. Forsaken by all and totally helpless, Poland's Jews—three and a half million of them—were about to begin their last exodus from the ghettoes to gas chambers." This passage was footnoted: "For an eyewitness testimony as to conditions in the Warsaw and Belzec ghettoes, see Karski, *Story of a Secret State*."[98]

Karski the academic used classic archives; when he quoted himself, it was with regard to the fate of Poland—his dissertation subject—and that of the Polish Jews. In the ensuing years, however, the extermination of the Jews disappeared completely from his academic and public discourse. For it was the prisoner who had escaped the Soviets and the Polish exile who interested Radio Free Europe and other activist audiences: "Jan Karski will present the methods of Soviet indoctrination in satellite countries."[99] Karski used his oratorical talents for the CIA on a lecture tour across Asia and Europe. In 1956, he testified in front of the House Un-American Activities Committee, where he presented himself as an academic expert with direct experience of the war. The former resister and author of *Story of a Secret State* went to testify about "Communism and the Soviet methods of conquest in the Eastern European area" during the year of uprising and revolts in Poland and Hungary. He found the committee too discreet, acknowledged its "very, very good work," and promised to speak out even more.[100]

Karski continued to tell the story of his meeting with Roosevelt in 1943, from which he excerpted only the passages on the Poles, the war, and the resistance. In 1957, he wrote to the newspapers, as he would do often, about the "false election in Poland" after the disturbances of 1956. He pointed out that this nonelection hid the true aspirations of the "Polish nation, which has not experienced such misery in half a century and has no hope for the future." He saw a clear paradox: "There is certain confusion, strangely enough, caused by a combination of communist propaganda and American traditional sympathy for the Polish People."[101] This concerned a different Poland, one that no longer existed.

In 1961, Karski, an anticommunist so virulent that his students nicknamed him "McCarthski," was invited to the Maxwell Air Force Academy. A photograph shows him equipped for flight at the side of an instructor, a colonel. Then he gave a lecture on communism. He introduced himself this way: "In 1943, I personally reported to President Roosevelt and other British and American officials."[102] In 1943, during World War II, what had he "reported"?

Karski, the new American, with his strong accent and particular habits, left no doubt about where his heart belonged. Thus he described himself, in French and not without humor, at the time he was undertaking a tour for the CIA:

I am a Catholic by religion, believing and practicing. I completed my university studies in Poland, in the faculty of law. . . .

During the war, I fought as a soldier against the Germans and became a prisoner of war. . . . in Russia. In 1939, Stalin's Russia collaborated with Hitler's Germany. The two countries attacked Poland from two sides.

I escaped, and once back in Poland I joined the resistance against the Nazis. . . . I traveled around Europe a number of times, naturally in secret. In 1940, I was arrested by the Gestapo. I escaped, without my teeth and with several ribs broken during torture. In 1943, I was sent to the United States to inform President Roosevelt and the American government about the situation in Poland. When the English and American governments recognized the communist regime in Poland, in 1945 . . . I left the embassy and suddenly I became an immigrant. I was alone, with no money, in a foreign country. I had to start my life over.[103]

6

Becoming Karski,
Becoming Lemkin

1978–2018

The losses of war may be repaired, but the losses of genocide are irreparable.[1]

—Lemkin

The messengers had borne witness. By his invention of the term "genocide" and his fight for the UN convention, Lemkin built a memorial for the annihilated through his writings. Karski, the Catholic resister, never failed to remember the Jewish origins of his wife, Pola Nirenska, and her people wiped out in the catastrophe: "But I reported what I saw."[2] In the late 1970s, he began to take part in public commemorations of the destruction of the Jews in Europe.

"There is no testimony without some involvement of oath . . . and without sworn faith. . . . The witness *promises* to say or to manifest something to another, his addressee: a truth, a sense which has been or is in some way present to him as a unique and irreplaceable witness."[3] Is it necessary to recall that the French word for "witness," *témoin*, is etymologically related to the word "martyr"?

"All murdered Jews have become my family"

Although Jan Karski's two days in front of the filmmaker Claude Lanzmann's camera took place in 1978, Lanzmann was still editing his film in the early 1980s. The filming of the interview probably catalyzed in Karski, who had remained more or less silent on the subject since the war, the desire to speak out once again. The psychiatrist Dori Laub acknowledged such desires in an essay titled "Not Knowing Is an Active Process of Destruction. Why the Testimonial Procedure Is of So Much Importance";[4] elsewhere, he wrote, "Memory leads to memory, perhaps even to an explosion of memories."[5] Karski was feeling a sense of urgency: fewer and fewer survivors were still alive, and what they had lived through was further and further in the past. The struggle against time was accompanied by a sense of guilt for not having testified earlier. In a *Washington Post* article titled "Holocaust: So Horrible No One Believed It Was True," Abe Karp, professor of Jewish studies at the University of Rochester, described a colloquium in which Karski participated in 1980: "'How would one know an event so horrible that a special term had to be fashioned to describe it?'" This referral to a "special term," "Holocaust," followed by two years the broadcast of the television series of the same name. Lemkin would not have been happy that the producers of the series had refused to use his neologism. Whether holocaust or genocide, Karp added that, even long after 1945, it remained impossible to believe that the event had occurred. It was a denial that Karski, now a professor at Georgetown University and "a Polish citizen during the war," confirmed, as he recounted yet again his mission to Washington and his meetings with Roosevelt and Frankfurter.[6]

Karski did not speak in a major public arena devoted to the extermination of the Jews until 1981, when he sat on a panel at "Discovering the 'Final Solution,'" also called the International Liberators' Conference, the first symposium organized by the forerunner of the United States Holocaust Memorial Museum.[7] On the first day, the organizer, Miles Lerman, recounted how he had survived, which meant that he was one of those alive in Poland in 1945, and described how he had come to be involved with this conference, which, even in 1981, was groundbreaking.

> On the day of my liberation, I returned to my hometown on the top of a tank of the advancing Soviet and Polish armies. I should have been jubilant, for Hitler's defeat was imminent, but I was not. How could I be? For of the 16,000 Jews who lived in my hometown before the Nazi onslaught, I found on my return home 11 surviving Jews, wandering around aimlessly, hoping to find some of their families alive. Unfortunately, most of them perished in the gas

chambers of the death camp of Belzec. Among them were my mother, my sister and her husband, three of her young boys—ages six, eight, and 13—plus 29 other members of my immediate family.[8]

Lerman then made two promises to the dead: to remember their fate on the site of their ordeal—whence his commitment to commemorating Belzec—and, above all, to speak history aloud: "We [are] to bear witness and tell the story of their agony and their torture and their painful deaths . . . to ensure that this shameful chapter in the history of mankind remains unaltered and undistorted forever and ever."[9]

"Shameful," "mankind": Lerman positioned himself as a moral witness, as did most of the delegates from the fourteen Allied nations who spoke: survivors, resisters, officers, war correspondents, doctors, and military chaplains, including many from the Eastern Bloc—a first in Washington. The conference was possible because Elie Wiesel had met General Vasily Petrenko, liberator of Auschwitz, in Moscow in 1979. It was Wiesel's wish that liberated and liberators would fight together against Holocaust denial, and he felt that testimony from Jewish survivors was necessary, even though he was not taken in by certain political agendas. In his own speech, Wiesel remembered the arrival of the first Americans in Buchenwald, where he had himself arrived, the only survivor of his family, after the death march from Auschwitz. Barely a teenager, he had seen these soldiers, grown men, crack; the experience of extermination overturned the generational pyramid, inverted values and meaning, as all life had been crushed: "You broke down, you wept. You wept and wept uncontrollably, unashamedly. You were our children then. . . . You wept. We could not. We had no more tears left. We had nothing left. In a way we were dead, and we knew it."[10]

Karski's speech made a big impression in the assembly hall of the State Department. So, this man was living in Washington? How was it that he wasn't known? He took his time, giving details on dates, places, people encountered, articles published, lectures given. He retraced every step of an eyewitness account that no one had listened to; he went so far as to replay scenes. Wiesel reported on his speech: "There was laughter when he imitated Roosevelt, and there were tears when he described the Warsaw ghetto and its misery."[11] Asked what he thought about the lack of action by those to whom he had spoken in London and Washington, Karski said that he no longer felt anything: "At that time, I was a recording machine. I was a tape recorder. If I had any human feelings—surprise, shock—I would have gone crazy a long time ago. I had no feelings at all. So, don't ask me was I surprised or not. I was not surprised about anything."[12]

Karski didn't ask "Who knew what?" He knew better than anyone what the answer was. On the other hand, his question was "When?" The precise instant when things became known transformed him the more he spoke. He began to reconstruct his identity, in a form of self-Judaization that he pursued until his death, twenty years later:

> Many of you at this conference gave testimony on the Jewish Gehenna. Respect is due to you.
>
> The Lord assigned me a role to speak and write during the war, when—as it seemed to me—it might help. It did not. . . .
>
> Furthermore, when the war came to its end, I learned that the governments, the leaders, the scholars, the writers did not know what had been happening to the Jews. They were taken by surprise. The murder of six million innocents was a secret. . . .
>
> Then, I became a Jew like the family of my wife, who is sitting in this audience—all of them perished in the ghettos, in the concentration camps, in the gas chambers—so all murdered Jews became my family.
>
> But I am a Christian Jew. I am a practicing Catholic. And, although not a heretic, still my faith tells me: the second Original Sin had been committed by humanity: through commission, or omission, or self-imposed ignorance, or insensitivity, or self-interest, or hypocrisy, or heartless rationalization.
>
> This sin will haunt humanity to the end of time.
>
> It does haunt me. And I want it to be so.[13]

Haunted by the sin of the abandonment of the Jews, the Catholic who had nevertheless testified for their survival since 1942 now proclaimed himself a Jew—an emotional, cultural, political Jew, not a religious one. It was not the term "Holocaust" that came to his mind to designate the catastrophe, however, but "Jewish Gehenna," an assumed pleonasm, a vision of hellfire both Christianized and harking back to the retributions of the Old Testament.

"Righteous Among the Nations"

Karski's prominence did not escape two Israelis present at the International Liberators' Conference: Gideon Hausner, the prosecutor at the Eichmann trial, and Yitzhak Arad, director of Yad Vashem. They invited him to Israel, where he received the title of Righteous Among the Nations the following year, in 1982.

In 1942, when Karski was in the Warsaw ghetto and Izbica and Lemkin was writing the first draft of *Axis Rule*, a Jew from the Yishuv, Mordecai Shenhabi, was already conceptualizing the commemoration of the killings and the rescuers by formulating the notion of "Righteous Among the Nations" coupled with a memorial to the extermination of the Jews, "Yad Vashem": "I will give them, in my house and within my walls, a memorial [*Yad*] and a name [*Shem*] . . . that will not be cut off" (Isaiah 56:5). Shenhabi proposed, in addition to a list of Jewish victims, a "list of the Righteous Among the Nations who saved souls or belongings" of destroyed Jewish communities.[14]

It would take almost ten years for the notion of the "Righteous" to become rooted in Israeli culture: "Rescuers came from all social strata. . . . All those who came to our aid are dear to us, and when the history of the Holocaust is written, an eternal monument will also be erected in honor of these Righteous among the Nations."[15] In the Martyrs' and Heroes Remembrance (Yad Vashem) Law passed in August 1953, the definition was founded on the idea of personal heroism: "The Righteous among the Nations who risked themselves to save Jews."

The extermination of the Jews, mentioned in the Constitution of Israel in 1948 (*Shoah* in Hebrew, *Holocaust* in English), did not become part of the nation's civic religion until the late 1970s. The Eichmann trial was one of the main steps in this evolution.[16] Ben Gurion wanted the victims of the genocide to be identified with the state of Israel, which was presented as rampart and recourse for all oppressed and persecuted Jews. The trial had barely gotten under way when it was suspended for the commemoration of Yom HaShoah[17]—the day of the Shoah—when, for the first time, the Righteous Among the Nations were named.

In his closing argument at the trial, Hausner "paid a tribute to these Gentiles who helped us" and listed the "non-Jews" who had rescued them:[18] "In the dark, horrible night which descended on Europe with Hitler's rise to power, there were also some rays of light. And the Jewish people will not forget its benefactors.[19] . . . And those kindly Poles who were hiding Jews right in the middle of the valley of death, under fearful danger, braving the wave of hellish hate which had enveloped all Poland; there were others also, there was the Polish underground, and there were ordinary people who helped, who concealed, who saved, who kept others alive [in Lithuania, Germany, Yugoslavia, Greece, Bulgaria, Romania]."[20] Hausner quoted Karski, who was not yet, in the strict sense of the term, a patented Righteous Among the Nations. Although he had suffered for and with Jews, although he had testified for their survival, he had not literally saved any. The eyewitness became the moral witness, the "courageous emissary of the Jewish resistance," thanks to whom "everyone had an account from a non-Jewish eyewitness."[21]

The state of Israel gradually transformed this individual recognition into a diplomatic tool. In 1962, David Alcalay, director of the bureau of testimony on Jewish victims, took over the Department of the Righteous. He alone was responsible for the two faces of Yad Vashem: the names of the victims, written, intoned, howled, and the names of the saviors, become the "Righteous," still very few in number at the time. The presiding judge at the Eichmann trial, Moshe Landau, was appointed to head the Commission for Designation of the Righteous. Later came the planting of trees—the roots of sacrifice—in the Garden of the Righteous and increasingly sophisticated ceremonies in Jerusalem as the perimeter of Yad Vashem expanded. Hausner was to be one of Jan Karski's sponsors—one of those who put together the dossier proposing him for the status of Righteous Among the Nations.

Jan Karski: The Righteous Among the Righteous

Like the processes involved in canonization, the dossiers of the Righteous Among the Nations contained testimonials. For instance, Irving Sorkin lauded Karski's exemplary life: "I am certain that you will consider Mr. Karski perfectly worthy of such an honor, as he is a rightful Gentile."[22] The biblical term "Gentile" was not chosen at random.

In 1982, Karski began to speak publicly about American affairs, particularly everything connected with World War II and the genocide of the Jews. Right after the war, he had been practically silent. Now, he talked and he wrote. In April 1985, during President Reagan's visit to Bitburg, Germany, Karski shared the opinion of a number of his compatriots: the necessary reconciliation with the Germans could not be concluded in a cemetery that contained the graves of SS soldiers, especially if Reagan did not go to visit an extermination site.[23] In the *Washington Post*, he recalled his war missions in London and Washington, concluding with a judgment that was unusually bitter for him:

> I brought information on the fate of Jews in Nazi-dominated Poland as well as desperate requests for help from Jews, addressed to the Allied governments, to save those who could still be saved. . . . The Jewish requests for help came to naught—the inactivity of the powerful Allied governments having been determined by war priorities, self-controlled ignorance, self-imposed disbelief or soulless rationality. Thus, 6 million Jews, helpless and abandoned by humanity, perished in agony. Today, some 40 years later, as an old man coming to the end of his earthly journey, I cannot but raise my voice. We must pursue peace, cooperation, justice and freedom. But our pursuit can never be based on *self-imposed forgetfulness* of what happened to the Jews during World War II.[24]

A few months later, *Shoah*, finally completed, was released worldwide, and Karski gave his point of view about being a character in the film in a letter to the editor in the *Washington Post* titled "Holocaust: The leaders knew." The letter was framed and placed in the middle of the page. Karski listed all those with whom he had met and concluded, "The widely spread opinion that the Western leaders were unaware of what happened to the Jews is no more than a myth. They knew."[25]

Claude Lanzmann's Karskis: 1978, 1985, 2010

Claude Lanzmann filmed Karski extensively in 1978. In his 1985 edit, he abandoned the heroic resister in the midst of his mission on behalf of Poland (Karski's choice in his memoir) and as the bearer of messages to the Allies trying to convince the president of the United States of the reality of the extermination. The second day of the interview, during which Karski described his missions outside Poland, was completely set aside, as was the account of his hallucinatory visit to Belzec-Izbica. Lanzmann assigned him only the task of reporting what he had seen with his own eyes in the ghetto, echoing what the Jews in Warsaw had asked of him in 1942: "You are going to deal with the English. Now you will give them your oral reports. I'm sure it will strengthen your report if you will be able to say 'I saw it myself.'"[26]

Lanzmann intended *Shoah* not only to show the uniqueness of the Shoah but also to stand as the only work on the uniqueness of the Shoah, through the "exemplarity of the singular."[27] In the spare narrative of the film, the former courier had only one role: to talk about his mission in the ghetto. It was up to him not to report everything he had gone through but to play his part in the symphony composed and orchestrated by Lanzmann, who had designed *Shoah* to start with the first death centers—Chelmno, Treblinka, Sobibor, and the gas chambers at Birkenau. This was why he left Karski's testimony about the ghetto to the end and retained only forty minutes of the rushes in the edit.[28]

> It was important to position the ghetto after the radical nature of the death was known, to show that extermination was included in the logic of the ghettos, in which people were dying of hunger. There was another reason: for there to be tragedy, and for there also to be suspense, the end had to be known from the beginning. Viewers had to know what would happen while at the same time having the feeling that it could not happen.[29]

However, Karski was resistant to Lanzmann's demands, just as he had refused to meet with him until after more than a year of Lanzmann's insistent correspondence.

Karski weeps. "Now, I go back thirty-five years. No, I don't go back no, no"—three nos. He leaves the couch, the library, the screen. Lanzmann is alone; a traveling shot down the empty hallway. Then Karski reappears, sitting: "I am ready." But he doesn't look at Lanzmann, and he still objects: "Even now I don't want . . . I understand your role. I am here. I don't go back in my memory. I couldn't tell any more."[30]

Karski mixes present and past: 1978: "I don't go back"; the war, "I couldn't tell any more."[31] He has a linguistic tic. Most of his sentences begin with "now," as if he were encouraging himself to speak—to make the past present. He sets out next to himself his cigarettes, notes, evidence of what he is advancing. Close by is the reassuring presence of his wife. Lanzmann edited all of this out. He did, however, exploit Karski's initial refusal to let himself be submerged in his memories, cutting from the dramatic "No!" to the serenity of the new citizen of the United States, land of liberty. In a telling illustration, a cutaway shot overflies the Statue of Liberty, the port of New York, and the south end of Manhattan, and then we discover, via the Stars and Stripes on the White House flagpole, the capital of the most powerful country in the world: the Lincoln and Jefferson memorials, the Washington Monument, and Capitol Hill.[32] Lanzmann's camera becomes Frank Capra's, and Karski's voice becomes James Stewart's; we fluctuate between *Mr. Smith Goes to Washington* and *Why We Fight,* in the democratic and valorous America that Karski had served. He was the only Polish Catholic whom Lanzmann interviewed at length, and he was presented as Righteous even before Yad Vashem recognized him as such.

Karski describes the ghetto on the soundtrack as images of Warsaw in the 1980s appear on screen: the buildings, both modern and decrepit, of a popular democracy, brick houses, empty lots. Close-up on a street sign, a backyard. At the back, in the basement, was there once a passage to the ghetto like the one on Muranowska Street through which Karski had gone? "Indeed, at that time, the building had become like a modern version of the River Styx which connected the world of the living with the world of the dead."[33]

Karski never went to Auschwitz. Yet, images from Birkenau and Auschwitz—piles of forks, spoons, pots, suitcases, shoes, glasses, shaving brushes, archives of objects, traces that reeked of evil, that cried out—formed a long montage that accompanied his words.[34] These heaps were substitutes for the archives that Lanzmann did not allow himself to use in his film. The items crammed into the showcases of the museum that Auschwitz I had become were now metonyms for the uniqueness of the Jewish catastrophe that, far from reifying it, offered a glimpse of the daily life of those who had been murdered.

Dialogue between Lanzmann and Karski:

> JK: It is one thing to know statistics. There were hundreds of thousands of Poles also killed—of Russians, Serbians, Greeks. We knew about it. But it was a question of statistics.
>
> CL: Did they insist on the complete uniqueness?
>
> JK: This was their problem: to impress upon me—and that was my mission— to impress upon all the people whom I am going to see that the Jewish situation is unprecedented in history.[35]

JK: The question could be asked—and at various stages of this film this question emerged—is there any comparison between what happened to the European Jews during the second world war, and any happening in past history? Whatever I know about history, it is totally unique. It was a problem in itself unprecedented historically.[36]

Lanzmann hoped that by having not only listened but also recorded and filmed, he would spur memories. By cutting together multiple testimonies that were so different and so similar, he hoped to encounter history between personal truth and heuristic value. And so he returned again and again to the same questions, trying to break down his interviewees to the point that a movie critic, though moved by the "terrible urgency of 'Shoah,'" lambasted him: "Lanzmann seems needlessly cruel. . . . While the length of the film is certainly justified by the subject matter, Lanzmann seems almost arrogant in protracting some sequences . . . reflect[ing] his sometimes unreasoning fanaticism. . . . The fourth night, when the subject turns mainly to the Warsaw Ghetto, is the weakest, except that it does include the riveting, eloquent testimony of Jan Karski."[37]

But why did Lanzmann not use all of Karski's words—in particular those on the Warsaw ghetto and Izbica—even though he was excited at the idea of meeting him? "I remember the strong feelings that washed over me when I realized . . . that Jan Karski was alive. . . . So, Karski was living, the emotion intensified when I saw him and began to shoot with him, forgetting how long it had taken to convince him to accept."[38] Lanzmann knew that Izbica, which Karski had visited, was not an extermination site with a gas chamber but a place of transit where people were murdered "incidentally." So why claim to have asked him about Belzec?

In later years, Karski became a Righteous Among the Nations. When he was interviewed for the Spielberg Archive, and then more and more often until his death in 2000, he affirmed the uniqueness of the extermination of the Jews: "The Holocaust is unique . . . the Holocaust is Jewish."[39] Although, as a professor of political science, Karski was aware of other genocides (Bosnia, Armenia, Poland), he always dwelled on the exceptional nature of the genocide of the Jews, extending the thought of Elie Wiesel: "Destruction of the Jews was a unique phenomenon of World War II. As Elie Wiesel said:

'All nations under Nazi domination were victims, but all Jews were victims.'[40] Thirty years after Lemkin's death, Karski fell short of his reflections on genocides by elevating the genocide of the Jews.

It is not surprising that in the new Yad Vashem museum—an imposing concrete triangle that leads from night to day, from death to life, from dark times in Europe to the bright light of Jerusalem—Karski appears in a filmed sequence.[41] The scene, chosen from the rushes of *Shoah* donated by Lanzmann, is that in which he described his meeting with Roosevelt. He creates a forceful presence on screen through his choice of tone of voice and gesture. He draws himself up in his seat to embody the "'Grand Seigneur' . . . the majesty of power and grandeur." Then he shrinks before the deluge of weighty words on the certain military defeat of Nazi Germany. But he is not satisfied. As he is about to leave, he knows that he has to talk about the Jews, as "it is not a secondary question." "I stood up and told him, Mr. President, I will return to Poland, I will say that I have met with President Roosevelt, I need a strong message, everyone will ask me, 'What did he say?'" Karski once again imitates Roosevelt: he draws himself up a bit more, takes a puff of an imaginary cigar, makes a hand gesture so that the smoke of his cigarette rises toward an infinite grandeur: "You tell them that we will win this war, the guilty will be punished for their acts, and justice will win out." This scene, which Lanzmann did not include in *Shoah*—deeming that Karski was overacting—became central to Yad Vashem.

In one section of the museum, Raphael Lemkin, his concept of genocide, and a 1944 aerial photograph of the Auschwitz-Birkenau complex before its deadly purpose was known are presented, along with this question: "Why wasn't Auschwitz bombed?"

Karski and Lemkin figure together in this staging of the "when" and "why." Why had the world not heard the cries of the murdered Jews? Why had it not listened to the messengers, and why had it let the Jews die? An essay by Avraham Levite is placed above the TV monitor on which Karski appears: "All of us [are] dying here in polar, ice-cold indifference of nations, forgotten by the world and its hustle and bustle."[42] Karski had understood; in 1978, evoking Lord Selborne, the master of propaganda who saw in his 1942 mission only the successful poisoning of minds, he said, with both humor and bitterness, "You would probably actually have to take Lord Selborne and place him in Belzec! Of course this is impossible—Lord Selbornes do not end their lives in Belzec, they end their lives in bed, regardless of whether war was won or lost."[43]

Late in life, Karski gave more and more interviews and attended many conferences; in Washington, DC, in 1999, he said, "Being a resister was very dangerous then. But I want to respond about the Jews. The Jews were abandoned by governments, by churches, by societies. But they were not abandoned by all of humanity. There were thousands of individuals in Poland, Denmark, Holland, France, Greece, and Hungary who tried to help. Most of them perished. I survived, with some luck." In his speech he repeated once again that his principal mission had been not for Poland but for the Jews: "abandonment of the Jews," "the example of the *St. Louis*," "the bombing of Auschwitz," "the resisters for humanity."[44]

Karski's popularity in the United States, and then in Europe, is easily explained. He embodied the questions that were being asked in the 1990s and 2000s. And people turned to him because he confirmed, rather than contradicted, their existing vision of the history of the Shoah. Karski also understood that people's ideas change over time. For instance, he expressed his admiration for Roosevelt, despite his immense disappointment in 1943: "The greatest president of the United States. He was an American president, not a Jewish or Polish or Estonian president. He acted for what he considered to be the interests of the American people."[45]

Wiesel and Karski were close friends at the time: "In truth, you have long ago become an honorary citizen of Jewish history, which will forever remember your courageous and noble activities on behalf of persecuted and doomed Jews during the German occupation of Europe," Wiesel said. "To me, you represent the tragic condition of the messenger whose message has been transmitted but not accepted."[46] He made the transition to witness, in the literal and figurative senses, a moral duty that was similarly incumbent upon those listening. At the inauguration of the Yad Vashem museum, in March 2005, five years after Karski's death, Wiesel said, "There is something more frightening than the messenger who tried to deliver the message and is unable to do so. . . . It is when the messenger has delivered the message and nothing has changed. . . . What is our role? We must become the messengers."[47]

Karski never embodied the tragedy better than when he became an honorary citizen of Israel in 1994, fifty-two years after he had arrived in England with his "message." The foreign minister, Shimon Peres, welcomed him with these words:

> You, sir, proved by your very actions that you rank High in the all too brief list of such great and unique personalities who stood out in the darkest age of Jewish history. Had the Jewish People been blessed with more courageous individuals such as yourself, with more "Righteous among the Nations," its decimation would certainly have been tempered yet further.[48]

Peres's use of a religious vocabulary did not escape Karski, who responded,

> This is the proudest and most meaningful day in my life. Through the honorary citizenship of the State of Israel, I have reached the spiritual source of my Christian faith. In a way, I have also become a part of the Jewish community. . . . And now I, Jan Karski—by birth Kozielewski—a Pole, and American, a Catholic, have also become an Israelite.[49]

Being Righteous had made him universal, he had saved "men and thus all humanity"; being an Israeli citizen returned him to his Christian—that is, Jewish—origins.

All those who visit his grave at the Mount Olivet cemetery in Washington share his convictions. At the grave, decorated with a cross, can be found fresh flowers—a Christian ritual—but also stones and candles—a Jewish ritual.

After Karski died, Karol Badyna, a Polish artist who specialized in likenesses of John Paul II, produced a sculpture of him sitting on a bench in Washington in 1943, as he had portrayed the scene in the final pages of his memoir. The bronze likeness is playing chess, the passion of Karski's life; the pieces on the board are configured in such a way that he wins no matter what play an adversary who sits down opposite him might make, in a synthesis of the metamorphosis of Jan Kozielewski into Jan Karski. Indeed, even in the face of strong opposition, he had always won: a pawn at the beginning of the war, a knight serving the resistance, then a court jester in his missions, he finally became Righteous Among the Nations and then Righteous of the Righteous, in an absolute moral coronation. The first Karski was that of World War II; the second Karski was the one discovered by Elie Wiesel and Claude Lanzmann; the third Karski, after his death in 2000, was at once American, Polish, Israeli, Catholic, and Jewish. When alive, he wanted to be everything at once; in death, he was instrumentalized by each identity in different ways.

Karski and Lemkin Enter the Realm of Literature

Bruno Tessarech and Yannick Haenel brought the character of Karski to French literature in 2009. The form of the novel allowed each author to deal with the polyphony of situations by offering multiple points of view. Tessarech's *Les Sentinelles* did not leave much open to debate, perhaps because the character of Karski was quite artificial—a highly romanticized version of the Catholic resister. Haenel was bolder in *Jan Karski*,[50] fashioning Karski as a new type of eyewitness who saw what others did not, without blind spots. Horrified, he watched the death of the Jews, the theophoric people, and touched God.

As an epigraph for his book, Haenel slightly shifted the meaning of Paul Celan's pessimistic "No one bears witness for the witness" to "Who witnesses for the witness?"[51] The question emphasized the fact that Karski narrated his own truth, that the images of him in the 1985 film were edited by Lanzmann, that chronology counts, and that 1943 was a long way from 1978—and an even longer way from 2009. In another of Haenel's novels, *Cercles*, a character actually refers to Shoah:

> I looked for traces of the ghetto. It was difficult because, in fact, there were no traces left. . . . There was nothing there, and yet he said that this was exactly where it had taken place. Was it possible that someone, in Warsaw, could designate a place, point to an empty lot, indicate a street, a part of a street, a hole in the street, and say, "There it is—that's where it took place"? Because even if you don't see anything—even if there's nothing to see—it was that nothing that I wanted to see.[52]

When *Shoah* was released, Lanzmann himself declared, in an American newspaper, "'That's the subject of the film, the fact that there's nothing left.'" As the article's author noted, "There are no pictures of gas chambers, of Auschwitz or Treblinka at their work of extermination. Many of the sites have been cleared, returned to pasture and silent woods. What Lanzmann

did was seek out those who saw the death machine: especially the few survivors of the Jewish *Sonderkommando.*" Remembering this "nothing" was
Karski's mission in the Warsaw ghetto: "Remember, Remember."[53]

Why had the world abandoned the Jews? Haenel's approach was quite
similar to that of the Yad Vashem museum. In returning to the meeting
with Roosevelt, he chose satire and parable. A disillusioned and wounded
Karski says again and again, in a long monologue, that the Jews of Europe
were not saved. In Arthur Nauzyciel's fascinating direction of the adaptation for the stage, Karski finds himself alone sitting, once again, in the lobby
of a large theater; soon, his Jewish wife will be dancing.[54] Dancing when
Jews are dead? The actor Laurent Poitrenaux, playing Karski, almost chants
his lines: the fate of six million Jews was sealed in 1942, despite Karski, Lemkin, Riegner, and the president of the United States. In this sense, Haenel
concurs with the greatest historian of extermination as a global phenomenon, Saul Friedländer, who observed that, although Hitler lost the war against
the Allies (a statement made by Roosevelt to Karski), he won the war against
the Jews by destroying not only six million human beings but also a civilization and a language: cultural genocide, Lemkin's term.[55] Lemkin also had
his turn in the spotlight in New York, in 2010, in a play by Catherine Filloux.
Haunted by the genocides of the Armenians and the Jews, Lemkin, who had
said sixty years earlier that "we will never be free of genocide," returns to the
world to discover, horrified, the killings of Bosnians and Tutsis.[56]

In France, the success of *Jan Karski*—which was translated into dozens
of languages—provoked bitter debate. Lanzmann, who considered the witnesses in *Shoah* to be his property, could not bear the idea that someone else
would use their words to subvert, as he saw it, the message of his film.[57]
Particularly insulted by the dialogue between Roosevelt and Karski as reinvented by Haenel, he decided to edit together an hour-long film from the
second day of the 1978 interview, which he titled *The Karski Report.* As he
had in *Un vivant qui passe*; *Sobibor 14 octobre 1943, 16 heures*; and *Le Dernier
des injustes*,[58] Lanzmann brought his "truth" to bear against the falsifiers.
Haenel, who had reconstructed much of both Karski and the content of his
message in his novel, was attacked severely for having made himself the ven-
triloquist of history—and for having taken liberties with Lanzmann's work.[59]

Lanzmann introduced his new edit on screen:

I decided as such, because it seemed absolutely essential to bring back the
truth. By relating the reactions to his reports from both his American and
British listeners, Karski makes us face a fundamental and deeply grave question: What does it mean to know? What does knowledge of an unfathomable
horror do to the person that's hearing about it for the first time—one who's
necessarily not ready to face a series of crimes that were unprecedented in the
history of mankind? Whatever has been said, the majority of Jews could not
be rescued once Hitler started to launch his war against them. Such is the
tragedy of History, which leaves no room for retrospective illusion hiding the
complexity, the heaviness, the opaqueness of an époque, veritable configuration of the impossible.[60]

If Haenel had engaged in a betrayal, Lanzmann, by invoking the absolute
truth of what the witness had said in front of his camera, was doing no different. In the 1985 version of *Shoah*, Karski's words had been edited with
other images, truncated, cut; now they were to become the historical truth,
without superimposed images of Warsaw or New York, with the intent of
raw testimony, so far from the sophisticated visual work of *Shoah*. And yet,
when one studies the rushes, one sees that editing choices—that is, cuts—
were made again in 2000. So, for Lanzmann, which were Karski's "true"
words? And which was the "true" Karski—that is, to which era did this Karski belong?

Indeed, Lanzmann recently revisited the meaning of his film: "The question of time is central to *Shoah*. The film is a struggle with time, against
time, and for time, too, from the beginning to the end, and even today."
The film was shot in the present: "The action takes place today"—that is, in
1985, when it was released—and it continues to be seen in the present. The
images came out of "a *treasure*, in the Greek sense of the word." Lanzmann,
the archeologist as filmmaker, spent days, even weeks, with some of his char-
acters, his "inventions" in the archeological sense—the sense of unearthing.
Karski, Murmelstein, and Lerner were part of it: "Their presence could not
be fit within the time of *Shoah*. Or else I would have needed hours and
hours more."[61] And so there were new edits of these figures beyond the

Shoah timeline. The time of the encounter between them and Lanzmann to retell the past time of their journey through the Shoah becomes the present time of the spectator. Was the filmmaker Lanzmann coming to resemble the novelist who wrote about his own deportation, Jorge Semprun? "We made this voyage in fiction, and I thus erased my solitude in reality. What good is writing books if one does not invent the truth? Or else, plausibility."[62] The witnesses did not claim to offer anything but the plausibility born of their memories. Philippe Mesnard has masterfully shown how Levi the survivor became Primo the witness by understanding how authenticity had to be reconciled with his readers' horizon of expectation.[63] And what is the writing of history if not another way of reconstructing such plausibility in another time, ours, the here and now? As Walter Benjamin put it,

> To articulate the past historically does not mean to recognize it "the way it really was." It means to seize hold of a memory as it flashes up at a moment of danger. . . . In every era the attempt must be made anew to wrest tradition away from a conformism that is about to overpower it. Only that historian will have the gift of fanning the spark of hope in the past who is firmly convinced that *even the dead* will not be safe from the enemy if he wins [this was written in 1940]. And this enemy has not ceased to be victorious.[64]

The "victory of the enemy" is that "nothing" remains in Warsaw, Poland. How can the traces be reconstructed? Far from "nothing"—from omission— Nathan Rapoport, creator of the first memorial to the Warsaw ghetto in 1948, chose an elegy on the pain of Jews faced with the destruction of the temple: "Could I have made a stone with a hole in it and said, 'Voilà! The heroism of the Jews.' . . . My task was to re-create the shadows of mother and fathers, young and old. Their tragic and epic end should stay in the memory of generations to come."[65] Today, the ghetto monument is no longer situated in front of "nothing," an immense empty lot. Constructed there, not without difficulty, was a contemporary building that houses the POLIN Museum of the History of the Polish Jews, covering centuries and not just the time of their extermination.[66] Between the monument and the museum, Karol Badyna created an elderly Karski, the book *Story of a Secret State* sitting on the arm of his armchair. This "talking" bronze Karski speaks of his mission in Polish, not in English as he did in his interviews. He who said he was a "machine" in the service of his message has been transformed into an automaton for posterity.

Karski: Polish Once Again

After 1945, Karski faced almost certain death, as did many resisters in the secret army, if he returned to Poland.[67] And so, he became an American. Until 1989, he was invisible in the country of his birth; then, when democracy returned, he was turned into a model citizen. Some leaders easily twisted the historical truth a bit to make his exceptional story the symbol of the true Poland; this was expressed, for instance, in a letter to him from the foreign minister, Andrzej Olechowski, congratulating him on becoming an honorary citizen of Israel: "Thanks to your extraordinary contribution, we have taken a new step toward eliminating false interpretations of the history of Polish–Jewish relations."[68]

Yet, some Polish associations, less scrupulous historians, and recent governments have tried to minimize or erase the aspect of Karski's mission in which he reported specifically on the fate of the Jews; instead, he is held up mainly as a hero of the resistance—which is true of the first Karski, but not the second one. It was in this spirit that he was recently awarded, posthumously, the title of colonel in the Polish army.

But these tributes can take another path: the hero is instrumentalized in a political combat that denies Polish collaboration in the genocide of the Jews—a collaboration minimized in the name of the suffering of all Poles. This new campaign began in 2012, when President Barack Obama posthumously awarded Karski the highest American civilian honor, the Presidential Medal of Freedom. In his announcement, made on April 23 while visiting the Holocaust Memorial in Washington with Elie Wiesel, Obama emphasized the need to tell young generations about a "crime unique in the history of humanity": "We must tell our children about how this evil was allowed to happen—because so many people succumbed to their darkest instincts; because so many others stood silent. But let us also tell our children about the Righteous Among the Nations. Among them was Jan Karski—a young Polish Catholic—who witnessed Jews being put on cattle cars, who saw the killings, and who told the truth, all the way to President Roosevelt himself."[69] At the medal ceremony on May 29, Obama used the term "Polish death camp," drawing fire from Polish authorities, who then went on to attack all those who did not specify that the death camps had belonged to the Nazis, who were occupying Poland, and that Auschwitz-Birkenau had been part of the Nazi Reich at that time. In early 2017, a German television network was sued for Holocaust denial for using the same term: "Do not mistake the victim for the killer. The death camps were Nazi, never Polish." The goal, obviously, was to insist upon the sole responsibility of the Nazis for the extermination of Jews—and for the unprecedented suffering of Poles during the war. There was no mention of the various types of complicity by Poles in the extermination of their Jewish neighbors; nor is the subject broached by the Institute of National Remembrance in Poland.[70]

Paradoxically, it was because he was not Jewish that Karski made such an impression on public opinion. In the era of the Righteous, he was the Righteous Among the Righteous. His likeness in sculpture can be seen in New York, in Lodz, at the University of Tel Aviv, and in the Krakow ghetto reconstructed for the shooting of Steven Spielberg's film on another Righteous of a very different type, Oskar Schindler. In the main square of the ghetto, Karski watches over Jewish and/or Israeli restaurants reinvented for tourists. And on book covers, in graphic novels, in movies, and on numerous websites, he has become *Karski: How One Man Tried to Stop the Holocaust.*[71]

Karski, Righteous Among the Righteous, paragon of moral integrity. In a vehement article, his American biographer and friend Tom Wood did not hesitate to use his voice to urge Americans to resist President Trump's anti-immigration measures: "Too many . . . of us . . . are silent in the presence of a malignant force. They shirk their duty. In the language of Holocaust scholarship, they are bystanders. Some, even, may turn out to be perpetrators." And Wood gave the final word to Karski, quoting him from their last meeting before Karski's death in 2000, seventeen years earlier: "People, all of us probably, we have infinite power to do good. And we have infinite power to follow evil. We are all schizophrenic, as I see our nature. We have a choice. We can choose to be robbers. We can choose to be good people. And our Lord left us the choice. Many people chose evil."[72]

Conclusion

Armenians, Jews, Tutsis

The perpetuation of the psychological scar: I realized that the function of
memory is not only to record past events but to stimulate human conscience.
—Lemkin, 1950

Who knows about Raphael Lemkin today, outside of a few intellectual and
legal circles? Despite his invention of the word "genocide," or because of
its problematic definition, the Polish Jewish lawyer, who died in the United
States, has not yet found his place in the global consciousness. Studied and
quoted mainly by those who advocated to have the catastrophe that befell
them called genocide, he often serves as a moral and intellectual cautionary
figure, for better or, sometimes, for worse.

In 2015, Armenian national and religious communities scattered around
the world commemorated the hundredth anniversary of the genocide. They
accorded a place of honor to Lemkin, who had begun his intellectual and
activist career with the Armenians and who returned to them always, including for cultural genocide:

> The cultural losses caused by the genocide of the Armenians in Turkey were
> stupefying. As the intellectual nucleus of Turkey, the Armenians owned in-
> valuable personal libraries, archives, and historical manuscripts, which have
> been dispersed and lost. Churches, convents, and monuments of great artistic
> and historical value were destroyed.[1]

The Armenian Genocide Museum-Institute in Yerevan offers Lemkin
Scholarship grants to students and researchers who specialize in genocide

studies. If Armenians are leaders in studying the legacy of the inventor of the word "genocide," it is because their own genocide is still being denied. It is not recurrently thrown into doubt, as is the genocide of the Jews, by those nostalgic for the Nazi order and by Islamist sycophants of the destruction of Israel, assassins, and "murderers of memory." In the case of the extermination of the Armenians, it is Turkey, which inherited and perpetuated the state that conducted the genocide, that stubbornly clings to denial.

"I transformed my personal disaster into a moral striking force. Was I not under a moral duty to repay my mother for having stimulated in me the interest in Genocide? Was it not the best form of gratitude to make a 'Genocide pact' as an epitaph on her symbolic grave and as a common recognition that she and many millions did not die in vain? I redoubled my efforts and found temporary relief from my grief in this work."[2] By inventing the word "genocide," Lemkin was able to make his personal sorrow universal. Beyond the inclusion of genocide in the legal field, its cultural and psychological ravages—no doubt its most lasting legacy—establish that it is impossible to compensate for: "After a lost war," Lemkin wrote, "a nation may reconstruct its technical and financial resources, restart a new life. But those who were destroyed in a genocide are lost forever. The losses of war may be repaired; the losses of a genocide are irreparable."[3] He also dwelled upon the "shame" and "sense of guilt" felt by those who survived, "often the only one from one's family or group of friends."[4]

How can it be proved that trauma, which is individual in nature, affects all victims as a community? Lemkin found himself in an intellectual situation somewhat similar to that of the sociologist Maurice Halbwachs, who tried in the 1920s to connect individual memory to group memory, later called collective or historical memory.[5] Anticipating what researchers such as François Fourquet have called "worldwide subjectivity," Lemkin wrote that all members of a group, at a particular time, share the same "emotional essence," which is transmitted through heredity.

The psychological impact of genocide on the victimized group is enormous. . . . Its psychological effect on the group is even bigger than on each individual, because every individual influenced by genocide conveys his feelings to members of his group. Every collectivization of emotions is more than the mathematical sum of those emotions. It creates a new and stronger emotional essence. To that must be added the refinement of pain, sorrow, the perception of injustice, and, above all, the impossibility of bringing those who have died back to life. This collective grief is hereditary; it is being transmitted to future generations not only by word of mouth between parents and children but also by songs, literature, and music.[6]

Once again, Lemkin took the example of the Armenians, who were divided between passing down the historical narrative to preserve their national identity and perpetuating the trauma as infinite torment: "[They] have tried to assemble names and historic facts relating to every community where genocide took place. . . . It would be morally unjust to think that these data are being collected for purely scientifically historical reasons. Each Armenian finds himself in every new document." And Lemkin added, "Members of the group who found themselves far from the scene of the genocide experienced it as victims."[7] With his encyclopedic mind, this original and attentive social sciences researcher had perceived very early the impact of genocide on members of the group, even those who were distant or absent from the time of the catastrophe. We have only to think, eighty years later, of the Americanization and Australianization of the Holocaust—which involves not only national political aspects but, even more, real identification with the group targeted: Jews.

Today, scholars of what is called postmemory concur with Lemkin; they show that genocides move through all generations because they break apart the basic unit, the family. Parents are "orphaned" of children, orphans are dispossessed of their parents, and extended family—uncles, aunts, cousins— are deprived of their close circle and thus of the possibility of belonging to a community of grief. A vanishing identity? As the Tutsis of Rwanda recover their voices after the prolonged abandonment, animalization, and reification that they have suffered, they are expressing themselves:

A genocide destroys everything, family ties included. . . . A void divides the families who have suffered. The memory of the dead drives them apart. Each member feels lonelier than the next. At school, when I hear classmates describe vacations with their grandparents, it tears at my heart. . . . But still, for me, the chance to become someone has passed. . . . I've pretty much lost my love of myself. I've known the filth of animals, I've seen the ferocity of the hyena and worse still—because animals are never as vile as that. I was forced by a brutal man. I was taken away, out there, to a place about which nothing can be said. But the worst is still there walking in front of me. My heart will always hold suspicions. It knows all too well that destiny can break its promises.[8]

Yet, the survivors struggle; one of them, Émilienne Mukansoro, speaks to all of her exterminated relatives: "I've spent more time with you than with my living family. I've tried to be my father and my mother."[9] Indeed, the survivors, and those who were born after, assume new family roles, replacing grandparents and even parents, brothers and sisters, uncles and aunts who have been killed. Sometimes they are much younger than those whom they are trying to protect in this way, as if inverting the generations could bring something back to life: hope. But it also brings back to life something from the time of the genocide: defeat.

Lemkin took the examples of both Armenian and Jewish survivors to illustrate his devastating idea: there is no future for victims of a genocide. He spoke once more for himself, for all Jewish victims, for all victims throughout the ages, and even for those in the future—as he did not believe in "never again" despite the "preventive" aspect of the 1948 convention. Even though the Tutsis in Rwanda had not read his words, they offer evidence of what he called "the perpetuation of the psychological scar." As Élise Rida Musomandera expressed it, "There are survivors, as the genocide was stopped, but do the survivors really exist?"[10] Or, in the words of the sociologist Esther Mujawayo, "The power of a genocide is exactly that: horror during, but still horror afterward. Within us there is no end to a genocide. There is just the stopping of murders, massacres, pursuits, but there is no end to the destruction."[11] Claudine, in Nyamata, said, "Thanks to the wedding, time wears a kind face at present, but only at present. Because I see clearly that the future has already been eaten up by what I lived through."[12]

As "eaten up" as the survivors who tried to return to live in their region that had been the site of genocide—the Jews in Poland and Ukraine after 1945—the Tutsis in Rwanda after 1994 had to confront, in addition to the denials, the perpetuation of the genocide in the constant presence of their murderous neighbors, with their sense of impunity: "Up to this day I am still living in this genocide that originated with you. . . . But it doesn't intimidate me, it doesn't keep me from talking about all my dead people, for I feel them all around me, even if they no longer speak."[13]

"No one, they can know what we've been through. No one."[14]

Genocide: the victims and the law finally on the same level: endless suffering, imprescriptible crime.

ACKNOWLEDGMENTS

This transnational project was possible thanks to the United States Holocaust Memorial Museum, the British National Archives, and the archives at the following institutions: Yad Vashem, United Nations in New York and Geneva, Stanford University, Columbia University, Georgetown University, and the Centre de documentation Juive contemporaine in Paris. I am particularly grateful to the Center for Advanced Holocaust Studies, directed by Paul Shapiro and Suzanne Brown-Fleming, which awarded me the Miles Lerman Fellowship so that I could work with its permanent and temporary researchers. My thanks to Jan Lambertz, who became the linchpin of the project—no article or archive escaped her—and Elizabeth Anthony, Omer Bartov, Rémy Besson, Mark Celinziak, Jo-Ellyn Decker, Rebecca Carter-Chand, Rebecca Erbelding, Martin Dean, Willa Johnson, Istvan Pal Adam, Emil Kerenji, Jürgen Matthäus, and Sybille Steinbacher, as well as the three wonderful librarians at the center, now the Jack, Joseph and Morton Mandel Center for Advanced Holocaust Studies: Ron Coleman, Megan Lewis, and Vincent Slatt.

In France, Poland, Israel, the United States, Great Britain, Switzerland, and Italy, colleagues and friends were unstintingly generous with their support: Philippe Mesnard (who suggested Jan Karski to me when I was already working on Raphael Lemkin), as well as Vincent Baudriller, Nicolas Beaupré, Georges Bensoussan, Luca Bernardini, Christian Biet, Aimée Brown-Price, Bernard Bruneteau, Bruno Cabanes, Sébastien Carney, the late David Cesarani, Evelyne Cohen, Dorota Dakowska, J. P. Daughton, Octave Debary,

Christian Delage, Bernard Delpal, Juliette Denis, Vincent Duclert, Jacques Ehrenfreund, Isabelle Ernot, Raphael Esrail, Yves Faure, Caroline Fontaine, Étienne Fouilloux, Jacky Fredj, Anne-Marie Gassier, Richard Goodkin, Jan Gross, Atina Grossman, Frédéric Gugelot, Gilles Heuré, the late Sarah Hirschmann and the late Albert Hirschmann, John Horne, Luba Jurgenson, Raymond Kevorkian, Audrey Kichelewski, Anaïs Kien, Alain Kleinberger, Anouche Kunth, Emmanuel Laurentin, Jean Lebrun, Annaig Lefeuvre, Jean-Claude Léon, Gaïdz Minassian, Claire Mouradian, Émilienne Mukansoro, Martine Morris and the late Terry Morris, Sophie Nagiscarde, Arthur Nauzyciel, Philip Nord, Nicolas Patin, Monroe Price, Andy Rabinbach, Nicole Rambourg, Louis Rimrodt, Habie Schwarz, Lior Smadja, Karen Taieb, Mark Tannenbaum, Yves Ternon, Dominique Varma, Paul Weindling, Nicolas Werth, Jay Winter, Alexandre Sumpf, and Slawomir Zurek.

Stéphane Audoin-Rouzeau, Hélène Dumas, Philippe Gumplowicz, the late Paulette Meyer-Moureaux, Renée Poznanski, Valérie Rosoux, Henry Rousso, Julien Serrousi, and Fabien Théofilakis read all or part of the manuscript; Sophie Hogg and Pauline Labey enthusiastically brought the project to Fayard, where it landed on the desk of Anthony Rowley a few days before his death.

I express my immense gratitude to all of you. This book is also yours; the choices remain mine.

This book was translated with extraordinary professionalism by Käthe Roth. My deepest thanks go to her, as well as the entire team in the George L. Mosse Program in History at the University of Wisconsin, starting with its energetic director, Skye Doney, who decided to publish this book and asked Käthe to translate it.

In fond memory of George Mosse, intellectual trailblazer and much more.

NOTES

Introduction

The reader may note that some texts that are cited as being originally in English have been retranslated from the French edition. This is because, despite our best efforts, these original texts remain buried deep in archives, not digitized, or unavailable for other reasons.

1. Charles Péguy, "Notre jeunesse," *Les Cahiers de la Quinzaine*, Cahier 12–11 (1910).

2. Jan Karski, *Story of a Secret State* (Boston: Houghton Mifflin, 1944).

3. Raphael Lemkin, "Destruction of Peoples as an International Crime, Genocide," *Polish Review* 18 (January 1945); *Axis Rule in Occupied Europe: Laws of Occupation, Analysis of Government, Proposal for Redress* (Washington, DC: Carnegie Endowment for International Peace, Department of International Law, 1944).

4. Rushes from *Shoah* conserved at the United States Holocaust Memorial Museum (USHMM) in Washington, DC, p. 61 of the typescript and audio tape, https://collections.ushmm.org/film_findingaids/RG-60.5006_01_trs_en.pdf.

5. Raymond Aron, *Mémoires* (Paris: Julliard, 1983), 176 (our translation). Claude Lanzmann quotes Aron from memory—thus in different words—in his introduction to the film *The Karski Report* (2010) and similarly in *Les Temps modernes* (January–March 2010). See chapter 6.

6. See Renée Poznanski, *Propagandes et persécutions: La Résistance et le "problème juif" 1940–1944* (Paris: Fayard, 2008).

7. Avishai Margalit, *The Ethics of Memory* (Cambridge, MA: Harvard University Press, 2002).

8. Robert Gerwarth, *The Vanquished: Why the First World War Failed to End, 1917–1923* (London: Allen Lane, 2016).

9. Saul Friedländer, *Réflexions sur le nazisme: Entretiens avec Stéphane Bou* (Paris: Seuil, 2016).

10. It was the transit center for Belzec that Karski saw, not the killing center in Belzec. Robert Kuwalek, *Belzec, le premier centre de mise à mort*, trans. Alexendre Dayet (Paris: Calmann-Lévy, 2013).

11. Raphael Lemkin, *Totally Unofficial: The Autobiography of Raphael Lemkin*, ed. Donna-Lee Frieze (New Haven: Yale University Press, 2013).

12. Samuel Beckett, *Worstward Ho* (1983); *The Unnamable*, 1959 (originally published as *L'innommable* [Paris: Minuit, 1953]).

Chapter 1. Karski the Soldier, Lemkin the Lawyer

1. Victor Zaslavsky, *Le Massacre de Katyn* (Paris: Perrin, "Tempus" imprint, 2007). See chapter 5 of this book.

2. Raphael Lemkin, *Totally Unofficial: The Autobiography of Raphael Lemkin*, ed. Donna-Lee Frieze (New Haven: Yale University Press, 2013), 59. This autobiography, edited together from fragments, was written in the 1950s.

3. Ibid., 79–80, 67.

4. Ibid., 70. The filmmaker Axel Corti portrayed this situation accurately in the first part of his trilogy *Welcome in Vienna*, "God Doesn't Believe in Us Anymore" (1982), on Jews trapped by Nazism as they tried to flee Europe.

5. Ibid., 80.

6. Raphael Lemkin, *La Règlementation des paiements internationaux* (Paris: Pedone, 1939).

7. Lemkin, *Totally Unofficial*, 51.

8. An Orthodox Jewish baker in Dubno in conversation with Lemkin, quoted in Lemkin, *Totally Unofficial*, 52.

9. Ibid., 52–54.

10. Ibid., 52.

11. Emanuel Ringelblum quoted in Samuel D. Kassow, *Who Will Write Our History? Emanuel Ringelblum, the Warsaw Ghetto, and the Oyneg Shabes Archive* (Bloomington: Indiana University Press, 2007), 11.

12. Nathan Weistock, "Simon Doubnov (1860–1941): Que faire quand sonne l'heure d'Haman? (1939)," *Revue d'histoire de la Shoah* 174 (2002): 11 (our translation).

13. Esther, III, 13, http://biblescripture.net/Esther.html.

14. The expression used was *Yiddishkeit.*

15. Weistock, "Simon Doubnov," 14–15 (our translation).

16. Varian Fry, "The Massacre of the Jews," *The New Republic* (December 21, 1942): 817.

17. Lepsius's first book, *Bericht über e Lage des armenischen Volkes in der Türkei* (Report on the Situation of the Armenian People in Turkey), was censored in August 1916, but twenty thousand copies had already been distributed. Werfel used the second edition, which included a 1915 interview with Enver Pasha, *Der Todesgang des Armenischen Volkes* (The Death March of the Armenian People).

18. Peter Stephan Jungk, *Franz Werfel: A Life in Prague, Vienna, and Hollywood*, trans. Anselm Hollo (New York: Grove Weidenfeld, 1990), 139.

19. Franz Werfel, *The Forty Days of Musa Dagh*, trans. Geoffrey Dunlop and James Reidel (Jaffrey, NH: Verba Mundi, 2012), 140. In his preface to the French edition, titled "Le crime de l'oubli" (The Crime of Forgetting), Elie Wiesel mentions "striking correspondences" between the fate of the Armenians and that of the Jews: "Is the author evoking a past experienced or a future prophesized? Is not the 'musa dagh' a sort of ghetto in which survivors, in a burst of pride and desperate courage, prepare to die in combat rather than perish in the bloodied dust of distant roads?" In Franz Werfel, *Les 40 jours du Musa Dagh*, trans. Paule Hofer-Bury (Paris: Albin Michel, 2015), 6 (our translation).

20. Werfel, *Forty Days*.

21. Quoted in Peter Stephan Jungk, *Franz Werfel: A Life in Prague, Vienna, and Hollywood*, trans. Anselm Hollo (New York: Fromm International, 1991), 165.

22. *Varian Fry: Mission américaine de sauvetage des intellectuels anti-nazis, Marseille 1940–1942*, exhibition catalogue (Arles: Actes sud, 1999). For another view of Fry, written by one of his assistants in Marseille, see Daniel Bénédite, *Un Chemin vers la liberté sous l'Occupation: Du Comité Varian Fry au débarquement en Méditerranée, 1940–1944* (Paris: Éditions du Félin-résistance, 2017 [1983]).

23. Quoted in the introduction by Otto Friedrich in Franz Werfel, *Cella, or, The Survivors* [1939, unfinished novel] (New York: Henry Holt, 1989).

24. Franz Werfel, "Our Path Continues" (December 27, 1940), in *Jewish Responses to Persecution*, vol. 2, *1938–1940*, ed. A. Garbarini, E. Kerenji, J. Lambertz, and Avinoam Patt (New York: Rowman & Littlefield, 2011), 485–88.

25. Peter Longerich, *Holocaust: The Nazi Persecution and Murder of the Jews* (Oxford: Oxford University Press, 2010); Omer Bartov, *Mirrors of Destruction: War, Genocide, and Modern Identity* (Oxford: Oxford University Press, 2002).

26. Lemkin, *Totally Unofficial*, 71.

27. Ibid., 72.

28. Kassow, *Who Will Write Our History? Oyneg Shabes*, "the joy of the Sabbath," was the code name chosen by Ringelblum for his archival collection in the ghetto. See Emanuel Ringelblum, *Oneg Shubbat, journal du Ghetto de Varsovie* (Paris: Calmann-Lévy/Mémorial de la Shoah, 2017).

29. Edward Raczynski to Lord Winterton, January 13, 1939, quoted in Bernard Wasserstein, "Polish Influences on British Policy Regarding Jewish Rescue Efforts in Poland 1939–1945," in *Polin: Studies in Polish Jewry*, vol. 11, *Focusing on Aspects and Experiences of Religion*, ed. Antony Polonsky (Liverpool: Liverpool University Press, 1998), 185.

30. Roberts quoted in Wasserstein, "Polish Influences," 187.

31. British National Archives (BNA), Kew, HO 213/347, Home Office, Aliens Department. Treatment of Jewish race, general question, January 6, 1942.

32. David Engel, "An Early Account of Polish Jewry under Nazi and Soviet Occupation Presented to the Polish Government-in-Exile, February 1940," *Jewish Social Studies* 45, no. 1 (1983): 1–16. See Joshua Zimmerman, *The Polish Underground and the Jews, 1939–1945* (Cambridge: Cambridge University Press, 2015).

33. Engel, "An Early Account," 6.

34. Ibid., 6–7.

35. Ibid., 8.

36. Jan Tomasz Gross, *Polish Society Under German Occupation: The General-gouvernement, 1939–1944* (Princeton: Princeton University Press, 1979).

37. Engel, "An Early Account," 9.

38. Ibid., 10 (emphasis in original).

39. On the ordeals suffered by Polish Jews at the hands of the Nazis and Soviets, see Julius Margolin, *Voyage au pays des Ze-ka* (Paris: Le Bruit du temps, 2010); Alain Blum, Marta Craveri, and Valérie Nivelon, eds., *Déportés en URSS: Récits d'Européens au Goulag* (Paris: Éditions autrement, 2012).

40. Engel, "An Early Account," 10.

41. Lemkin, *Totally Unofficial*, 57.

42. "The Outbreak of the German-Polish War," in *The Volkovysk Memorial Book* or *Wolkovisker Yizkor Book* or *Hurban Volkovysk*, ed. Moses Einhorn (New York and Tel Aviv: Committee of Volkovysk Émigrés, Katriel Lashowitz, USHMM Collection, 1946, 1947, 1988), chap. 5, p. 330 (our translation from the French; original is in Yiddish). This is a trilogy of three separate works: 1. *Sefer Zikaron Volkovysk*, ed. Moses Einhorn (New York, 1949); 2. *Volkovysk* (Tel Aviv: Committee of Volkovysk Emigres, 1946); 3. *Volkovysk* (Tel Aviv: Katriel Lashowitz, 1988). See http://www.taytsh.org/bibliography/volkovysk-memorial-book.

43. Letter from Moshe Kleinbaum (who arrived in Geneva after an odyssey lasting several months) to Nahum Goldmann, president of the Administration Committee of the World Jewish Congress, March 12, 140, reproduced in Jürgen Matthäus with Emil Kerenji, *Jewish Responses to Persecution, 1933–1946* (Lanham, MD: Rowman and Littlefield, 2017), 47–48.

44. Calel Perechodnik, *Am I a Murderer? Testament of a Jewish Ghetto Policeman*, trans. and ed. Frank Fox (Boulder, CO: Westview Press, 1996), 2. Perechodnik was writing in 1943, after his family was murdered by the Nazis.

45. *Volkovysk Memorial Book*, 330 (our translation).

46. Engel, "An Early Account," 9.

47. Ibid., 9–10.

48. Ibid., 14.

49. Ibid., 12.

50. Ibid., 14.

51. Jan Lanicek, "Governments-in-Exile and the Jews during and after the Second World War," *Holocaust Studies* 35, no. 2–3 (2012): 73–94.

52. George Orwell, "Antisemitism in Britain," *Contemporary Jewish Record*, London, April 1945.

53. Engel, "An Early Account," 11.

54. Jan Tomasz Gross, *Neighbors: The Destruction of the Polish Community in Jedwabne, Poland* (Princeton: Princeton University Press, 2001).

55. Jan Karski, *Story of a Secret State* (Boston: Houghton Mifflin, 1944), 82.

56. Reports quoted by Saul Friedländer in *Les Années d'extermination: L'Allemagne nazie et les Juifs, 1939–1945* (Paris: Seuil, 2008), 86–87 (our translation).

57. Raphael Lemkin, manuscripts, New York Public Library (NYPL), Collection 922, displaced scholars. I would like to thank Jan Lambertz for telling me about this invaluable archival collection.

58. Dr. Henry Rozenthal, letter on the letterhead of the Adult School of Jewish Studies, Young Men's Hebrew Association (our translation). Raphael Lemkin, manuscripts, NYPL, Collection 922, displaced scholars.

59. Letter from Ms. Drury to President Few of Duke University, July 3, 1940. Raphael Lemkin, manuscripts, NYPL, Collection 922, displaced scholars.

60. Lemkin, *Totally Unofficial*, 97.

61. Michael Ignatieff, "The Danger of a World without Enemies: Lemkin's Word," *New Republic* 226, no. 9 (February 2001): 26–28.

62. Lemkin, *Totally Unofficial*, 80.

Chapter 2. Karski Discovers the Annihilation of Lemkin's World

1. Marian Kozielewski, International Tracing Service file, Bad Arolsen. KZ Oswiecim, 14/8/40–4/4/41.

2. Jan Lanicek, "Governments-in-Exile and the Jews during and after the Second World War," *Holocaust Studies* 35, no. 2–3 (2012): 73–94.

3. Polish Underground Labor Movement, *The Camp of Disappearing Men: A Story of the Oswiecim Concentration Camp, Based on Reports from the Polish Underground Labor Movement* (Office of War Information, Poland Fights, 1944).

4. Ibid., 33–34.

5. Ibid., 43.

6. Prime Minister Winston Churchill's Broadcast to the World about the Meeting with President Roosevelt, August 24, 1941, https://www.ibiblio.org/pha/timeline/410824awp.html.

7. See Catherine Collomp, *Résister au nazisme: Le Jewish Labor Committee, New York, 1934–1945* (Paris: CNRS éditions, 2016).

8. Holocaust Memorial, Washington, DC, Archives, Prm-70, "Memorandum Submitted to the President of the United States . . . by a Delegation of Representative of Jewish Organisations," December 8, 1942.

9. The *New York Times* reported on December 17, 1942, "A joint declaration by members of the United Nations was issued today condemning Germany's 'bestial policy of cold-blooded extermination' of Jews and declaring that 'such events can only strengthen the resolve of all freedom-loving peoples to overthrow the barbarous Hitlerite tyranny.'"

10. British National Archives (BNA), C1240/61/18, December 15, 1942 (our translation).

11. BNA, Kew, letter sent on June 30, 1942, different service stamps, up to July 17, 1942 (our translation).

12. BNA, Kew, report of June 29, 1942.

13. BNA, Kew, Fo. 371, 31097.

14. The same photographs are found in the collections of the United States Holocaust Memorial Museum in Washington, DC, at Yad Vashem in Jerusalem, in the archives of the Polish government in exile at the Hoover Institution, and in Warsaw; archivists have acquired copies of microfilms carried by people smugglers that were prepared and preserved in Poland at the risk of many resisters' lives. Dr. Emil Apfelbaum, in particular, worked at the hospital in Czyste and conducted research on the famine in the Warsaw ghetto in 1942. His working photographs formed the basis for this series.

15. Published following the demonstration on July 22, 1942, in a leaflet by Alfred J. Dobbs et al., *German Atrocities in Poland and Czechoslovakia: Labour's Protest* (London: Liberty Publications, 1942), http://pbc.gda.pl/Content/72811/Labours_pro test.pdf.

16. BNA, Kew, six-page speech (our translation).

17. BNA, Kew, note by D. Allen, September 11, 1942 (emphasis added).

18. Richard Bolchover, *British Jewry and the Holocaust* (Cambridge: Cambridge University Press, 1993); Pamela Shatzkes, *Holocaust and Rescue: Impotent or Indifferent? Anglo-Jewry 1938–1945* (Basingstoke: Palgrave, 2002).

19. Daniel Blatman, "On a Mission against All Odds: Samuel Zygielbojm in London (April 1942–May 1943)," *Yad Vashem Studies* 2 (1990): 237–72.

20. Printed in boldface on the back cover of *Stop Them Now: German Mass Murder of Jews in Poland* (London: Liberty Publications, September 1942), https://www.marxists.org/subject/jewish/stop-murder.pdf.

21. Ibid., 11, 12, 13.

22. Ibid., 5.

23. Ibid.

24. Ibid. (emphasis in original).

25. Ibid., 7.

26. Ibid., 15.

27. Ibid., 9. The cemetery on Okopowa Street was identified through another series of photographs, taken by Heinrich Jöst, a sergeant in the German army, on September 19, 1941. These photographs remained in his possession until 1982 and then were donated to Yad Vashem. In some cases, victims and executioners took similar pictures, for radically different purposes. See the exhibition *Regards sur les ghettos* and its eponymous catalogue (Paris: Mémorial de la Shoah, 2014). Imre Kertesz, for example, describes these carts in *Être sans destin* (Arles: Actes sud, 1998).

28. Jan Karski, *Story of a Secret State* (Boston: Houghton Mifflin, 1944), 332.

29. Samuel Golfard's diary describing an *Aktion* in Galicia. Written January 30, 1943, relating the events of 1942, in *The Diary of Samuel Golfard and the Holocaust in Galicia*, ed. Wendy Lower, USHMM series Jewish Responses to Persecutions, gen. ed. Jürgen Matthäus (Lanham, MD: AltaMira Press, 2011), 64.

30. Marcel Cohen, interview in *Europe* (January 2016): 214.

31. Jacob Sloan, ed., *Notes from the Warsaw Ghetto: The Journal of Emanuel Ringelblum* (New York: McGraw Hill, 1958), 295, 297–98.

32. Jan Karski, *Mon témoignage devant le monde: Histoire d'un État clandestin* (Paris: Robert Laffont, 2010), 275 (our translation).

33. Republic of Poland, Ministry of Foreign Affairs, *The Mass Extermination of Jews in German Occupied Poland: Note Addressed to the Governments of the United Nations on December 10th, 1942, and Other Documents* (London, New York, and Melbourne: Hutchinson and Co., 1942). The Mémorial de la Shoah in Paris recently acquired a copy of this brochure, one of the three copies in the Library of Congress in 1943. It is possible to imagine that Lemkin and Karski consulted this very copy in Washington, DC.

34. George Orwell, *Chroniques du temps de la guerre (1941–1943)* (Paris: Éditions Lebovici, 1988), 245, broadcast of December 12, 1942 (our translation).

35. At least in some form. Ibid., December 17, 1942, 248–49 (our translation).

36. "Défi, l'ordre nouveau en Pologne," *Les Cahiers du Témoignage chrétien*, no. 13–14 (January–February 1943): 12 (emphasis in original; our translation).

37. Our translation. Feiner's second report was probably dated August 31. Daniel Blatman, *Notre liberté et la vôtre: Le mouvement ouvrier juif BUND en Pologne, 1939–1949* (Paris: Cerf, 2002), 185.

38. Karski, in London, sent a message from the Jewish resistance to Sikorski on this subject. Joshua D. Zimmerman, *The Polish Underground and the Jews, 1939–1945* (Cambridge: Cambridge University Press, 2015), 301.

39. Feiner, quoted in Karski, *Story of a Secret State*, 324.

40. Ibid.

41. BNA, Kew, text of telegram of December 12, 1942, copy of the British Censor. The original telegram is available at https://codoh.com/library/document/3336/?lang=en.

42. BNA, Kew, Shmuel Zygielbojm, telegram to Churchill, December 15, 1942.

43. BNA, Kew, telegram of December 4, 1942, to Tartakower and Miller, World Jewish Congress, New York, copy of the British Censor; copy of telegram viewable at http://www.deathcamps.org/reinhard/pic/stupp.jpg.

44. Rushes for *Shoah*, USHMM, reels 310 and 311, typescript, 44–45, https://collections.ushmm.org/film_findingaids/RG-60.5006_01_trs_en.pdf. These reels were devoted entirely to Zygielbojm.

45. Ibid., 48.

46. Nowak wrote his memoir much later, in 1978, but before Karski returned to the spotlight. Logically, he cites Karski in his account of being in London in 1942–43. Jan Nowak, *Courier from Warsaw* (Detroit: Wayne State University Press, 1982).

47. I consulted the proofs of *Story of a Secret State* in the Karski archives in Georgetown. Karski carefully edited every word that he felt inappropriate.

48. Transcription of the radio program in which Karski participated anonymously in London: "The Jewish Mass Executions: Account by an Eye-Witness," in Alexei Tolstoy, *Terror in Europe: The Fate of the Polish Jews* (London: National

Committee for Rescue from Nazi Terror, n.d. [1943]), reprinted in *PL.IT/rassegna italiana di argomenti polacchi* (May 2014): 136–41. I am grateful to one of the foremost experts on Karski, Luca Bernardini, for having found this text for me in the excellent online journal *PL.IT/rassegna italiana di argomenti polacchi.*

49. Ibid., 139.

50. Karski, *Story of a Secret State*, 321 (introduction to the chapter "The Ghetto").

51. *Polish Fortnightly Review*, no. 82 (December 15, 1943): 9.

52. "Le Massacre des Juifs en Pologne: Récit d'un témoin oculaire," *Fraternité*, special issue (September 1943) (our translation). (Translator's note: this text has now undergone one further translation into English.) "Nouvelles arrestations massives et déportations des Juifs de France vers les camps de la torture et de la mort," article on page 1, lower right, and page 2. At the same time, the emissary from the Polish government in exile in unoccupied France, S. Zabiello, was sending accurate reports on deportations of Polish Jews from France to London. *Le Gouvernement polonais en exil et la persécution des Juifs en France en 1942 d'après les documents inédits*, compiled and edited by Pawel Korzec and Jacques Burko (Paris: Cerf, 1997); *Pardès*, no. 16 (1992): 121–33.

53. Alexei Tolstoy, *Terror in Europe: The Fate of the Polish Jews* (London: National Committee for Rescue from Nazi Terror, n.d. [1943]), 139.

54. In Berlin, at the site, destroyed after the war, a memorial—very judiciously transparent for those who do not want to see it—was erected only in 2014.

55. Lemkin Archives, NYPL, loose sheet, 1949 (our translation).

56. *Volkovysk Memorial Book*, 3 vols., ed. Moses Einhorn (New York, 1949); the Yiddish version was published by the Committee of Volkovysk Emigres in Tel Aviv in 1949. The work was reprinted and expanded in English in 2002 (Mahwah, NJ: Jacob Solomon Berger, 2002) with a list of donors, including a number of descendants of Lemkin's brother, Elias. At the time, he stated that he was the only survivor of the family. The Yiddish version has this dedication, in English: "In memoriam dedicated in Love and reverence to the sacred memory of my Family and the Jewish Community of Wolkowysk."

57. Bradfisch quoted in Peter Longerich, *Holocaust: The Nazi Persecution and the Murder of the Jews* (Oxford: Oxford University Press, 2010), 198.

58. Nebe quoted in Peter Longerich, *Heinrich Himmler*, trans. Jeremy Noakes and Lesley Sharpe (Oxford: Oxford University Press, 2012), 525.

59. Quoted in Longerich, *Holocaust*, 152.

60. Ibid., 222.

61. *Volkovysk Memorial Book*, 933 (our translation)

62. Quoted in Raphael Lemkin, *Totally Unofficial: The Autobiography of Raphael Lemkin* (New Haven: Yale University Press, 2013), 55.

63. Izaak Goldberg, *The Miracles versus Tyranny* (New York: Philosophical Library, 1978), 128.

64. Vassili Grossman, "The Hell of Treblinka," translated from Russian by Molly Godwin-Jones and Maxim D. Shrayer, in *Voices of Jewish-Russian Literature: An Anthology*, ed. Maxim D. Shrayer (Boston: Academic Studies Press, 2018), 433.

65. Goldberg, *The Miracles versus Tyranny*, 130. This Czech doctor's wandering through labor camps and ghettos was very typical of the few unlikely survivors—whence the title of his memoir.

66. Grossman, "Hell of Treblinka," 444–45.

67. *Volkovysk Memorial Book*, 918 (our translation).

68. Zalmen Gradowski, "In the Heart of Hell," in *The Literature of Destruction: Jewish Responses to Catastrophe*, ed. David G. Roskies (Philadelphia: Jewish Publication Society, 1988), 563–64.

69. *Volkovysk Memorial Book*, 945 (our translation).

70. Ibid., 929 (our translation).

71. Handwritten letter from Szlamek on the Belzec camp sent to Hersz Wasser, April 1942 (original in Polish and Yiddish), http://www.memorialdelashoah.org/upload/minisites/ringelblum/shoah/documents/document11-en.htm. See Samuel Kassow, *Who Will Write Our History? Rediscovering a Hidden Archive from the Warsaw Ghetto* (New York: Vintage Books, 2009); Kassow, *Who Will Write Our History? Emanuel Ringelblum, the Warsaw Ghetto, and the Oyneg Shabes Archive* (Bloomington: Indiana University Press, 2007).

72. The Yiddish publication *Oyneg Shabes Mitteilungen* reported, in its April 1942 issue, deportations from Lublin to Belzec and the "rumor" of "asphyxia by gas as in Chelmno." Quoted at length in Daniel Blatman, *En direct du ghetto: La presse clandestine juive dans le ghetto de Varsovie, 1940–1943* (Paris: Cerf, 2005), 454–57.

73. Kassow, quoting a report, written in Polish, in the Oyneg Shabes in *Who Will Write Our History?*, 296.

74. Rushes for *Shoah*, reel 305, typescript, p. 32.

75. Karski, *Story of a Secret State*, 324–25.

76. Ibid., 322.

77. Ibid., 330.

78. *The American Mercury* (November 1944): 567–75.

79. Karski, *Story of a Secret State*, 330.

80. George Creel, a veteran newsman—he ran the Committee on Public Information, an American propaganda organ, during World War I—sent the text to Karski to check his reconstruction of Karski's words. That is why the Karski archive at Stanford University contains a document called "Poland's Underground," by "Mr. X," as told to George Creel. The episode was also described more succinctly in another article in *Collier's Weekly*, Martha Gellhorn's "Three Poles," radioed from London in 1943 and published on March 18, 1944. Specific dates did not seem terribly important; articles on the situation in Poland were being published with information that was already quite out of date.

81. Mr. B., as told to George Creel, "Revenge in Poland," *Collier's Weekly*, November 6, 1943, 34.

82. Ibid., 32–33. See also Mr. X, "Poland's Underground." Karski's decision to discuss homosexuality—it seems that he was unaware that it was punishable by death or imprisonment in a concentration camp in the Reich—is striking. Karski is

talking freely to an American journalist and presenting himself as a paragon of Catholic morality in the Polish underground that he is representing. I would like to thank Jean Lebrun for making me aware of the encounter between the playwright Pierre Barillet and Karski in Paris in 1946, when Karski returned to that city to collect Polish underground documents to take to the United States. Barillet recounted their liaison and kept to the end of his life the book that Karski dedicated to him. Pierre Barillet, *À la ville comme à la scène* (Paris: Fallois, 2004), 33–34.

83. "Défi, l'ordre nouveau en Pologne," *Cahiers du Témoignage chrétien*, no. 13–14 (January–February 1943): 11 (our translation).

84. Mr. B., "Revenge in Poland," November 6, 1943, 34.

85. Ibid., 32.

86. Ibid., 20, 32.

87. Mr. B., "Revenge in Poland," October 30, 1943, 11, 69.

88. Robert Kuwalek, *Belzec, le premier centre de mise à mort*, trans. Alexendre Dayet (Paris: Calmann-Lévy, 2013).

89. Samuel Golfard, in *Diary of Samuel Golfard*, went even further, accusing those whom he called the "Jewish Gestapo," the ghetto police officers, of participating in the same system of corruption.

90. Karski, *Story of a Secret State*, 342.

91. Mr. B., "Revenge in Poland," November 6, 1943, 20.

92. Krüger was not killed but replaced; he committed suicide in 1945. I am grateful to Nicolas Patin for these details. See his *Krüger, un bourreau ordinaire* (Paris: Fayard, 2017).

93. David Engel, "An Early Account of Polish Jewry under Nazi and Soviet Occupation Presented to the Polish Government-in-Exile, February 1940," *Jewish Social Studies* 45, no. 1 (1983): 8.

94. USHMM Collection, no. 32057 (our translation).

95. Karski, *Mon témoignage*, 296–97 (our translation).

96. I extend my warmest thanks to Slawomir Zurek, director of the Polish-Jewish Literature Studies Centre at the John Paul II Catholic University of Lublin, who took me to Izbica and Belzec. In both cases, the train tracks were still in the same place. In 1942, these two small towns had an 80 percent Jewish population.

97. Golfard, *Diary of Samuel Golfard*, 56 (Eastern Galicia, August 1942). Electrocution was also mentioned in the report "The Mass Extermination of Jews in German-Occupied Poland," report sent by the Polish Ministry of Foreign Affairs to the United Nations, December 10, 1942.

98. In fact, small gas chambers had been used in the late nineteenth century to suffocate stray dogs in Paris, and then in Mexico. Arnaud Exbalin, *La grande tuerie des chiens. Enquête sur les canicides dans le Mexique colonial* (Ceyzérieux: Champ Vallon, 2021), chapter 3, "Décanisations."

99. *The Ghetto Speaks*, no. 20, February 1, 1944 (our translation).

100. "Le Massacre des Juifs en Pologne," 2 (our translation). The French underground newspaper *Fraternité* was relaying the BBC's interview with Karski. We see that the resistance in France was well informed via London—even if it was, in this

case, a year late—and supported actions against mass deportations from France. See Renée Poznanski, *Propagandes et persécutions: La Résistance et le "problème juif,"* *1940–1944* (Paris: Fayard, 2008).

101. Karski, *Story of a Secret State*, 348–49.

102. "Le Massacre des Juifs en Pologne" (our translation).

103. Karski, *Story of a Secret State*, 349–50.

104. I am grateful to Martin Dean, who opened so many avenues to me and answered my questions with all of his formidable knowledge of the extermination of the Jews.

105. Yitzhak Arad, *The Operation Reinhard Death Camps* (Bloomington: Indiana University Press, 1987), 350–51.

106. "Memorandum Submitted to the President of the United States," December 8, 1942, n.p., https://www.jewishvirtuallibrary.org/memo-from-jewish-leader -press-president-roosevelt-to-act.

107. Republic of Poland, Ministry of Foreign Affairs, *Mass Extermination*, 9.

108. Karski quoted in Frank Baron, "The 'Myth' and Reality of Rescue from the Holocaust: The Karski-Koestler and Vrba-Wetzler Reports," in *German-Speaking Exiles in Great Britain*, vol. 2, ed. Anthony Grenville (Amsterdam and Atlanta: Editions Rodopi B.V., 2000), 173.

109. Testimony of Myeczyslaw Sekiewicz, forced Sonderkommando laborer, after the war, in Patrick Montague, *Chelmno and the Holocaust: The History of Hitler's First Death Camp* (London and New York: I. B. Tauris, 2012), 44 (translation adapted).

110. Captain Witold Pilecki, *Witold's Report from Auschwitz*, trans. Karolina Linda Potocka and Witold Wybranski (Zabki, Poland: Apostolicum Publishing House, 2017), 5. The report was written in 1945. http://rtmpilecki.eu/wp-content/ uploads/2018/05/RAPORT_WITOLDA_GB_WWW.pdf.

111. The organ of the American Representation of the General Jewish Workers' Union of Poland. I consulted this issue at the Princeton University library, where it was received on July 21, 1943. It is likely that intellectuals at Princeton, such as Albert Einstein and Jacques Maritain, read issues of *The Ghetto Speaks*. In the British National Archives, it can be seen that by August 1942 there were questions about the use of gas and about the accounts that had come from Poland. Diplomatic prudence, apparently, was called for: "I think we shall surely have to return a very guarded reply on the lines that our attention has been drawn to the report in question, but that H.M.G. has no means of confirming it" (BNA, Kew, September 7, 1942). This is around the date when Karski arrived in Izbica.

112. *The Ghetto Speaks*, no. 2 (August 5, 1942), 2.

113. This scene was cut from the final edit of *Shoah*. It can be found in the film rushes at USHMM, Washington, DC.

114. Rushes for *Shoah*, USHMM, 43.

115. Karski, *Story of a Secret State*, 349.

116. Ibid., 354.

117. Ibid., 321–22.

118. Arthur Koestler, *Arrival and Departure* (New York: Macmillan, 1943), 69. The French-language version of the book was titled *Croisade sans croix* [Crusade without a Cross] (Paris: Calmann-Lévy, 1946)—a rather inaccurate translation, although it referred to the almost Christ-like figure of the hero of the book. Koestler referred to what he also called "the great anti-Fascist crusade which, with drums and fanfares, advanced from defeat to defeat."

119. Koestler quoted in Baron, "The 'Myth' and Reality," 174. See also David Cesarani, *Arthur Koestler: The Homeless Mind* (Cambridge: Free Press, 1999), 202–3.

120. Koestler, *Arrival*, 69.

121. Ibid., 71.

122. Ibid., 71–72.

123. Ibid., 75–78.

124. George Orwell, "Arthur Koestler," *New York Times*, 1944. Reprinted in George Orwell, *Critical Essays* (London: Secker and Warburg, 1946). This was not only the opinion of British critics; in his review of the book for the *New York Times* on November 21, 1943, the Jewish American author Saul Bellow spoke of it only in terms of political morals and made no mention of the specific fate of the Jews in the train episode.

125. *Manchester Evening News*, December 9, 1943, reproduced in George Orwell, "Arthur Koestler," in *George Orwell: The Collected Essays, Journalism & Letters*, vol. 3, *As I Please, 1943–1946*, ed. Sonia Orwell and Ian Angus (Boston: Nonpareil Books, 2000), 234 (emphasis in original).

126. George Orwell, "Arthur Koestler," http://orwell.ru/library/reviews/koestler/english/e_ak.

127. Bottome quoted in Cesarani, *Arthur Koestler*, 208.

128. "Arthur Koestler" [late 1943], reprinted in *Hiéroglyphes* [1944] (Paris: Les Belles Lettres, 2012) (our translation). Koestler is in fact citing three million Jews killed. Sitwell was gay, whence Koestler's snide allusion to Proust.

129. Osbert Sitwell, quoted in Cesarani, *Arthur Koestler*, 208.

Chapter 3. Flashback

1. George Orwell [1943], "Looking Back on the Spanish War," in *Orwell: My Country Right or Left, 1940–1943*, vol. 2, *Essays, Journalism & Letters*, ed. Sonia Orwell and Ian Angus (Jaffrey, NH: Nonpareil, 2000), 253.

2. NYPL, Manuscripts, Col. 922, Displaced Scholars, Marc Bloch (our translation). Bloch, an illustrious historian to whom an American visa was immediately granted in 1940, refused it because his mother and oldest son were excluded; instead, he entered the French resistance.

3. The legacy of the Great War has been rediscovered from the executioners' point of view. This recent past has also been explored from the point of view of the victims and "witnesses," or "accomplices," on site or very far away. See Gerd Krumeich, ed., *Nationalsozialismus and Erster Weltkrieg* (Essen: Klartext-Verlag,

2010); Christian Ingrao, *Croire et détruire: Les intellectuels dans la machine de guerre nazie* (Paris: Fayard, 2009).

4. Charles de Gaulle, London Radio, September 18, 1941, in *De Gaulle: Discours et messages*, vol. 1, *Pendant la guerre* (Paris: Plon, 1970), 102–3 (our translation).

5. British National Archives (BNA), Kew, Sikorski, June 9, 1942, speech, 6 (our translation).

6. *The Times* (London), December 4, 1942, 3.

7. "Nazi War on Jews. The New Barbarism. Response of Civilized World," *The Times* (London), December 5, 1942.

8. Professors of Germany, "To the Civilized World," *North American Review* 201, no. 765 (August 1919): 285, https://www.jstor.org/stable/25122278.

9. Among them Roger Casement, who wrote the "Casement Report" (1903), in *Correspondence and Report from His Majesty's Consul at Boma Respecting the Administration of the Independent State of the Congo* (London: His Majesty's Stationery Office), 21–81, https://archive.org/details/CasementReport/page/n1. A testimonial in *The Times* (London) read as follows: "[The rubber] is collected by force. The soldiers drive the people into the bush. If they will not go they are shot down, and their left hands cut off and taken as trophies to the commissaire. The soldiers do not care who they shoot down, and they more often shoot poor helpless women and harmless children. These hands, the hands of men, women, and children, are placed in rows before the commissaire, who counts them to see that the soldiers have not wasted the cartridges. The commissaire is paid a commission of about 1d. a pound upon all the rubber he gets. It is therefore to his interest to get as much as he can" (November 18, 1895).

10. The African American journalist and legal expert Washington Williams, in a letter written in 1890 to the Secretary of State of the United States, was the first to use the term "crimes against humanity" in relation to the atrocities committed in the Congo under King Leopold II of Belgium.

11. Roundell Palmer, 3rd Earl of Selborne, an officer during World War I, was a personal friend of Winston Churchill's. In 1942, he was supposed to be minister of economic warfare but instead became the chief of the Special Operations Executive, which was tasked with countering anticommunist propaganda in Eastern Europe, and thus in Poland, in parallel with the fight against the Nazis.

12. Rushes for *Shoah*, USHMM, reel 316, typescript, 62–63, https://collections .ushmm.org/film_findingaids/RG-60.5006_01_trs_en.pdf.

13. See the pioneering book by John Horne and Alan Kramer, *German Atrocities, 1914: A History of Denial* (New Haven: Yale University Press, 2001). See also Annette Becker, *Les Cicatrices rouges, 14–18: France et Belgique occupées* (Paris: Fayard, 2010). Even as experienced a historian as Deborah Lipstadt thought, at the time she wrote *Beyond Belief: The American Press and the Coming of the Holocaust (1933–1945)* (New York: Free Press, 1986), that the atrocities of World War I were pure propaganda, that they had not taken place. Contemporary historiography contradicts her.

14. Marc Bloch, "Réflexions d'un historien sur les fausses nouvelles de la guerre," *Revue de synthèse historique*, 33 (1921): 32 (our translation).

15. *Evening Standard*, October 15, 1942.

16. Bloch, "Réflexions," note 24 (our translation).

17. Annette Becker, *Voir la Grande Guerre, un autre récit* (Paris: Armand Colin, 2014).

18. This was a common practice, as shown in a 1917 film by the Section cinématographique des armées in which French soldiers made candles, with this description: "Making candles with fat from military abattoirs to light up the foxholes." A German promotional film shows a woman rubbing her hands with glycerin extracted from animal bones. Beside her is the Eiffel Tower: the pride of producing substitutes to win the war.

19. *The Times* (London), April 17, 1917, 5, cited in Joachim Neander and Randal Marlin, "Media and Propaganda: The Northcliffe Press and the Corpse Factory Story of World War I," *Global Media Journal—Canadian Edition* 3, no. 2 (2010): 73–74, https://core.ac.uk/download/pdf/26945870.pdf.

20. Adrian Gregory, *The Last Great War: British Society and the First World War* (Cambridge: Cambridge University Press, 2008), 57.

21. Bertrand Russell, "Government Propaganda," in *These Eventful Years*, vol. 1, *The Twentieth Century in the Making, as Told by Many of Its Makers* (Encyclopaedia Britannica, 1924). See Neander and Marlin, "Media and Propaganda."

22. Adolf Hitler, *Mein Kampf* (New York: Reynal & Hitchcock, 1940), 237–38.

23. Victor Klemperer, *The Language of the Third Reich, LTI—Lingua Tertii Imperii: A Philologist's Notebook*, trans. Martin Brady (London: Athlone Press, 2000), 26–27.

24. Report cited in chapter 2. BNA, Kew, Poland, C 8789, September 11, 1942.

25. *New York Times*, November 26, 1942, 16; Rafael Medoff, *The Anguish of a Jewish Leader: Stephen S. Wise and the Holocaust* (Washington, DC: David S. Wyman Institute for Holocaust Studies, 2015).

26. Our translation. Three *Christian Century* editorials from 1942 to 1944 returned to this theme: "Horror Stories from Poland" (December 9, 1942); "Polish Atrocities Are Entered in the Books" (December 30, 1942); "Biggest Atrocity Story Breaks in Poland" (September 13, 1944).

27. Raymond Arthur Davies, "The Human Soap Factory," in *The Truth about Poland* (1946), chapter 5 (our translation). "Raymond Arthur Davies" was a pseudonym used by Rudolph Shohan, convicted of fraud in Canada and likely a Soviet agent. I would like to thank the Canadian Holocaust scholar Mark Celinscak for this information.

28. J. Neander, "The Danzig Soap Case: Facts and Legends around 'Professor Spanner' and the Danzig Anatomic Institute 1944–1945," *German Studies Review* 29, no. 1 (February 2006): 63–86.

29. Victor Gollancz, *"Let My People Go": Some Practical Proposals for Dealing with Hitler's Massacre of the Jews and an Appeal to the British Public* (London: Victor

Gollancz Ltd., 1943), 10, 1 (emphasis in original). The text was dated "Christmas Day, 1942"—a date deliberately chosen.

30. Jacques Maritain, "Anti-Semitism as a Problem for the Jew," *The Commonweal*, September 25, 1942, in Jacques Maritain and Raissa Maritain, *Œuvres complètes*, vol. 8, *1944–1946* (Fribourg: Éditions Universitaires, 1989) (our translation). See also Jacques Maritain, "Le Droit raciste à l'assaut de la civilization," in *Le Droit raciste à l'assaut de la civilisation*, ed. E. Hamburger, M. Gottschalk, P. Jacob, J. Maritain, and B. Mirkine-Guétzevitch (New York: Éditions de la Maison française, 1943), 111.

31. William Shirer, "The Propaganda Front," *Washington Post*, February 14, 1943, https://www.justice.gov/sites/default/files/criminal/legacy/2010/04/11/ezra-pound -p4.pdf.

32. Gollancz, *"Let My People Go,"* 29.

33. William L. Shirer, "The Propaganda Front," *Washington Post*, January 3, 1943, B7.

34. William L. Shirer, "The Propaganda Front: No Atrocity Stories, Facts," *Washington Post*, March 21, 1943, B7.

35. Gerhart M. Riegner, *Never Despair: Sixty Years in the Service of the Jewish People and the Cause of Human Rights*, trans. William Sayers (Chicago: Ivan R. Dee, 2006), 56–57.

36. Raymond Aron, *Memoirs: Fifty Years of Political Reflection*, trans. George Holoch (New York: Holmes & Meier, 1990), 122.

37. Varian Fry, "The Massacre of the Jews," *New Republic* (December 21, 1942): 816. See also Thomas Weber, *La Première Guerre d'Hitler* (Paris: Perrin, 2012).

38. Fry, "Massacre of the Jews," 818. See Becker, *Les Cicatrices rouges, 14–18.*

39. Eleanor Roosevelt asked Welles on September 12, 1942, cited by Andy Marino in *A Quiet American: The Secret War of Varian Fry* (New York: St. Martin's Press, 1999). In her daily column, "My Day," Roosevelt in fact did not mention Fry. On December 5, 1942, she mentioned the extermination of two-thirds of the Jews in Poland, the exact information that had come to her. She added that protesting was useless and that Hitler would have to be punished by death. Eleanor Roosevelt, *My Day: The Best of Eleanor Roosevelt's Acclaimed Newspaper Columns, 1936–1962*, ed. David Emblidge (Cambridge, MA: Da Capo Press, 2009).

40. Raphael Lemkin, *Totally Unofficial: The Autobiography of Raphael Lemkin*, ed. Donna-Lee Frieze (New Haven: Yale University Press, 2013), 113. Lemkin's use of the word "genocide" here is an anachronism, as he had not yet invented the term at this time.

41. Raphael Lemkin, *Axis Rule in Occupied Europe: Laws of Occupation, Analysis of Government, Proposals for Redress* (Washington, DC: Carnegie Endowment for International Peace, 1944). The preface was written in 1943, and the book was published in the fall of 1944.

42. Hayim Nahman Bialik, "City of the Killings," in *Songs from Bialik: Selected Poems of Hayim Nahman Bialik*, ed. and trans. Atar Hadari (Syracuse: Syracuse University Press, 2000), 1.

43. The term was first used in the United States to describe what was happening in the wars in the former Yugoslavia in the 1990s.

44. Abel Pann, *Autobiographie: Le roman d'un Juif* (Paris: Cerf, 1996), 119–20 (our translation). See also Abel Pann, *In the Name of the Czar: 24 Original Pictures* (American Jewish Chronicle, 1918); Becker, *Voir la Grande Guerre*, 89–91.

45. Simon Dubnow, *Le Livre de ma vie: Souvenirs et réflexions, matériaux pour l'histoire de mon temps* (Paris: Cerf, 2000), 720–22 (our translation); the passage was written May 16–17, 1915. The word "Judeophobia" appears in the Russian original; Dubnow also used the expression "hate of the Jew." I thank Alexandre Sumpf for these linguistic details.

46. Alexandre Sumpf, *La Grande Guerre oubliée: Russie, 1914–1918* (Paris: Perrin, 2014); Nicolas Werth, "Dans l'ombre de la Shoah, les pogroms des guerres civiles russes," introduction to *Livre des pogroms: Antichambre d'un génocide, Ukraine, Russie, Biélorussie,1917–1922* (Paris: Calmann-Lévy, 2010), 36–37, and "Les Déportations des 'populations suspectes' dans les espaces russes et soviétiques, 1914–1953," *Communisme*, no. 78–79 (2004): 11–43. This was the third wave of pogroms in Russia, after those in 1884 and 1908. My warm thanks to Nicolas Werth, who, more than cited here, is followed to the letter.

47. *Volkovysk Memorial Book*, 107–9.

48. Mark von Hagen, "The Moral Economy of Ethnic Violence: The Pogrom in Lwow, November 1918," *Geschichte und Gesellschaft* 31 (2005): 203–26.

49. *La Baïonnette*, September 7, 1916 (our translation).

50. Turkish document sent to Pope Benedict XV, Vatican Archives (VA), asV, guerra 14–18, 244, fasc. 110. Author unknown, *Vérité sur le mouvement révolutionnaire arménien et les mesures gouvernementales* (Constantinople, 1916).

51. *Hilal*, March 14, 1918 (our translation). Copy conserved in the VA, secretariat of state, guerra 14–18, 244, fasc. 112.

52. Philippe Burrin, *Ressentiment et apocalypse: Essai sur l'antisémitisme nazi* (Paris: Seuil, 2004), 71–75.

53. Jean Jaurès, speech to the Assemblée, December 3, 1886 (our translation). Vincent Duclert, *La France face au génocide des Arméniens* (Paris: Fayard, 2015), 140–49.

54. Paul Painlevé quoting René Pinon (our translation).

55. Quoted in Richard Breitman and Allan J. Lichtman, *FDR and the Jews* (Cambridge, MA: Belknap Press of Harvard University Press, 2013), 214.

56. Annette Becker and Jay Winter, "Le Génocide arménien et les réactions de l'opinion internationale," in *Vers la guerre totale: Le tournant de 1914–1915*, ed. John Horne and the Centre international de recherche de l'Historial de la Grande Guerre (Paris: Éditions Tallandier, 2010).

57. Breitman and Lichtman, *FDR and the Jews*, 214. As president, Roosevelt discussed the Armenians with his secretary of the treasury, Henry Morgenthau Jr.—none other than the son of Henry Morgenthau Sr., the American ambassador to the Ottoman Empire and real-time witness to the massacres. I shall return to this. See

Keith Pomakoy, *Helping Humanity: American Policy and Genocide Rescue* (Lanham, MD: Lexington Books, 2011).

58. Elisabeth Kontogiorgi, *Population Exchange in Greek Macedonia: The Rural Settlement of Refugees 1922–1930* (Oxford: Oxford University Press, 2006), 54. Kontogiorgi attributes the quotation in a footnote to Martin Gilbert, *Winston S. Churchill*, vol. 4, *World in Torment, 1916–1922* (Hillsdale, MI: Hillsdale College Press, 1975), 854.

59. Charles Graves, *Mr. Punch's History of the Great War* (New York: Frederick A. Stokes, 1919), 270.

60. Heinrich Vierbücher, *Arménie 1915: Ce que le gouvernement impérial a caché aux sujets allemands: le massacre d'un peuple civilisé par les Turcs*, 1930 (our translation).

61. UK Parliament, House of Lords Hansard, December 17, 1942, https://hansard.parliament.uk/Lords/1942-12-17/debates/af4d15ee-1598-4a11-a46e-ae0af28460 64/PersecutionOfTheJewsAlliesDeclaration.

62. See the different works by Dzovinar Kevonian and Sevane Garibian, in particular "Ailleurs, hier, autrement, connaissance et reconnaissance du génocide des Arméniens," *Revue d'histoire de la Shoah*, no. 277–78 (2003); Taner Akçam, *A Shameful Act: The Armenian Genocide and the Question of Turkish Responsibility*, trans. Paul Bessemer (New York: Metropolitan Books, 2006). Akçam recently wrote another remarkable book, in which he proves the intention and the responsibility of the Young Turks, and especially Talaat Pasha, in the extermination of the Armenians: *Killing Orders: Talaat Pasha's Telegrams and the Armenian Genocide* (London: Palgrave Macmillan, Palgrave Studies in the History of Genocides imprint, 2018). This book has been translated into French, with an original preface by Annette Becker (Paris: CNRS Editions, 2020).

63. Lemkin, *Totally Unofficial*, 19.

64. Vahakn N. Dadrian and Taner Akçam, *Judgment at Istanbul: The Armenian Genocide Trials* (New York and Oxford: Berghahn Books, 2011). At the time, Armenian activists were on a mission to eliminate former perpetrators.

65. Lemkin, *Totally Unofficial*, 20.

66. Joseph Kessel, "Témoignage de M. Joseph Kessel au procès Schwartzbard," in *Reportages, Romans*, ed. Gilles Heuré (Paris: Gallimard, Quarto imprint, 2010), 635 (our translation).

67. Lepsius's testimony was drawn from his *Report on the Situation of the Armenian People in Turkey*, published in 1916.

68. Half-hour interview with Lemkin by Quincy Howe, broadcast 1949, CBS archives. Quotation from http://www.armeniapedia.org/wiki/Lemkin_Discusses_ Armenian_Genocide_In_Newly-Found_1949_CBS_Interview.

69. Lemkin, *Totally Unofficial*, 20.

70. Wolf Gruner, "'Peregrinations into the Void?' German Jews and Their Knowledge about the Armenian Genocide during the Third Reich," *Central European*

History 45 (2012): 1–26. See also Stefan Ihrig, *Atatürk in the Nazi Imagination* (Cambridge, MA: Harvard University Press, 2014).

71. Klemperer quoted in Gruner, "'Peregrinations into the Void?,'" 2 (Gruner's translation).

72. *Convention (II) with Respect to the Laws and Customs of War on Land*, The Hague, 1899, Preamble, https://ihl-databases.icrc.org/applic/ihl/ihl.nsf/ART/150-11 0001?OpenDocument.

73. The clause was included, with slight changes, in the 1907 preamble to the convention, which was to become, once ratified in 1909, the basis for international law on warfare in 1914. Rupert Ticehurst, "The Martens Clause and the Laws of Armed Conflict," *International Review of the Red Cross* 37, no. 317 (1997): 125–34; Vladimir Pustogarov, "Fyodor Fyodorovich Martens (1845–1909)—A Humanist of Modern Times," *International Review of the Red Cross* 36, no. 312 (1996): 300–314.

74. Raphael Lemkin, "Acts Constituting a General (Transnational) Danger Considered as Offences against the Law of Nations," trans. Jim Fussell, http://www.pre ventgenocide.org/lemkin/madrid1933-english.htm; "A Report on Terrorism," trans. Vincent Chanethom, http://watchersofthesky.com/wp-content/uploads/2014/10/ lemkins-madrid-report-in-1933.pdf.

75. Lemkin, "Acts Constituting."

76. Lemkin, "Report on Terrorism," "Acts Constituting."

77. Lemkin, "Report on Terrorism" (emphasis added).

78. Provisions for minimal protection of cultural assets had existed since the Hague Convention (IX) of 1907. Following the suggestion by the Russian painter and lawyer Nicholas Roerich, the Roerich Museum in New York asked Georges Chklaver, of the Institut des hautes études internationales at the Université de Paris, to draft a convention for discussion by international bodies. The Roerich Pact (also known as the Treaty on the Protection of Artistic and Scientific Institutions and Historic Monuments) was signed on April 15, 1935.

79. Lemkin cited Pella's book *The Repression of the Crimes against the Personality of the State* (1930), which became a legal classic. Ironically, Pella would be accused—rightly or wrongly—of anti-Semitism after World War II, and he and Lemkin had a falling-out.

80. Lemkin, "Report on Terrorism" (emphasis added).

81. A term used by Hugo Grotius but also a reference to the Torah and the Talmud that Lemkin, former student in the *heder* (Jewish school), knew well. Intention of the evil act: Exodus 21, 12–14.

82. Lemkin, "Acts Constituting" (emphasis in original).

83. Ibid.

84. Jan Karski, *The Great Powers and Poland, 1919–1945: From Versailles to Yalta* (Lanham, MD: University Press of America, 1985). I consulted the typewritten manuscript at Georgetown University.

85. Lemkin, "Acts Constituting" (emphasis in original).

86. NYPL, microfilm 2, notes from the 1950s (our translation).

87. *Washington Post*, December 3, 1944 (our translation).

88. Jan Karski, *Story of a Secret State* (Boston: Houghton Mifflin, 1944), 384. This was one of the numerous passages that Karski added or modified when the first edition was published. See the proofs in the Georgetown University archives. Chapter 33, "My Report to the World," is one of the most heavily marked up in the entire book, proving its importance to the publication in the United States in wartime.

89. Stephen Wise, *The Personal Letters of Stephen Wise* (Boston: Beacon Press, 1956), 166.

90. Ibid., 260.

91. Calel Perechodnik, *Am I a Murderer? Testament of a Jewish Ghetto Policeman*, trans. Frank Fox (Boulder, CO: Westview Press, 1996).

92. Emanuel Ringelblum cites Maxence Van der Meersch's *Invasion 14*, published in 1935 (published in English as *Invasion*, trans. Gerard Hopkins [New York: Viking, 1937]) in *Chronique du ghetto de Varsovie* (Paris: Payot, 1958), 312–13 (our translation). Seven hundred thousand Poles emigrated to work in the mines in northern France after World War I, giving rise to their interest in the period of occupation in 1914–18.

93. Library of Congress, Pehle, John, memorandum for the Secretary's Files, 1944 January 16; the Morgenthau Diaries (microfilm Publication Bethesda, MD: University Publications of America, c. 1995–97) (our translation). Microfilm 23, 392–73P, volume 694, document 190–192. I am grateful to Rebecca Erbelding of the USHMM, who tracked down all references to Armenians and to Lemkin in the archives of the War Refugee Board for me. Her doctoral dissertation, "About Time: The History of the War Refugee Board," has been published by UMI Dissertation Publishing (2015). (See chapter 4.)

94. Letter from Randolph Paul to Bruce Bliven, February 4, 1944, Papers of the War Refugee Board (Bethesda, MD: University Publications of America, 2002) (our translation). Microfilm LM0305, reel 25, Folder 7, documents 692–695, USHMM.

95. Frankfurter participated as a Zionist, although an ambivalent one—a view he always held. H. N. Hirsch, *The Enigma of Felix Frankfurter* (New York: Basic Books, 1981).

Chapter 4. Naming a Nameless Crime

1. British National Archives (BNA), Kew, Fo. 371 1942. Germany. *Treatment of War criminals*, telegram no. 7686. For the chronology, see chapter 2.

2. USHMM, copy of the archives of the Polish government in exile deposited at Stanford University, dossier 70, 19–20.

3. Chaim Weizmann, speech given at Madison Square Garden, New York, March 1, 1943 (our translation).

4. Quoted in "35,000 Slain Jews Honored at Rally. Speakers Condemn Warsaw Persecutions as the Most Barbarous in History," *New York Times*, June 20, 1943, 34.

5. BNA, Kew, Shmuel Zygielbojm, telegram to Churchill, December 15, 1942. See chapter 2.

6. Shmuel Zygielbojm's letter published in the *Polish Review*, June 14, 1943, https://www.marxists.org/subject/jewish/zygielbojm-suicide-letter.pdf. The October 4, 1943, issue of the *Polish Review* began with a series of poems "to the Jews, to the memory of Shmuel Zygielbojm."

7. Adolph Held, quoted in "35,000 Slain Jews."

8. Jan Ciechanowski, *Defeat in Victory* (New York: Doubleday, 1947), 179.

9. General Sikorski, 9, I 1943, File 111, government in exile, Polish archives, USHMM.

10. *Memorandum*, Assistant Secretary, Department of State, July 10, 1943, USHMM (our translation).

11. Jan Karski, *Story of a Secret State: My Report to the World* (London: Penguin Books, 2012), 419.

12. Rushes for *Shoah*, USHMM, reel 313. Lanzmann did not use in *Shoah* the material from the second day of his interview with Karski, during which he spoke about his meetings at the White House with Roosevelt and at the Supreme Court with Justice Frankfurter. In 2010, he used some parts of this 1978 interview in a new film, *The Karski Report*. See chapter 6.

13. Ibid.

14. Ibid., reel 314.

15. Library of Congress, Manuscript Division.

16. Rushes for *Shoah*, USHMM, reel 315. Understandably, Lanzmann did not keep these remarks, even in his new edit in 2010.

17. Ibid. On the "nos" of Karski and Frankfurter, see the introduction and chapter 6.

18. *Minutes of Meeting of Representation of Polish Jewry, on Occasion of the Visit of Mr. Jan Karski*, Cincinnati, American Jewish Archives, August 9, 1943, 1 (our translation).

19. Whom he had met in London; see chapters 2 and 6.

20. *Minutes of Meeting of Representation of Polish Jewry*, 5 (our translation).

21. Schwarzbart quoted in E. Thomas Wood and Stanislaw M. Jankowski, *Karski: How One Man Tried to Stop the Holocaust* (New York: Wiley, 1994), 178.

22. *Minutes of Meeting of Representation of Polish Jewry*, 8 (our translation).

23. Ibid., 5, 7.

24. *Oswiecim* (*Camp of Death*) (New York: Poland Fights [Polish labor group], 1944), 41–48, https://archive.org/details/OswiecimCampOfDeath. The original Polish-language version was published by the resistance in 1942. The 1944 translation was conserved by Karski, Georgetown University archives.

25. "Jewish evacuation," internal verbatim record, Treasury Department, in the presence of Henry Morgenthau Jr., Treasury Secretary, December 19, 1943, USHMM archives, 14 and 21. See Rebecca Erbelding, "About Time: The History of the War Refugee Board," PhD dissertation, George Mason University, 2015, published as *Rescue Board: The Untold Story of America's Efforts to Save the Jews of Europe* (New York: Penguin Random House, 2019).

26. "Jewish evacuation," 13.

27. Letter from the World Jewish Congress dated April 13, 1944, signed by its president, Nahum Goldmann, including a memo from December 3, 1943 (our translation). Copy at the USHMM. I will not discuss here the well-known issue of negotiations between the Nazis and the Hungarian Jewish aid organizations. See Z. Vagi, L. Csosz, and G. Kadar, *The Holocaust in Hungary: Evolution of a Genocide*, trans. Zsofia Zvolensky (Lanham, MD: AltaMira Press, 2013).

28. Vagi, Csosz, and Kadar, *The Holocaust in Hungary*, 11.

29. The report was dated January 13, 1944. It is reproduced in Michael Mashberg, "Documents Concerning the American State Department and the Stateless European Jews, 1942–1944," *Jewish Social Studies* 39, no.1–2 (Winter–Spring 1977): 163–82. The quotation is on 164.

30. Ibid., 167 (emphasis in original).

31. Richard Breitman, *Official Secrets: What the Nazis Planned, What the British and Americans Knew* (New York: Farrar, Straus and Giroux, 1999).

32. Mashberg, "Documents Concerning the American State Department," 174.

33. Message from President Roosevelt to the president of the World Jewish Congress, July 31, 1944, Truman Library, Jta no. 176 (emphasis added).

34. It is also what John Pehle would wonder all his life. In 1981, he said, "But by and large, I am afraid that the American effort to save the oppressed people of Europe was too little and too late." In *The Liberation of the Nazi Concentration Camps 1945: Eyewitness Accounts of the Liberators*, ed. Brewster Chamberlin and Marica Feldman (Washington, DC: United States Holocaust Memorial Council, 1987), 175.

35. USHMM archives, Board of Economic Warfare (our translation).

36. Raphael Lemkin, *Totally Unofficial: The Autobiography of Raphael Lemkin* (New Haven: Yale University Press, 2013), 114.

37. Ibid., 115.

38. Ibid., 115, 117.

39. *The Diary of Samuel Golfard and the Holocaust in Galicia*, ed. Wendy Lower, USHMM series Jewish Responses to Persecutions, gen. ed. Jürgen Matthäus (Lanham, MD: AltaMira Press, 2011), 94–95.

40. Isaac Schneersohn, Foreword, in *La Persécution des Juifs dans les pays de l'Est présentée à Nuremberg*, a collection of documents edited by Henri Monneray, preface by General Telford Taylor, introduction by René Cassin (Paris: Éditions du Centre, CdJC, 1949), 8 (our translation).

41. *New York Times*, February 7, 1943, section M, pp. 1, 16.

42. Arthur Koestler, *New York Times*, January 9, 1944, reprinted in his *The Yogi and the Commissar, and Other Essays* (New York: Macmillan, 1945), 90.

43. This is the "rule" of the distance-compassion ratio that contemporary humanitarian experts often denounce: the farther away the evil is, geographically or socially, the less one is interested in it. Only events within one's close circle can arouse compassion.

44. Koestler, *The Yogi and the Commissar*, 91.

45. Ibid., 93.

46. Lemkin, *Totally Unofficial*, 58.

47. Lemkin, note in the Collection of the NYPL.

48. Lemkin, *Totally Unofficial*, 115, 116.

49. NYPL, Lemkin Papers, microfilm no. 2, n.d. Some words are crossed out or illegible, and the text was probably written under huge stress and at a time when Lemkin had not fully mastered English.

50. Raphael Lemkin, "Le crime de génocide," *Notes documentaires et études*, no. 417, La documentation française (1946) (our translation).

51. Title of chapter 7 in the provisional outline of *Totally Unofficial*.

52. Several fragments at the NYPL.

53. Lemkin, *Totally Unofficial*, 1.

54. Raphael Lemkin, *Axis Rule in Occupied Europe: Laws of Occupation, Proposals for Redress* (Washington, DC: Carnegie Endowment for international Peace, Division of International Law, 1944), 77. Articles 46 and 52 (confiscations and forced labor) of The Hague Conventions were cited.

55. Ibid., 78.

56. Ibid., 79 (emphasis added).

57. Raphael Lemkin, *Key Laws, Decrees, and Regulations Issued by the Axis in Occupied Europe* (Board of Economic Warfare, Blockade and Supply Branch, Reoccupation Division, December 1942), typescript, USHMM.

58. Johann Chapoutot, *La Loi du sang: Penser et agir en nazi* (Paris: Gallimard, "Bibliothèque des Histoires," 2014).

59. Lemkin, *Key Laws*, 8800.

60. Lemkin, "Le crime de génocide," *Notes documentaires et études*, no. 417 (September 24, 1946), 3 (emphasis added; our translation).

61. Abram de Swaan, *Diviser pour tuer: Les régimes génocidaires et leurs hommes de main* (Paris: Seuil, 2016); Christian Ingrao, *La Promesse de l'Est: Espérance nazie et génocide, 1939–1943* (Paris: Seuil, 2017).

62. "Bits of This and That," *Washington Post*, September 16, 1943. Lemkin probably wrote this notice himself.

63. Lemkin, *Axis Rule*, 338.

64. Ibid.

65. Ibid., 128.

66. "Report of Minister Whitlock," in *German War Practices*, part 1, *Treatment of Civilians*, ed. D. C. Munro, G. C. Sellery, and A. C. Krey (Committee on Public Information, 1918), 78. See also James Wilford Garner, *International Law and the World Order* (New York: Longmans Green, 1920), 184n1, in which he quotes the "opinion of the American minister to Belgium in a report to the department of state in April 1917."

67. General Ludendorff, *The General Staff and Its Problems*, vol. 1, 156, 157, quoted in Lemkin, *Axis Rule*, 67n2. Lemkin also quoted Roosevelt at the conference of the

International Labor Organization on November 6, 1941, reminding his audience that two million foreign forced laborers were replacing Germans who had left for the front.

68. Lemkin, *Axis Rule*, 67.

69. French-language manuscript, NYPL, 4 (our translation). See Annette Becker, "La 'Grosse Bertha' frappe Saint-Gervais," in Annette Becker et al., *La Très Grande Guerre* (Paris: Le Monde Éditions, 1994).

70. Lemkin to Jackson, May 4, 1945, Lemkin Archives, NYPL.

71. "Secret Field Marshal v. Reichenau Order, Subject: Conduct of Troops in Eastern Territories, October 10, 1941," https://phdn.org/archives/www.ess.uwe.ac.uk/genocide/USSR2.htm. Lemkin cited the order in a letter dated October 12, 1941 (Office of US Chief Committee for War Crimes), in *The Holocaust: Selected Documents*, vol. 10, *The Einsatzgruppen or Murder Commandos* (New York and London: Garland, 1982), 6, document 2. See also Telford Taylor, "Cross-Examination of von Rundstedt at Nuremberg by General Telford Taylor," in *The Anatomy of the Nuremberg Trials: A Personal Memoir* (London: Bloomsbury, 1993), 520–21.

72. Von Rundstedt quoted in Raphael Lemkin, "Genocide—A Modern Crime," *Free World* 4 (April 1945): 39.

73. Ibid. In a *Washington Post* article titled "Retribution," no doubt inspired by Lemkin, von Rundstedt was quoted again about the punishments that awaited the Germans.

74. Letter from Wallace to Lemkin, February 11, 1946, Library of Congress Archives, Wallace fonds. In 1944, Wallace was involved mainly in deliveries of matériel to the Soviet Union in a lend-lease arrangement, whence his visit to the Kolyma gulag, where he saw Potemkin Village–type experiments on detainees (whom he took for actual laborers) subjected to extreme forced labor. Related by Varlam Shalamov in *Kolyma Tales*, trans. John Glad (London: Penguin Books, 1994). Wallace obviously did not understand the meaning of mass violence.

75. Taken from the title of chapter 7 of Lemkin, *Totally Unofficial*.

76. *Washington Post*, December 3, 1944.

77. Norman Bentwich, "The Law of War Crimes," *Palestine Post*, November 23, 1945.

78. Lemkin's response in the *Washington Post* on December 14, 1944, to a letter to the editor in that newspaper written by "army officer, Virginia," dated December 3, 1944, and published on December 10. We see the use that different prosecutors of the post–World War II trials might have made of Lemkin's clear response.

79. Sterling North, *Washington Post*, December 24, 1944.

80. Otto D. Tolischus, "Twentieth-Century Moloch: The Nazi-Inspired Totalitarian State, Devourer of Progress—and of Itself," *New York Times Book Review*, January 21, 1945.

81. P. O. Douglas, "Genocide," *Washington Post*, December 29, 1944 (letter written December 20).

82. Letter to the editor, *Washington Post*, December 29, 1944.

83. Review of Jan Karski's book *Story of a Secret State* (Boston: Houghton Mifflin, 1944), in *Polish Review*, January 18, 1945.

84. Advertisement in the *New York Times*, February 4, 1945.

85. *New York Times*, December 3, 1944.

86. Advertisement in the *Chicago Tribune*, December 3, 1944.

87. "Poland's 'Underground State' Exhibition," *Polish Review*, September 4, 1944.

88. New York exhibition, May 10–June 8, 1944, *Polish Review* (our translation).

89. For example, in the *Polish Review*, March 28, 1944, and in all sorts of underground leaflets exhibited or reproduced. Karski's archives contain a large number, which he collected in Europe in 1946.

90. Sterling North, "The Post's Book of the Week," *Washington Post*, December 31, 1944, section S, p. 5.

91. *Chicago Daily* (in Polish), January 25, 1945.

92. Karski, *Story of a Secret State* (2012), 320.

93. Unsigned book review of *Story of a Secret State* in the Ogden [Utah] *Standard-Examiner*, January 7, 1945, 18, https://www.newspapers.com/clip/31390595/the-ogden-standard-examiner/ (emphasis added).

94. There was just about no one to liberate, whence the choice of the word "opened." In fact, "liberate" would signify a political will, that of making the camps central to the war. This was never the case for the Allies.

95. Daniel Blatman, *The Death Marches: The Final Phase of Nazi Genocide*, trans. Chaya Galai (Cambridge: Belknap Press, 2011).

96. *New York Times*, January 9, 1944, p. sm5.

97. Exhibition catalogue for *Filmer la guerre: Les Soviétiques face à la Shoah 1941–1946* (Paris: Mémorial de la Shoah, 2014).

98. Canadians were also present at Bergen-Belsen. See Mark Celinsack, *Distance from the Belsen Heap: Allied Forces and the Liberation of a Nazi Concentration Camp* (Toronto: University of Toronto Press, 2015).

99. Elie Wiesel, *Night*, trans. Marion Wiesel (New York: Hill and Wang, 2012); originally published in Yiddish in 1955. See chapter 6.

100. John Dower, *War without Mercy: Race and Power in the Pacific War* (New York: Pantheon Books, 1986).

101. Paul Winkler, "Torture Camps," *Washington Post*, February 12, 1944, p. 6.

102. Cartoon by Garner Rea, *Colliers*, February 19, 1944.

103. Cartoons by Helen Hokinson, *The New Yorker*, May 13 and May 20, 1944.

104. Edmund Wilson, *The New Yorker*, November 25, 1944, p. 92.

105. "Gallup Finds Most Believe Atrocity Tales," *Washington Post*, December 3, 1944.

106. Edward T. Folliard, "Skeptic Yanks See Proof of Nazi Atrocities," *Washington Post*, April 16, 1945, p. 1.

107. William L. Shirer, "The Propaganda Front," *Washington Post*, January 3, 1943, p. B7 (our translation).

108. "Atrocities of World War One," *Washington Post*, May 6, 1945, p. B4 (our translation). Wittenberg, Luther's city, was a military prison camp during World War I. On the reality of and propaganda about these camps, see Heather Jones, *Violence against Prisoners of War, in the First World War, Britain, France and Germany, 1914–1920* (Cambridge: Cambridge University Press, 2013).

109. "Gazing into the Pit," *The Christian Century*, May 9, 1945.

110. Marcel Cohen, "Faire avec presque rien ou le métier d'un écrivain stupéfait," *Europe*, January 2016, p. 207 (our translation).

Chapter 5. The War Is Over

1. Lemkin, critical reading of *Les Mémoires de Mgr Jean Naslian*, 2 vols. (Imprimerie mechithariste, 1955) (our translation).

2. United Nations General Assembly, "Resolution 96 (1). The Crime of Genocide," December 11, 1946.

3. Jan Gross, *Fear: Anti-Semitism in Poland after Auschwitz* (New York: Random House, 2007); Gross, *Golden Harvest: Events at the Periphery of the Holocaust* (Oxford: Oxford University Press, 2012); Aude Kichelewski, *Les Survivants: Être juif en Pologne de 1945 à nos jours* (Paris: Vendémiaire, 2016).

4. Translator's note: *Survivant* is, directly, a survivor. *Rescapé* has the additional nuance of "being safe, uninjured."

5. Henry Rousso, ed., *Après la Shoah, rescapés, réfugiés, survivants, 1944–47*, catalogue for an exhibition, curated by Henry Rousso at the Mémorial de la Shoah in Paris, 2016.

6. USHMM archives, report of Earl G. Harrison to President Truman, August 24, 1945, https://www.ushmm.org/exhibition/displaced-persons/resourc1.htm.

7. The amateur film is in the USHMM archives.

8. Letter in the file of Raphael Lemkin at the International Tracing Service, Bad Arolsen, No. 228134 (our translation).

9. "All wiped out. No more family." File of the International Tracing Service, Bad Arolsen. Elias Lemkin, No. 3763; Lea, No. 690424; Samuel, No. 696053; Sholom/Saul, No. 794 636.

10. I am grateful to Juliette Denis, expert in the wartime USSR, for these details. See Catherine Gousseff, *Échanger les peuples: Le déplacement des minorités aux confins polono-soviétiques, 1944–1947* (Paris: Fayard, 2015).

11. Memo of December 19, 1943, USHMM, p. 26 (our translation).

12. See chapter 4.

13. Files of the International Tracing Service, Bad Arolsen, Daniel Lemkin, No. 474146.

14. Anonymous, "Retribution," *Washington Post*, May 6, 1945 (our translation).

15. Raphael Lemkin, "The Legal Case against Hitler, Part I," *The Nation*, February 24, 1945, p. 206.

16. In 1942, Franz Neumann wrote a prescient book on Nazism, *Behemoth: The Structure and Practice of National Socialism* (Oxford: Oxford University Press,

1942). He was later Raul Hilberg's dissertation adviser at Columbia University, New York.

17. Telford Taylor, *The Anatomy of the Nuremberg Trials: A Personal Memoir* (London: Bloomsbury, 1993), 49.

18. Ibid., 50.

19. Ibid., 103.

20. Hersch Lauterpacht, *An International Bill of the Rights of Man* (New York: Columbia University Press, 1944). He criticized *Axis Rule* in the *Cambridge Law Journal*. See Philippe Sands, *East West Street: On the Origins of Genocide and Crimes against Humanity* (London: Weidenfeld and Nicolson, 2016).

21. Interview with Professor Lemkin at United Nations Radio, June 12, 1957, p. 1. World Jewish Congress Collection, box H276, file 10.

22. Our translation.

23. Alexander also wrote the Nuremberg code on ethical medical experiments. "Science under dictatorship," he wrote, "becomes subordinated to the guiding philosophy of the dictatorship." Leo Alexander, "Medical Science under Dictatorship," *New England Journal of Medicine* 241, No. 2 (July 14, 1949): 39.

24. Paul Julian Weindling, *Nazi Medicine and the Nuremberg Trials: From Medical War Crimes to Informed Consent* (Basingstoke: Palgrave Macmillan, 2004), 85. I am grateful to Paul Weindling for confirming my hypothesis of barbarism assumed by Lemkin.

25. Raphael Lemkin, "The Significance of the Concept of Genocide in the Trial of War Criminals," 1946, Lemkin Archives, Columbia University, New York City, box 4, file 4.

26. Letter from Egon Schneller to Raphael Lemkin to thank him with ten copies of his article "International Film for Discovery of War Criminals," Lemkin Archives, Columbia University, New York City, box 5, file 5. See Christian Delage, *La Vérité par l'image, de Nuremberg au procès Milosevic* (Paris: Denoël, 2006).

27. Quoted by Mark Lewis, *The Birth of the New Justice: The Internationalization of Crime and Punishment, 1939–1950* (Oxford: Oxford University Press, 2014) 205.

28. Letter from Lemkin to David Maxwell Fyfe, assistant general prosecutor, August 26, 1946, AJHS, Lemkin Papers, quoted in Anson Rabinbach, "Raphael Lemkin et le concept de génocide," *Revue d'histoire de la Shoah* (July 2008): 541 (our translation).

29. Sands, *East West Street*, 301.

30. Melchior Palyi, book review of *Axis Rule*, *American Journal of Sociology* 51, no. 5 (March 1946): 496–97. See also Melchior Palyi, *Papers*, Special Collections Research Center, University of Chicago Library. We may admire Palyi's scholarly prescience, as it would not be until the 1980s that the Nazism of the occupation would be studied in this way, via the local and regional decisions more or less arbitrated by Berlin.

31. Ibid., 497.

32. Eugène Aroneanu, "Les Nations Unies et le crime contre l'humanité," *Le Monde*, December 10, 1948 (our translation).

33. Jacob Robinson, "The International Military Tribunal and the Holocaust: Some Legal Reflections," *Israel Law Review* 7, no. 1 (January 1972): 7.

34. Jacob Robinson cited by Mark Lewis in *Birth of the New Justice*, 155, 159.

35. Robinson, text written in 1945, quoted in Michael Marrus, "A Jewish Lobby at Nuremberg: Jacob Robinson and the Institute for Jewish Affairs, 1945–1946," *Cardozo Law Review* 27 (April 2006): 1654.

36. Quoted in David Cesarani, *Final Solution: The Fate of the Jews 1933–1949* (New York: St. Martin's Press, 2016), 786. See, for example, Benjamin Fondane [1942], "Préface en prose," in *L'Exode: Super Flumina Babylonis* (Paris: La Fenêtre ardent, 1965).

37. Sigrid Arne, "Nazi Victim Helps Repay Debt," *Portland Press Herald*, March 16, 1947, quoted in Raphael Lemkin, *Totally Unofficial: The Autobiography of Raphael Lemkin* (New Haven: Yale University Press, 2013), xxi.

38. Sigrid Arne, interview with Raphael Lemkin, *Washington Post*, March 16, 1947, section B, p. 3.

39. American report for the United National Relief and Rehabilitation Administration, July 29, 1946, UN Archives, New York.

40. Hirad Abtahi and Philippa Webb, *The Genocide Convention: The Travaux préparatoires*, vol. 1 (Boston: Martinus Nijhoff, 2009), 459. The quotation is by Mr. Durdenevsky (USSR), speaking at the 123rd plenary meeting, November 21, 1946.

41. Lemkin, *Totally Unofficial*, 80.

42. Raphael Lemkin, *Axis Rule* (Washington, DC: Carnegie Endowment for International Peace, 1944), 84–85. Lemkin is quoting *Le Frankfurter Zeitung*, March 28, 1941.

43. Lemkin, "Le Crime de génocide," *Notes documentaires et études*, no. 417 (September 24, 1946) (our translation).

44. Letter from Raphael Lemkin to the Emergency Committee in Aid of Displaced Foreign Scholars, June 21, 1944, NYPL.

45. Quoted in Lewis, *Birth of the New Justice*, 204.

46. Genet [pen name of Janet Flanner], "Letter from Paris," *The New Yorker*, October 16, 1948, p. 111.

47. Raphael Lemkin, "Encyclopédie des génocides," French-language manuscript, in *Caractères juridiques du genocide*, chap. 2, p. 5 (our translation).

48. "Observations Concerning the Articles," in Abtahi and Webb, *Genocide Convention*, 636.

49. Radio-Lille, December 1948, French-language transcript in the Lemkin Archives, Jacob Rader Marcus Center, Cincinnati (our translation).

50. Mark Mazower, *No Enchanted Palace: The End of Empire and the Ideological Origins of the United Nations* (Princeton: Princeton University Press, 2009).

51. Raphael Lemkin, "Totally Unofficial Man," in *Pioneers of Genocide Studies*, ed. Samuel Totten and Steven Leonard Jacobs (New Brunswick, NJ: Transaction Publishers, 2002), 392–93.

52. Our translation.

53. Letter to Eleanor Roosevelt, February 1, 1950, Lemkin Archives, Cincinnati (Lemkin reminds E. Roosevelt of the past).

54. Lemkin to Léon Blum, February 18, 1950, Lemkin Archives, Cincinnati (our translation).

55. Letter to François de Menthon, January 3, 1950. Quoted in Lewis, *Birth of the New Justice*, 182.

56. Eugene Holmes, "Anti-Semitism," review of *Must Men Hate?* by Sigmund Livingston, *Journal of Negro Education* 15, no. 2 (Spring 1946): 207.

57. "US Accused in UN of Negro Genocide," *New York Times*, December 18, 1951, p. 13.

58. Letter from Oakley Johnson, of New York, June 24, 1953, Lemkin Archives, Cincinnati. See Guillaume Mouralis, *Le Moment Nuremberg: Le procès international, les lawyers et la question raciale* (Paris: Les Presses de Sciences Po, 2019). An English translation is to be published in 2021 by Oxford University Press.

59. See the works by Myriam Cottias, in particular "La Traite et l'esclavage racialisé comme genocide," in *Rapport de la Mission d'étude en France sur la recherche et l'enseignement des génocides et des crimes de masse*, ed. Vincent Duclert (Paris: CNRS Éditions, 2018).

60. Lemkin added "regrettable" by hand on the typescript.

61. NYPL, sparse notes from the 1950s, microfilm 4 (our translation).

62. Lemkin, *Totally Unofficial*, 128. In fact, Vyshinsky had written a short book in the 1930s on the interference of international criminal law in the internal politics of the Soviet Union.

63. Text written November 16, 1949, for the International Labour Conference, London, Lemkin Archives, Cincinnati (our translation).

64. "Charge of US Genocide Called Red Smoke Screen," *Washington Post*, December 16, 1951, p. m6.

65. "Communist Genocide Campaign," notes by Lemkin, Reel 4, Lemkin Archives, NYPL, 1951.

66. Ibid.

67. "Berle Chides U.S. on Genocide Issue," *New York Times*, January 13, 1951, p. 2.

68. Raphael Lemkin, NYPL, Manuscripts and Archives Division, Reel 3. Published in L. Y. Luciuk, ed., *Holodomor: Reflections on the Great Famine of 1932–1933 in Soviet Ukraine* (Kingston, ON: Kashtan Press, 2008), 237–38.

69. Cf. Nicolas Werth's conclusion in *Les Grandes Famines soviétiques* (Paris: Que sais-je, 2020). For a more journalistic approach, see Ann Applebaum, *Red Famine: Stalin's War on Ukraine* (London: Penguin, 2018).

70. *Haratch*, no. 208, December 9, 1945, in Chavarche Missakian, *Face à l'innommable, avril 1915* (Marseille: Éditions Parenthèses, 2015) (our translation).

71. Chavarche Missakian, "La Grande Crise," excerpts of letters written in August 1915, translated by Krikor Beledian, *Europe*, special issue *Témoigner en littérature*, ed. Frédérik Detue and Charlotte Lacoste, no. 1041–42 (2016): 57, 58.

72. Letter to Thelma Stevens, member of the Council of Methodist Women, July 26, 1950, NYPL. Numerous priests, in particular, were deported to Dachau.

73. CBS, "U.N. Casebook," documentary series, broadcast February 13, 1949. Interview with Lemkin on the UN convention and the Armenian genocide. A partial transcript is available at http://www.armeniapedia.org/wiki/Lemkin_Discusses_Armenian_Genocide_In_Newly-Found_1949_CBS_Interview. Part of the interview can be viewed at https://vimeo.com/125514772.

74. Raphael Lemkin, "Prolongement de la cicatrice psychologique," manuscript, NYPL, n.p. (our translation).

75. Quoted in Tanya Elder, "Documenting Lemkin's Life by Exploring His Archival Papers," in *The Origins of Genocide: Raphael Lemkin as a Historian of Mass Violence*, ed. Dominik J. Schaller and Jürgen Zimmerer (London and New York: Routledge, 2009), 45.

76. Raphael Lemkin, 1958 review of *Les Mémoires de Mgr Jean Naslian*, 2 vols. (Imprimerie mechithariste, 1955) (our translation), Lemkin Archives, Cincinnati.

77. John Cooper, *Raphael Lemkin and the Struggle for the Genocide Convention* (Basingstoke: Palgrave Macmillan, 2008).

78. The meetings were on October 27 and November 9, 1948: "I spoke for an hour with Professor Raphael Lemkin, who told me about 'genocide,' in which I was very interested. . . . Received Professor Lemkin, of the genocide." Angelo Giuseppe Roncalli, *Journal de France*, vol. 1, *1945–1948* (Paris: Cerf, 2006), introduction and annotation by Étienne Fouilloux (to whom I extend my warm thanks), 563–69 (our translation).

79. Lemkin, *Totally Unofficial*, and *Lemkin on Genocide*, ed. Leonard Jacobs (Lanham, MD: Lexington Books, 2012).

80. *Investigation of the Psychological Reactions of Three Areas: The Victimized Group / The Genocidist / The Outside World.* Manuscript, Lemkin Archives, NYPL.

81. Here, I use the word "neighbor" as defined by Jan Gross in *Neighbors: The Destruction of the Jewish Community in Jedwabne, Poland* (Princeton: Princeton University Press, 2000).

82. The concept was "invented" by Niederland in 1961. See Bruno Cabanes, "Le Syndrome du survivant: Histoire et usages d'une notion," in *Retour à l'intime au sortir de la guerre*, ed. Bruno Cabanes and Guillaume Picketty (Paris: Tallandier, 2009), 199–211.

83. Lucien Febvre, "Face au vent" (1946), in *Combats pour l'histoire* (Paris: Armand Colin, 1953), 41 (our translation).

84. Anouche Kunth, *Exils arméniens, du Caucase à Paris, 1920–1945* (Paris: Belin, 2016).

85. Quoted in Steven L. Jacobs, ed., *Raphael Lemkin's Thoughts on Nazi Genocide: Not Guilty?* (Lewiston, NY: Edwin Mellen Press, 1992), xx.

86. Soazig Aaron, *Le Non de Klara* (Babelio, 2002).

87. Lemkin Archives, Cincinnati (our translation).

88. British National Archives, Kew, 1532 Kar, 19/5/1944 (our translation).

89. Ad in the *New York Times*, November 28, 1944.

90. Quoted in E. Thomas Wood and Stanislaw M. Jankowski, *Karski: How One Man Tried to Stop the Holocaust* (Hoboken: John Wiley & Sons, 1994), 240.

91. Eve Grot, "Not the Whole Story," *Soviet Russia Today*, March 1945, p. 28.

92. Annette Becker, "Avoir faim/ravitailler," in *Les Cicatrices rouges, 14–18: Belgique et France occupées* (Paris: Fayard, 2010), 131–58; Bruno Cabanes, "The Hungry and the Sick: Herbert Hoover, the Russian Famine, and the Professionalization of Humanitarian Aid," in *The Great War and the Origins of Humanitarianism, 1918–1924* (Cambridge: Cambridge University Press, 2014), 189–247.

93. Poor Lemkin suffered a similar disaster with his archives—due in this case to American liberalism: he had stored nine boxes of documents in Washington and was unable to go to retrieve them. They were "put up for auction for scrap." By a stroke of luck there was in the auction hall a "Mr. Blondell who knew Dr. Rafael Lemkin's achievements"; he bought the papers for twenty dollars and found Lemkin, who was "delighted" to recover them. "They are of great sentimental value for me. They are not worth much money now, I guess. Just documents. But perhaps after I'm dead, someday, they may be worth something." "Owner Will Regain Genocide Documents," *Washington Post*, October 14, 1953, p. 15.

94. Council of Polish Political Parties, *Poland Accuses: An Indictment of the Major German War Criminals* (London: The Montgomery Printing & Stationery Co., 1946).

95. Rousso, *Après la Shoah*; Hasia Diner, *We Remember with Reverence and Love: American Jews and the Myth of Silence after the Holocaust, 1945–1962* (New York: New York University Press, 2009), and "Origins and Meanings of the Myth of Silence," in *After the Holocaust: Challenging the Myth of Silence*, ed. David Cesarani and Eric J. Sundquist (London and New York: Routledge, 2012), 192–201; Simon Perego, *Pleurons-les. Les Juifs de Paris et la commémoration de la Shoah (1944–1967)* (Paris: Champvallon, 2020).

96. Jan Karski, "The Great Powers and Poland, 1919–1945," PhD dissertation, Georgetown University, 1953, 415. Also available in Jan Karski, *The Great Powers and Poland: From Versailles to Yalta* (Lanham, MD: Rowman and Littlefield, 2014), 357.

97. Ibid., 461. Quotation taken from Karski, *Great Powers*, 365–66.

98. Ibid., 415.

99. *Washington Post*, March 3, 1952, section B, p. 5 (our translation).

100. Monday, October 29, 1956, US House of Representatives, Committee on Un-American Activities, International Communism (Revolt in the Satellites), testimony of Dr. Jan Karski, Library of Congress, https://babel.hathitrust.org/cgi/pt?id=uc1.$b654273&view=1up&seq=11.

101. Jan Karski, "Poland's Election: Results Rejected as Not Reflecting Desires of the Nation," "Letters to the Times," *New York Times*, January 20, 1957.

102. Jan Karski, personal archives, Georgetown University.

103. Handwritten note in French, n.d. (around 1956), Karski Archives, Georgetown University (our translation).

Chapter 6. Becoming Karski, Becoming Lemkin

1. Raphael Lemkin, NYPL, microfilm reel no. 2, *Perpetuation of the Psychological Scar*, 1950s typescript.

2. Claude Lanzmann, *Shoah, an Oral History of the Holocaust: The Complete Text of the Film* (New York: Pantheon Books, 1985), 174.

3. Jacques Derrida, "A Self-Unsealing Poetic Text," trans. Rachel Bowlby, in *Revenge of the Aesthetic: The Place of Literature in Theory Today*, ed. Michael P. Clark (Berkeley: University of California Press, 2000), 194.

4. Dori Laub, "Not Knowing Is an Active Process of Destruction. Why the Testimonial Procedure Is of So Much Importance," in *Trauma Research Newsletter* 1, Hamburg Institute for Social Research, July 2000. Laub, an American psychiatrist, was one of the founders of the Fortunoff Video Archive for Holocaust Testimonies at Yale University, named after Alan A. Fortunoff, who made a generous endowment gift.

5. Dori Laub, "Psychoanalysis and Genocide: Two Essays," Genocide Studies Program, Yale University, 2002, https://gsp.yale.edu/sites/default/files/gs20_21_-_psychoanalysis_and_genocide_two_essays.pdf.

6. Marjorie Hyer, "Holocaust: So Horrible No One Believed It Was True," *Washington Post*, March 28, 1980, https://www.washingtonpost.com/archive/local/1980/03/28/holocaust-so-horrible-no-one-believed-it-was-true/9501ed7c-b463-45e6-8e04-88c0f94100b4/.

7. President Jimmy Carter appointed Elie Wiesel to chair the President's Commission on the Holocaust, which gave rise to the United States Holocaust Memorial Museum. Housed in a building designed by the architect James Ingo Freed, it was inaugurated in 1993. Miles Lerman was the project's linchpin.

8. Miles Lerman, foreword to chapter 1, "Opening," in *The Liberation of the Nazi Concentration Camps 1945: Eyewitness Accounts of the Liberators*, ed. Brewster Chamberlin and Marcia Feldman (Washington, DC: United States Holocaust Memorial Council, 1987), 12. Lerman, who arrived in the United States from a displaced persons camp in 1947, was the executive director of the United States Holocaust Memorial Council.

9. Ibid.

10. Elie Wiesel, chapter 1, "Opening," in Chamberlin and Feldman, *Liberation of the Nazi Concentration Camps*, 14.

11. Wiesel quoted in E. Thomas Wood and Stanislaw Jankowski, *Karski: How One Man Tried to Stop the Holocaust* (New York: J. Wiley & Sons, 1994), 255.

12. Jan Karski, participant in panel discussion, "Discovering the 'Final Solution,'" in Chamberlin and Feldman, *Liberation of the Nazi Concentration Camps*, 191.

13. Jan Karski, presentation, in Chamberlin and Feldman, *Liberation of the Nazi Concentration Camps*, 181. The passage is cited by Raul Hilberg in the chapter

titled "Messengers" in his *Perpetrators Victims Bystanders: The Jewish Catastrophe, 1933–1945* (New York: HarperCollins, 1992), 224. Thereafter, Karski repeated these words often. "Righteous" file, Yad Vashem archives. Hilberg was the only historian featured in the film *Shoah*.

14. Yad Vashem website, https://www.yadvashem.org/yv/en/exhibitions/righteous /milestone02.asp.

15. Yona Kesse, elected representative of the Mapai Party, quoted in Sarah Gensburger, *National Policy, Global Memory: The Commemoration of the "Righteous," from Jerusalem to Paris, 1942–2007*, trans. Katharine Throssell (New York: Berghahn, 2016), 9.

16. David Cesarani, *Eichmann: His Life and Crimes* (London: William Heinemann, 2000).

17. The commemoration took place on April 13, 1961. From 1951, when it was created, until 1959, the "Day of Commemoration of the Genocide and the Ghetto Uprising" took place on the date of 27 Nissan in the Jewish calendar. The transition from the notion of celebrating heroism to that of commemorating the catastrophe for Jewish victims is notable.

18. Gideon Hausner, *Justice in Jerusalem* (New York: Harper & Row, 1966), 397. The book was published simultaneously in many languages in 1966, and "the world knew" once more through it. Lanzmann, however, did not mince his words: "The Eichmann trial would be of no use to me. Reading the transcripts, it became clear to me that the trial had been conducted by ignorant people: the historians at the time had done too little research, the president and the judges were poorly informed; Hausner, the chief prosecutor, thought that pompous, moralizing flights of rhetoric compensated for what he lacked in knowledge . . . the tearful witnesses gave a kind of show, making it impossible to recreate what they had truly experienced." Claude Lanzmann, *The Patagonian Hare: A Memoir*, trans. Frank Wynne (New York: Farrar, Straus and Giroux, 2012), 425. I would like to thank Fabien Théofilakis, a foremost Eichmann scholar. See his "Adolf Eichmann à Jérusalem, 1960–1962: La Shoah en France devant la justice," in *Gestapo et polices allemandes: France Europe de l'Ouest, 1939–1945*, ed. P. Arnaud and F. Théofilakis (Paris: CNRS éditions, 2017), and *"Un jour, c'est l'histoire qui jugera"—Eichmann à Jérusalem: La Shoah vue de la cage de verre* (Paris: Odile Jacob, forthcoming).

19. Hausner then listed examples of countries that had been among the Just—Denmark, Belgium, Sweden, France, the Netherlands, Italy—which, Hausner said, "we shall never forget" or "we shall always remember."

20. Hausner quoted in Gensburger, *National Policy, Global Memory*, 16–17. The list of countries at the end of the quotation is included in the original text but was not included in the translation.

21. Hausner, *Justice in Jerusalem*, 236. Translator's note: The translation in this work changes "Jewish resistance" to "Polish underground." We have amended the translation to retain the author's original meaning.

22. Yad Vashem Archives, Karski file.

23. The Bitburg affair was one of the reasons that the United States was pushed to ratify the 1948 convention on genocide. See Ansom Rabinbach, "Raphael Lemkin et le concept de genocide," *Revue d'histoire de la Shoah* (July 2008): 511–54. As most of the extermination sites were situated in Poland or the Soviet Union, Reagan obviously could not visit them during this G7 meeting in West Germany.

24. Jan Karski, *Washington Post*, letters to the editor, April 22, 1985 (emphasis added).

25. Jan Karski (Washington), *Washington Post*, letters to the editor, December 1, 1985.

26. Lanzmann, *Shoah*, 171.

27. Expression by the German philosopher Andris Breitling.

28. See the writings by Rémy Besson: his dissertation, "La Mise en récit de Shoah" (EHESS, adviser: Christian Delage, 2012), "Le Rapport Karski, une voix qui résonne comme une source," *Études photographiques*, no. 27 (May 2011); *Shoah une double référence? Des faits au film, du film aux faits* (Paris: Éditions MkF, 2017).

29. Lanzmann quoted in Aline Alterman, *Visages: Shoah, le film de Claude Lanzmann* (Paris: Cerf, 2006) (our translation). See C. Lanzmann, "Le Lieu et la parole," in Claude Lanzmann, Bernard Cuau, and Michel Deguy, *Au sujet de Shoah, le film de Claude Lanzmann* (Paris: Belin Éditeur, 2011), 304.

30. Lanzmann, *Shoah*, 167, 174.

31. Ibid.

32. The camera literally falls upon the White House by sliding down the flagpole in a camera movement similar to that sliding down a dead tree in the Birkenau camp.

33. Karski, *Story of a Secret State*, 338. In the film, Nowolipki Street, most of which was in the ghetto, is shown. The etymology of the name is no doubt related to the gardens that bordered the street in the seventeenth century (*nowy* means "new" and *lipa* means "linden"). The street's name became known through a 1930s social novel by Pola Gojawiczynska, *Dziewczeta z Nowolipek* (The Girls of Nowolipki), which was adapted for film several times. I would like to thank Dorota Dakowska for her valuable assistance.

34. On the suitcases from the Auschwitz Museum shown elsewhere in the film, see Éric Marty's reflections in *Le Débat* (December 2010), reprinted in *Sur Shoah de Claude Lanzmann (Le marteau sans maître)* (Paris: Éditions Manucius, 2016).

35. Lanzmann, *Shoah*, 168.

36. Rushes for *Shoah*, USHMM, reel 318, p. 70. See "Franklin Delano Roosevelt, un leader du monde," *Les Temps modernes, Le Rapport Karski* (2010): 20.

37. Tom Shales, "Bearing Witness to Horror" (review of the PBS broadcast of *Shoah*), *Washington Post*, April 27, 1987.

38. Claude Lanzmann, "*Jan Karski* de Yannick Haenel, un faux roman," *Les Temps modernes* (January–March 2010): 2 (our translation).

39. The archive created by Steven Spielberg in 1994 is housed at the University of Southern California. It should be noted that although the Tutsi genocide in Rwanda

in 2000 is not on the archive's list of genocides, that of Bosnia, in 1994—the year of the archive's creation—is.

40. Jan Karski, "Foreword," in Ewa Kurek, *Your Life Is Worth Mine: How Polish Nuns Saved Hundreds of Jewish Children in German-Occupied Poland (1939–1945)* (New York: Hippocrene Books, 1997), 9.

41. Inaugurated in March 2005, the museum was designed by Moshe Safdie. See Moshe Safdie, Joan Ockman, and Diana Murphy, *Yad Vashem: Moshe Safdie—The Architecture of Memory* (Zurich: Lars Müller, 2006).

42. Levite's text, written in January 1945, is presented in a new translation by David Suchoff in his "A Yiddish Text from Auschwitz: Critical History and the Anthological Imagination," *Prooftexts* 19, no. 1 (January 1999): 59–69. The quotation is on 63.

43. Rushes for *Shoah*, USHMM, 70. On Lord Selborne, see chapter 3.

44. Speech lasting twenty-three minutes plus questions, USHMM, February 4, 1999 (our translation), Fulbright ceremony, USHMM oral archives.

45. Ibid. (our translation).

46. Elie Wiesel to Jan Karski, May 10, 1994. Yad Vashem archives, Karski file. Also quoted in part in Annette Becker, "Jan Karski from Eye Witness to Moral Witness: What to Do with Your Senses?," in *Modern Conflict and the Senses*, ed. Nicholas J. Saunders and Paul Cornish (Abingdon: Routledge, 2017), 234.

47. Elie Wiesel at the inauguration ceremony for Yad Vashem, March 15, 2005, https://www.yadvashem.org/events/15-march-2005/ceremony.html.

48. Letter from Shimon Peres to Jan Karski, May 12, 1994. Yad Vashem archives.

49. Jan Karski, speech in Washington, May 12, 1994. Yad Vashem archives.

50. Yannick Haenel, *Jan Karski* (Paris: Gallimard, L'Infini imprint, 2009).

51. In the original German, "Niemand zeugt für den Zeugen." Paul Celan, "No One Bears Witness for the Witness," from *Breathturn*, in Paul Célan, *Breathturn into Timestead: The Collected Later Poetry*, trans. Pierre Joris (New York: Farrar, Straus and Giroux, 2014), 65.

52. Yannick Haenel, *Cercles* (Paris: Gallimard, 2007), 485–86 (our translation). See also Yannick Haenel, *The Messenger: A Novel*, trans. Ian Monk (Berkeley, CA: Counterpoint, 2012).

53. Anthony Lewis, "Abroad at Home; 'Remember, Remember,'" *New York Times*, December 2, 1985, section A, p. 15.

54. Karski's second wife, Pola Nirenska, a survivor of the Shoah, was a dancer and then a dance teacher. I extend my warmest thanks to Arthur Nauzyciel (today the director of the Théâtre national de Bretagne), who has involved me since the beginning in this magnificent theatrical adventure. The play, *Jan Karski (mon nom est une fiction)*, has been performed throughout France and in Switzerland and Poland. Nauzyciel has not drawn the critical fire of Lanzmann and revisionist historians; yet, the play is based on Haenel's novel.

55. Saul Friedländer, *The Years of Extermination: Nazi Germany and the Jews, 1939–1945* (New York: HarperCollins, 2007).

56. Catherine Filloux, *Lemkin's House* (2005). The play has nowhere near the strength of Haenel's novel, but its timeliness makes it of great interest.

57. Lanzmann returned to this polemic in 2016, when Elie Wiesel died. Lanzmann rebuked Wiesel for not praising his film enough, which he regarded as a betrayal.

58. Claude Lanzmann, *Un vivant qui passe*, 1997, 1 h 5 m: 1979 interview with Maurice Rossel, delegate from the International Red Cross committee to Theresienstadt in June 1944; *Sobibor 14 octobre 1943, 16 heures*, 2001, 1 h 35 m; *Le Dernier des injustes*, 2013. The transcripts of these films have been published by Gallimard.

59. "These young writers are complaining . . . as distance allows them, they believe, all the indifference and the worst distortions, in the name of a tearful and retrospective moralism," Lanzmann wrote in "*Jan Karski* de Yannick Haenel: Un faux roman," *Les Temps modernes* (January–March 2010), 1 (our translation).

60. Claude Lanzmann, *Le rapport Karski*, 2010, 48 m.

61. Claude Lanzmann, "Autoportrait à quatre-vingt-dix ans," interview with Franck Nouchi and Juliette Simont, in Juliette Simont, ed., *Claude Lanzmann: Un voyant dans le siècle* (Paris: Gallimard, 2017), 278–80 (our translation).

62. Jorge Semprun, *L'Écriture ou la vie* (Paris: Gallimard, 2002), 188 (our translation).

63. Philippe Mesnard, *Primo Levi: Le passage d'un témoin* (Paris: Fayard, 2011).

64. Walter Benjamin, "Theses on the Philosophy of History," in *Illuminations: Essays and Reflections*, trans. Harry Zohn, ed. Hannah Arendt (Boston and New York: Mariner Books, 2019), 198–99 (emphasis in original). In December 2010, Haenel responded to a letter that I had sent him regarding my intentions for this book: "Like you, I think that the name of Jan Karski is one of a becoming—a metamorphosis—that gives us a huge amount to think about in terms of how the twentieth century fits into history. It is an issue essential to understanding, working out, and testing what is the nerve center of our censures. Not only did he bear within himself overlapping temporalities (and you have noted that his interview with Lanzmann in *Shoah* is constantly shaped by shifts between past and present), but he was in himself a palimpsest. Karski was a man of secrets—as such, he was a fiction, his own fiction (starting with the invention of his name)—a fiction that told the truth, that of a formulation (and constant reformulation) of what the world after 1945 was capable of hearing and accepting. . . . Like you, I think that the essential thing is not Jan Karski's message, but the resistance that this message provoked, the discourses that it started, the changes that it revealed in the slow construction of 'what we know' or, rather, 'what we want to know.' Unfolding Karski through time, through transformations of the image that we have of him, and also through the transformations in Karski himself (and his spiritual evolution) is, I believe, your subject: it inverts the rather weighty certainties . . . [of those who] do not want to know how much of what took place under the name of Jan Karski has been kept back and played out through time—that is, up to the present" (our translation). Annette Becker, personal archives.

65. Henry Rousso, ed., *Après la Shoah: Rescapés, réfugiés, survivants (1944–1947)* (Paris: Mémorial de la Shoah, 2016), 134 (our translation). Nathan Rapoport, a refugee in the USSR, had wanted to create a monument to the destruction of the ghetto in 1943; his proposal was deemed too romantic and nationalistic by the Soviets. After the war, he immigrated to France. The Warsaw monument was judged sufficiently important for a replica to be placed at the entrance to the Yad Vashem complex in Jerusalem. See also James Young, *The Texture of Memory: Holocaust Memorials and Meaning* (New Haven: Yale University Press, 1994), 168; Annette Becker, *"War and Faith": The Religious Imagination in France, 1914–1930*, trans. Helen McPhail (Oxford and New York: Berg, 1998), 132.

66. Designed by the Finnish architects Rainer Mahlamäki and Ilmari Lahdelma and inaugurated in stages between 2013 and 2015.

67. For instance, Witold Pilecki, the author of one of the most remarkable eyewitness accounts on Auschwitz, where he organized the resistance, was executed by the communists in 1948; he was rehabilitated in 1990. See Witold Pilecki, *The Auschwitz Volunteer: Beyond Bravery*, trans. Jarek Garlinski (Los Angeles: Aquila Polonica (US) Ltd., 2012).

68. Letter from Andrzej Olechowski to Jan Karski, May 4, 1994, Yad Vashem archives.

69. "President Obama Announces Jan Karski as a Recipient of the Presidential Medal of Freedom," https://obamawhitehouse.archives.gov/the-press-office/2012/04/23/president-obama-announces-jan-karski-recipient-presidential-medal-freedo.

70. Whence the various accusations of antipatriotism made against the historian Jan Gross. The Order of Merit of the Republic of Poland that he received in 1996 was withdrawn after his book *Neighbors: The Destruction of the Polish Community in Jedwabne, Poland* (Princeton: Princeton University Press, 2001) was published.

71. The title of the first biography, written by E. Thomas Wood and Stanislaw M. Jankowski, *Karski: How One Man Tried to Stop the Holocaust* (Hoboken: John Wiley & Sons, 1994). A film made by Slawomir Grünberg in 2015 featured Wood's interviews of Karski in 1996.

72. Tom Wood, "When Silence Is a Sin: A Hero of the Holocaust Leaves Us Lessons about Duty," Medium.com, January 31, 2017, https://medium.com/@tomwood_94144/when-silence-is-a-sin-88a7853fb230. Ten Karski groups on Facebook reposted the article.

Conclusion

1. Lemkin, critical reading of *Les Mémoires de Mgr Jean Naslian*, 2 vols. (Imprimerie mechithariste, 1955) (our translation).

2. Raphael Lemkin, *Unofficial Man* (unpublished autobiography), quoted in S. L. Jacobs, "Genesis of the Concept of Genocide According to Its Author from the Original Sources," *Human Rights Review* 3, no. 2 (2002): 103.

3. Lemkin, NYPL, typescript pages, 1950s (our translation).

4. Raphael Lemkin, NYPL, microfilm reel no. 2, *Perpetuation of the Psychological Scar*, typescript from the 1950s (our translation).

5. Annette Becker, *Maurice Halbwachs, un intellectuel en guerres mondiales, 1914–1945* (Paris: Noêsis, 2003).

6. Raphael Lemkin, "Perpetuation of the Psychological Scar," n.d., Manuscripts and Archives Division, NYPL, Box 2, Folder 4, Reel 3 (our translation). See also Charlotte Kiechel, "Legible Testimonies: Raphaël Lemkin, the Victim's Voice, and the Global History of Genocide," *Genocide Studies and Prevention: An International Journal* 13, no. 1 (2019): 42–63.

7. Lemkin, "Perpetuation of the Psychological Scar" (our translation).

8. Jean Hatzfeld, *Blood Papa: Rwanda's New Generation*, trans. Joshua David Jordan (New York: Farrar, Straus and Giroux, 2018).

9. Interview in Mushubati, Rwanda, 2016 (our translation). Annette Becker, personal notes.

10. Élise Rida Musomandera, *Le Livre d'Élise* (Paris: Les Belles Lettres, 2014), 72 (our translation).

11. Quoted in Catherine Bedarida, "Il n'y a pas de fin à un genocide," *Le Monde*, May 19, 2005 (our translation). See also Esther Mujawayo and Souad Belhaddad, *SurVivantes* (La Tour d'Aigues, France: L'Aube, "Poche Essai" collection, 2005).

12. Quoted in Jean Hatzfeld, *The Strategy of Antelopes: Living in Rwanda after the Genocide*, trans. Linda Coverdale (New York: Farrar, Straus and Giroux, 2009), 4.

13. Joséphine Kampiré, quoted in Hélène Dumas, *Le Génocide au village: Le massacre des Tutsi du Rwanda* (Paris: Seuil, 2014), 277, 290 (our translation). See Stéphane Audoin-Rouzeau, *Une initiation* (Paris: Seuil, 2017).

14. I quote with affection the French mixed with Yiddish of Philippe Gumplowicz's mom (our translation).

INDEX

George L. Mosse Series in the History of European Culture,
Sexuality, and Ideas

STEVEN E. ASCHHEIM, SKYE DONEY,
MARY LOUISE ROBERTS, AND DAVID J. SORKIN

Series Editors

Of God and Gods: Egypt, Israel, and the Rise of Monotheism
JAN ASSMANN

*Messengers of Disaster: Raphael Lemkin, Jan Karski, and
Twentieth-Century Genocides*
ANNETTE BECKER; translated by KÄTHE ROTH

*Respectability and Violence: Military Values, Masculine Honor,
and Italy's Road to Mass Death*
LORENZO BENADUSI; translated by ZAKIYA HANAFI

The Enemy of the New Man: Homosexuality in Fascist Italy
LORENZO BENADUSI; translated by
SUZANNE DINGEE and JENNIFER PUDNEY

*The Holocaust and the West German Historians:
Historical Interpretation and Autobiographical Memory*
NICOLAS BERG; translated and edited by JOEL GOLB

Collected Memories: Holocaust History and Postwar Testimony
CHRISTOPHER R. BROWNING

Cataclysms: A History of the Twentieth Century from Europe's Edge
DAN DINER; translated by WILLIAM TEMPLER with JOEL GOLB

*Fascination with the Persecutor:
George L. Mosse and the Catastrophe of Modern Man*
EMILIO GENTILE; translated by JOHN and ANNE TEDESCHI

La Grande Italia: The Myth of the Nation in the Twentieth Century
EMILIO GENTILE; translated by SUZANNE DINGEE and
JENNIFER PUDNEY